RUTH PURTILO, R.P.T., Ph.D.

Associate Professor,
Department of Medical Jurisprudence and Humanities,
University of Nebraska Medical Center
Omaha, Nebraska

HEALTH PROFESSIONAL/PATIENT Interaction

3RD EDITION

1984   W.B. SAUNDERS COMPANY

Philadelphia / London / Toronto   Mexico City / Rio de Janeiro / Sydney / Tokyo

W. B. SAUNDERS COMPANY
Harcourt Brace Jovanovich, Inc.

The Curtis Center
Independence Square West
Philadelphia, PA 19106

Library of Congress Cataloging in Publication Data

Purtilo, Ruth

Health professional/patient interaction.

Includes bibliographies and index.

1. Medical personnel and patient.   I. Title.
[DNLM: 1. Allied health personnel.   2. Patients.
3. Professional-Patient relations.   W 21.5 P986a]

R727.3.P87 1984   610.69'6   83–20196

ISBN 0–7216–1115–X

Cover illustration courtesy of H. Armstrong Roberts, Inc.

Health Professional/Patient Interaction   ISBN 0–7216–1115–X

Last digit is the print number: 9   8   7   6   5

To
DAVID T. PURTILO,
whose contributions to my personal
life and professional development are many

FOREWORD

Concern for the quality of their personal relationships with the patients they serve has characterized the health professions since their varied beginnings as full-time specialties.

Initially, the importance attached to personal relationships in the work situation was reflected principally in the practical ethics of each group—a collection of rather specific rules of behavior which spelled out the "shalls" and "shall nots" of interaction with clients and colleagues: "Never let a patient call you by your first name"; "take time to listen to your patients, but don't become personally involved"; "stand up when you are addressed by your supervisor." Professional socialization of the student during this period consisted largely of learning and coming to believe in these no-nonsense commandments. Questions of rationale were few, and commitment to the importance of these rules in maintaining the comfort of the patient and the professional status of the practitioner was generally widespread.

As curricula in many health fields became incorporated in academic degree programs, concern for the psychosocial aspects of health care received a second, very different form of attention. The students' required programs came to include a much larger number of courses in the behavioral sciences. Study in areas ranging from general Psychology and Sociology to more health-oriented fields such as Psychology of the Handicapped, Social Gerontology and Child Development was added in the expectation that knowledge of theory in these areas would improve the graduates' ability to understand and cope with the personal problems of their patients. There was, however, discouragingly little organized effort to relate this new component of the curriculum to the professions' practical rules for on-the-job behavior. The specific components of the professional role were seldom challenged, analyzed or defended in terms of psychosocial theory; the two varieties of professional instruction simply coexisted without basic integration.

More recently still, the practical commandments of the professions have encountered the challenge and pervasive mood of rejection to which most arbitrary rules of social behavior have been subjected since the 1950's. Study of behavioral science has continued and been expanded, but commitment to a clear-cut set of professional-role behaviors has atrophied and become uncertain. It seems likely that much of the graduate professional's knowledge of psychosocial theory remains largely unused in the practical world of day-to-day relationships with patients and co-workers, for few conceptual bridges have been built to allow practical guidelines for social interaction to be derived from the principles of behavioral science.

Until very recently, the situation has been, at best, wasteful and, at worst, chaotic. Now, however, there are promising signs of change in the pattern of unstructured reliance on individual intuition in the practical situation, and in the squandering, through disuse, of the knowledge gained through study of behavioral science. The nursing profession, in particular, has taken a strong lead in examining role expectations in the light of theory. Using concepts suggested by Talcott Parsons, nurses have, for example, classified their responsibilities to patients as *instrumental* (acts which give the patient technical assistance to help solve a specific health problem; acts designed to get the patient well) and *expressive* (acts designed to help the patient reduce and tolerate the psychological discomfort of illness and of the healing process; acts which treat the patient as a person rather than as a case). Working from this classification, nursing and other health specialties have given greater attention to the expressive component of their work, and have begun a searching analysis of the patterns of interaction through which expressive goals are generally met.

In this book, Ruth Purtilo makes a landmark contribution to the effort to build effective bridges between theory and practice of effective interaction for the health professional. Through analyses which are both utilitarian and eloquent, she has provided a fine model for continuing efforts to derive new commandments—guidelines for interaction which are rationally based on theory, and sensibly flexible in application. This book should provide both immediate help to faculty and students in health fields and a stimulus to these professions to give even higher priority to future extension of this analysis.

NANCY T. WATTS, R.P.T., PH.D.
Massachusetts General Hospital

PREFACE

This book is designed for the student in the health professions. Soon after entering a health profession, students discover that professional goals can be realized only when they learn to combine their skills with those of their professional allies, and when, together, they effectively interact with the person needing their skills—the patient.

This book, which explains the basis for and methods of achieving effective interaction with the patient, should aid the student by (1) enhancing his or her self-understanding; (2) helping to clarify the dynamics of the health professional–patient relationship; and (3) developing an awareness of the complementary roles of other health professionals. Addressing itself to a wide variety of situations, this book should be especially useful in seminars that examine human relationships, and in introductory professional courses. General principles of human interaction are combined with practical suggestions for solving specific problems confronting the health professional. Factual data based on studies in the biomedical and behavioral sciences are supplemented with lively illustrations from literature and the humanities to direct attention to the diverse sources influencing human interaction. The purpose of this book is not to discuss every topic in depth but rather to stimulate the student to explore the topics further.

At the outset of this project, it was necessary to decide to whom the book should be directed. To a large extent the term "health professional" is loosely used to designate any person providing health services, from the technician with six weeks of on-the-job training to the person with a doctoral degree or beyond. Total health care does depend on many disciplines, and the techniques described in this book are basic enough to be useful to anyone providing health services. However, the book addresses itself primarily to the person whose preparation includes studies in the liberal arts, basic sciences, and the theory and techniques of a health professional, and who pursues full-time formal education beyond high school for a minimum of three to five years.

Few books or articles are directed to the "health professional" per se. Therefore, the reader will find that in this book excerpts quoted often reflect the terminology of one particular group. However, it will quickly become apparent that an excerpt originally directed to the nurse, technologist, physician, or therapist is equally relevant to other groups as well. Therefore, part of the unintended function of this book is to show the extent to which different groups share common dilemmas and insights.

In some instances, it was necessary to assign meanings to key terms: (1) *Patient*—the person needing a health service, whether it be diagnosis, evaluation, or treatment. (2) *Clinical education*—the extra-classroom portion of the health professional's formal education, which takes place in a setting similar to that in which he or she will eventually seek employment. Clinical education usually begins early in professional preparation and may progress from two or three hours a week to a full-time assignment. The term "clinical education" was chosen to distinguish it from "internship," because the latter is often confined to the period following completion of classroom education, suggesting several years of preparation at the graduate school level. (3) *Clinical experience*—the composite of learning experiences to which the student is exposed during clinical education.

Other terms that may cause confusion are defined before use. The situations described and the names of patients, health professionals, and other persons in case studies, appearing as examples or in the "Questions for Thought and Discussion" section, are fictitious. When the last word of a manuscript has been typed, its life has but begun. In sharing my ideas with you, the reader, I hope that, in turn, you will be stimulated to share yours with others, thus making us all more knowledgeable in the exciting venture of human interaction.

RUTH PURTILO

ACKNOWLEDGMENTS

A cardinal joy of preparing all three editions of this book has been the opportunity to share its development with a group of friends and professional colleagues. They clarified, corrected, suggested, and encouraged, knowing full well that the end product would be identified as my own. While they have become too numerous to mention individually, I do want to acknowledge them collectively and to extend my warmest thanks.

In the ten years since the first edition appeared, I have also been the fortunate recipient of numerous letters in which readers have offered responses, suggestions, and critiques. Furthermore, I have discussed issues examined in the book with a large number of health professions students and faculty around the country. I thank them for the growth I experienced during those encounters, and they will recognize portions of those discussions that have been incorporated into the second and third editions.

Three persons in my personal life deserve the first line of thanks:

My husband, David Purtilo, consistently affirms by his example that it is possible to combine high-quality patient care, complex cancer research, and a full measure of human compassion. He also has been my constant source of personal encouragement and stimulation, demonstrating the link between effectiveness in one's professional and in one's personal relationships.

My parents both suffered strokes since the time the first edition was published. Their struggles, courage, and continual concern for those they love during this period, and my mother's subsequent death, provided a look at some aspects of older persons' lives from a perspective that was sometimes painfully close. Their encouragement, even during the times of their own struggle, has provided much inspiration for me and I am ever grateful to them for this gift.

Several persons at W. B. Saunders have been outstanding in their guidance and support. I owe special gratitude to Brian Decker for his assistance in the development of Edition One, Marie Low for hers in Edition Two, and Baxter Venable for his help in the preparation of this edition. Also, over the years many persons have asked who provided the excellent line drawings; it is with many thanks that I acknowledge Grant Lashbrook for this contribution.

The manuscript preparation of Editions One and Two was completed largely by me. The tediousness of having to tackle Edition Three alone at the typewriter in the wee hours was alleviated by the able and efficient assistance of Ms. Pamela Polsley. Her skill and cheerfulness made the preparation of Edition Three a pleasure. Accordingly, I express my deep thanks to her.

RUTH B. PURTILO

CONTENTS

Part I

THE HEALTH PROFESSIONAL

Part I

This book, written for the health professions, begins with an emphasis on the health professional because the key to all successful human interaction lies in understanding oneself. People entering these professions bring with them a unique combination of abilities, needs, values, and fantasies that they expect to incorporate into the positions they assume as health professionals. They are sometimes surprised that patients and others with whom they interact fail to see them primarily as individuals and instead respond only to outward characteristics and behaviors—to images. The astute health professional will identify those behaviors, characteristics, and images and learn to use them constructively during interaction.

Part I is written with the health professional as an individual in mind.

Chapter 1 focuses on the health professional as he or she exhibits the behaviors and projects the image of a student. The questions asked in this chapter are fundamental to furthering one's understanding of oneself in the health professions: "What *is* professional education?" "What is expected of me during this period of professional preparation?" "How does it affect me as a *person*?"

Chapter 2 focuses on the health professional as he or she projects the image of helper. In this chapter, the person is viewed in a patient–health professional relationship. A health professional's attitudes toward and understanding of such a relationship directly influence the effectiveness of interaction with patients.

Chapter 3 zeroes in on the whole person who is assuming the roles and functions of a health professional, emphasizing ways to remain healthy and satisfied with one's choice of profession. Included are sections on how to make time for oneself, how to develop reasonable work habits, and how to utilize the strengths of the community of persons with whom one works. Teamwork is explained in some detail. The mechanisms of peer review and whistle-blowing are treated as means of helping to assure professional growth while maintaining the high standards of one's profession. By the end of Part I, readers should be better able to visualize themselves as others do in the many roles of a health professional. Understanding one's own actions and attitudes is thus the first step toward effective interaction.

Chapter 1

FOCUS: STUDENT

The Act of Becoming

"Would you tell me please, which way I ought to go from here?"
"That depends a good deal on where you want to get to," said the Cat.
ALICE IN WONDERLAND[1]

Persons like yourself, who take a leap into the unknown of preparation for a career in the health professions, sometimes feel like Alice in Wonderland, plummeting headlong into studies but uncertain of where the path is leading.

One reason for wonder is that in some ways preparation for work in the health fields seems different from that for other fields. While those in other programs of study are partying on Friday afternoon, the health professions student is in full uniform at the workplace, carrying out a clinical education requirement; while roommates are still trying to get out of bed, it's not unusual for the health professions students to be on the way out the door; and while most careers do not require students to adopt a given set of "professional" attitudes, behaviors, and ethical guidelines, the health professions do.

One can think of an education in the health professions as preparation for carrying out a lifelong commitment and for realizing a certain type of lifestyle. Identity as a health professional carries with it expectations on the part of society as well as privileges and responsibilities. In choosing to be a health professional, one is in essence deciding the types of activities that will take up the best energy of the best days of one's life. The preparation, then, is central not only to what one will do but also to who one will become.

What can a health professions student expect during the years of formal education? Three types of learning experience will predominate: the acquisition of basic concepts and theories, the mastery of professional skills, and the attainment of attitudes appropriate to one's role as a health professional. Each will have its place in the preparation for effective interaction with patients.

The following pages discuss these three areas of learning: knowledge (theoretical concepts and ideas), skills, and attitudes—to help the student understand more fully why he or she is asked to pursue particular learning activities in the classroom or clinical setting.

KNOWLEDGE (THEORETICAL CONCEPTS)

What knowledge does a person need in order to become a competent health professional? Knowledge in the basic sciences provides a foundation for understanding the body and the natural forces acting upon it. Knowledge in the behavioral sciences of psychology, sociology, and anthropology provides understanding of people's needs and behaviors and of how these needs and behaviors affect interaction. Mathematics, statistics, and instruction in computer technology furnish a baseline for problem-solving techniques and research. Knowledge in the liberal arts exposes one to the great political, religious, and philosophical ideas and establishes one's own link with history. Theoretical knowledge underlying the techniques relevant to one's profession lays the foundation for applying specific professional skills.

At times it appears that one is getting only glimpses of what one finally needs for an adequate knowledge base. However, the student who does not become overly discouraged early on soon begins to assimilate the knowledge from these various sources into a working base of information.

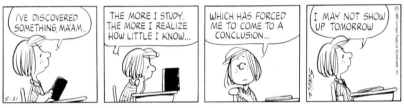

© 1980 United Feature Syndicate, Inc.

Knowledge can probably most effectively and efficiently be acquired and integrated in a classroom setting. There large numbers of people can listen to one lecturer impart information and answer questions, and discussions may readily follow. Each individual can then supplement the lecture and discussion material with as much outside study as he or she deems necessary. The student's grasp of the material can be determined by written or oral examination. If the only type of learning needed for professional competence were acquisition and integration of knowledge, there would be no need to include extensive laboratory experience or clinical education in the preparation of health care providers.

SKILLS

At the time they enter their professional curriculum, students are usually more accustomed to classroom learning than to laboratory and clinical learning. In the years of professional preparation, more time in the laboratory and clinic is required for the acquisition of skills.

Consider the skills needed for competence in a health profession.

Technical Skill. This is the ability to apply safely a given technique to secure a diagnosis or conduct an evaluation or treatment. The medical technologist obtains a sample of blood and analyzes its contents. The physical therapist applies proper stabilization or resistance to restore optimal functioning of a body part. The inhalation therapist mixes and regulates the output of the proper balance of gases. In each case, the intricate coordination of mind and body is needed, as well as sound judgment. The application of techniques requires effective management of oneself, the patient, equipment, and time.

Skill in Interpersonal Relationships and Communication. This is the ability to interact with a wide variety of people during the course of one's working day: other health professionals, supportive personnel, patients and their families, students, visitors, administrators, and business contacts such as professional-equipment salesmen. This skill demands that the health professional understand the dynamics underlying different types of human relationships, especially the authority-dependency relationship that characterizes so much interaction in the health care environment. It means being able to accept responsibility as a supervisor and constructive criticism as one who is supervised. It involves caring, sharing, and listening and demands tact, diplomacy, consistency, and forthrightness. Much of this book focuses on the means whereby the health professional can gain maximal benefit from mastery of interpersonal and communication skills.

Teaching and Administrative Skill. This is the ability to (1) instruct a patient, his or her family, students, other health professionals, and supportive personnel; (2) organize and implement workable solutions to problems; (3) communicate effectively by both written and oral means; (4) evaluate oneself and others objectively; and (5) utilize equipment and supplies wisely.

Research Skill. This is the ability to formulate a hypothesis and collect data that will help to determine whether or not the hypothesis is correct. Highly specialized or simple equipment available within a health facility may be utilized. Honest, accurate reporting of findings is imperative in order to assure high standards of practice.

The acquisition of skill often requires long, tedious hours of practice. The frustration that sometimes accompanies mastering a skill was illustrated recently in a story related by a friend who was trying to teach her 7-year-old daughter how to ski cross-country. They came to a hill, and the mother gave the child explicit instructions about how to position her body, hold the poles, and maneuver the skis in order to succeed in this new challenge. Next the mother demonstrated the process. The child, who had been watching intently, pushed off down the slope and immediately fell. Reflecting on the experience, the mother said, "I forgot to tell her, 'If you do everything exactly as I do it, *and then fall the first few times you try it,* you'll be able to do it.'" Likewise, a student who observes an apparently simple skill may find that it takes weeks of repetition to master that skill and avoid regrettable mistakes.

In order to understand better how a student acquires a skill, consider the following steps. The student

1. acquires background knowledge related to the skill (the cognitive learning described above).
2. experiences the skill applied to himself or herself.
3. applies the skill to a classmate.
4. observes a professional person using the skill.
5. assists the professional person in using it.
6. is closely supervised in the first attempts to use it alone.
7. satisfactorily uses it in a variety of situations, without direct supervision.
8. is tested for mastery of the skill.

Note the progression from classroom to clinical setting in this process. Number 1 can easily take place in a classroom or with the help of a programmed text. Numbers 2 and 3 take place in the laboratory. Then, numbers 4 through 8 all take place where supervision and a variety of situations are available. Thus, the mastery of professional skills requires that part of the training be in the clinical setting.

ATTITUDES

In order to begin thinking about how attitudes can determine effectiveness of interaction in the health professions, the student should consider the following groups of questions related to attitudes.

1. How do you feel about helping people? Do you ever resent having to help? How do you expect people to respond to you after you have done your best to help them?
2. How do you react to a person who is physically deformed? Do you feel pity? embarrassment? compassion? all of these?
3. What qualities of life give a person "dignity"? Are most older people more ready to die than younger people? Would some people be better off dead? What type of illness or deformity do you dread most?
4. Would you compromise your convictions if it meant the difference between keeping your job and losing it? Can you think of any circumstances in which you would compromise your convictions?

The development of attitudes that will best further the fundamental purposes of the health professions is an important aspect of professional preparation. Questions about helping, qualities that make life worth living, and the role of one's convictions highlight the way in which attitudes are central to effective functioning. Many of these and similarly difficult questions are discussed in later chapters.

One important attitude to acquire or refine is a love of learning itself: It ought to be cultivated during this period. A recent report by the United States National Commission on Excellence in Education suggested that the primary payoff for learning is the activity of learning itself, pursued and cultivated through a lifetime. Unfortunately, the "drive" instilled in many young people today to accumulate knowledge and other types of "information" takes the joy out of the process and replaces it with an urgent, stressful, competitive motive. As Meg Greenfield noted in *Newsweek*,

> Schooling needs to be saved from . . . the punishers, the opportunists and the exploiters who profess an undying devotion to the old-fashioned virtues and the life of the mind. . . . [2]

The inquisitiveness and sense of adventure in discovering the contours of an unknown horizon can help to keep health professionals not only competent but also imaginative in their approach to patients.

Integration of Classroom and Clinical Education

The reader is now familiar with three kinds of learning that take place during professional preparation: knowledge, skills, and attitudes. In addition, he or she knows the environments in which each kind of learning most efficiently and effectively takes place. With this baseline, the nature of the relationship between classroom and clinical education can be explored briefly.

Clinical education introduces the student to the peculiarities of the work environment. The quality and quantity of teaching that takes place are determined by such wide-ranging factors as the availability of patients or clients and the familiarity of other professionals in the environment with the student's capabilities and limitations. The learning environment is much less controlled than in the classroom. New smells, sounds, and sights combine with new tasks to present a weighty challenge to the best of classroom students. Most students find it the most exciting of their educational experiences. Everyone recognizes this phase as crucial for moving toward full clinical competence.[3] Some educators consider the clinical aspect of learning to be the most important. In an article entitled "The Allied Health Student as a Hospital Employee," the author proposed the following:

> The internship [clinical education] phase of the health science programs is the "heart" of the student's educational experiences. . . .
> The concept of learning as the dissemination, understanding and implementation of knowledge is exemplified in health career programs. Dissemination of information is carried out in the classroom, understanding is reinforced in the seminar which accompanies the internship, and implementation takes place in the internship situation. Undoubtedly the internship affords the student an opportunity to significantly implement the knowledge he acquires from his classroom work and from the hospital sponsor's tutorship.[4]

Refinement is one of the most important functions of clinical education. Refinement implies that the person has the basic materials with which to work but the new materials may be introduced to complete the refining process. The basic materials consist of the person's own individual qualities and previous learning. The new materials include (1) large numbers of patients with different problems, (2) several manifestations of a single pathological condition, (3) time limitations, (4) multiple professional responsibilities related to the particular situation, and (5) assimilation of particular techniques into workable evaluation or treatment programs. The desired end product in the kaleidoscope is the competent professional person.

In summary, the student is actively involved in formal learning for several years. During this time he or she is exposed to many formative influences. Among these influences are the instructors' personalities and philosophies, the particulars of the classroom and clinic environments, and the life experiences of the student. These combine to produce a unique professional *person*.

Anticipation and Anxiety

Until now this chapter has focused on the role of the student as a participant in formal professional preparation. Consider now the anticipation and the anxiety inherent in the student role.

ANTICIPATION AS MOTIVATOR

Especially during the clinical aspects of professional preparation, a student becomes aware of the potential he or she has for "making a difference" in the lives of persons who have been struck down by illness or injury. This sense of anticipation about the value of one's future role is a great motivator for many students to try to make the best of their preparation period.

Because as a student one often is working with incomplete training in the techniques and skills required for professional judgment, sometimes there is a tendency to distrust one's own assessment of a situation. A close working relationship with the clinical instructor greatly diminishes the likelihood of error, however. Students, with their anticipation, fresh outlook on the profession, and newly acquired knowledge, often become articulate and committed advocates for patients.

During this period of preparation, students are exposed to many situations that illustrate that being a health professional is not limited to applying clinical skills. One becomes an integral part of the health care setting. For example, consider the following incident.

> A very elderly woman, who speaks only Yiddish, is admitted to a semi-private room to await major surgery next week. The first night, at the customary evening hour, the members of her family are required to leave. Her fear begins to mount and she becomes progressively worse during the night, until she is in great physiological as well as psychological distress. The sedation given seems to do little to relax her or to reduce her anxiety. She receives exactly the same amount

of nursing attention as the other patient. No one stays with her or attempts to comfort her. The other patient tries to reassure her but, without a knowledge of the language, is able to do little. When you come into their room the next morning to check on the English-speaking patient, she tells you about the occurrences of the night before and says, "I hope you can do something to comfort this woman. I feel just terrible!"

What can you do in this situation? To whom can you speak? How far should you go in getting involved in this matter?

A purpose of this book is to help students think more clearly about how they might serve as wise and sympathetic advocates while maintaining the necessary acuity and perspective.

ANXIETY: A FORM OF STRESS

Although students are filled with anticipation about their future role as health professionals, they sometimes also experience anxiety. Anxiety can best be thought of as a type of *stress*. A person experiences stress when he or she feels suspended in a gray zone between impossibility and resignation. That is, if one either believes that something is impossible to achieve or is resigned to not achieving it, one usually does not feel stress with regard to it. Stress results from a person's inability to reach a goal that is believed to be attainable. It is a feeling of being "out of control," and the tension arises from attempts to figure out how to get back in control of the situation (and subsequently reach the desired goal).

How does stress affect a person? First, it distorts a situation. Everyone sometimes experiences a situation in which some aspect becomes blown out of proportion. Have you ever felt that your whole life depended on getting a particular position, or on winning the affection of a particular person? In *Moby Dick*, Ahab's whole life centered on seeking revenge on the great white whale. Achievement of that goal became so all-consuming that Ahab's own safety, as well as the comforts and enjoyments of life, became a secondary consideration. Because people like Ahab overemphasize the importance of realizing some particular goal, we say that they are "driven," being controlled by some external force.

Second, stress takes its toll on a person's body and energies. Many disorders thought of as classically "psychosomatic" are believed to be ways in which the body responds to stress. For example, in recent years much attention has been given to the type of person who responds aggressively by striking out. This "Type A" person is believed to be more prone to cardiovascular problems, especially heart attacks. Research to evaluate the effects of stress on those who internalize all tension is also now being conducted, and there is evidence that this mode of response, too, exacts a heavy toll.

Often, when a person feels anxious it is because he or she is aware of being under stress but is not aware of the source. Therefore, some common sources of stress that the student experiences as anxiety are discussed here. Once the source is identified, the student has taken the first step in knowing how to assess the situation and decide if, and how, the tension can be relieved.

ANXIETY RELATED TO STUDENT LIFE

Most anxiety related to student life is temporary, arising from the usual personal pressures experienced by everyone, such as anticipation of an examination. However, there are at least three questions that raise their fearsome heads from time to time during one's student experiences.

The first is, "Am I good enough?" This type of insecurity is most evident just before an exam, but when one can attach the anxiety to something as concrete as an exam, it is possible to deal with it (usually we test whether we are indeed good enough by actually taking the exam!). Much more troublesome is a somewhat diffuse feeling that the other students and one's professional models have qualities that seem to be lacking in oneself.

The second question, "Do I have what it takes?," is rather like the first. Whereas the first question usually relates to one's moral or intellectual capacities, the second concerns one's physical or emotional limits. It is a question that is often asked by students who experience the rather common reaction of feeling faint the first time they see a badly injured patient, watch surgery, or are unexpectedly overwhelmed by a noxious odor.

A third, somewhat different question is, "Can I pay?" Many students feel burdened by the financial demands that an education places on them and their families. Anxiety about having to take another loan or find a job, or the possibility of having to drop out of school altogether, is more common than is sometimes supposed.

Some anxieties are related to student life only insofar as they affect one's performance as a student. That is, anxieties arising from nonstudent issues become student-related when one fails an exam or cannot concentrate on course work or must miss important sessions. An impending divorce, either one's own or that of parents, an unwanted pregnancy, the news that a loved one is seriously ill—all of these and many other problems can influence one's performance as a student. In such instances it is important to identify the source of the anxiety so that one's feelings at the moment can be placed in the proper perspective.

In addition to these sources of student-related anxiety, there are some anxieties that are more directly related to choice of profession.

ANXIETY RELATED TO CHOICE OF PROFESSION

Anxiety about one's choice of profession may be rooted in one of the following three sources: The choice was made (1) when the person was too young, (2) without many valid reasons, or (3) to the exclusion of several other alternatives. None of the three sources need imply that the choice was wrong (rarely does a student find that he or she made the wrong choice), but it does provide some insight into the bases for anxiety.

Each of the three sources should be considered separately to understand better why it breeds anxiety.

1. Pressures on young people to decide what they are going to be lead many to choose a career early in life, sometimes as early as junior high school. Actually, the game starts at age 2 or 3, when adults ask their toddlers, "What are you going to be when you grow up?" To gain approval, the toddler tells what he or she wants to be.

My 3½-year-old nephew has already learned the game. He recently reported to me that he is going to be a policeman or a "mommy" when he grows up. What he does not know is that the game follows him through grade school and junior high school. Then without warning, he, like others, will become aware that the adult questioning has ceased to be a game. At this point, his high school counselor will ask, "Have you decided yet what you are going to be? You know, it will make a difference in the courses you will have to take next year." By the time he begins college, the student feels he should have a well-definied career in mind! The choice is made. Then suddenly the student is preparing for the profession in which he likely will be engaged for the rest of his life. The realization hits like a sledgehammer, and he asks himself, "Is this what I *really* want?"

2. Closely related to any early choice is the possibility that the choice may have been made without many valid reasons. This does not mean that it was necessarily the wrong choice, but the realization does sometimes lead to anxiety. Many decisions are made on the advice of friends or family members, and many others on the assumption that one can be helpful to people. Still others are influenced by a book, a magazine article, or a television program. Subjective decisions such as these offer insight into why some students must later reconsider their choice of profession.

3. Finally, one reason students become anxious about their choice of profession is that the choice was made to the exclusion of other viable alternatives, a dilemma faced by able, highly qualified students in every field. The student thus not only asks, "Is this what I want?" but also ponders the far more difficult question: "Is this what I want more than the other good opportunities open to me?" The decision dilemma is aptly illustrated by the frustration felt by the student when an English composition instructor assigns a paper "on any topic"—any topic at all in the wide world of ships, cabbages, kings, and sealing wax. How much easier (but how much more confining) it is when the alternatives are limited!

RESPONDING TO ANXIETY

It was suggested previously that one of the most important steps in dissipating the tension associated with anxiety is to identify the source of the anxiety. The sources just listed are only a few examples of the types of anxiety experienced, but they do help the reader gain an idea of how wide the scope of anxiety is!

Identifying the source of anxiety is not always easy. One method is to share feelings with a friend or trustworthy classmate. The sting of anxiety is that it alienates a person from others, who know that the person is acting strangely but do not know why. If the person discusses the anxiety and tries to get at the root of it, he or she has overcome the aloneness of the experience. An amazing side effect of this process is that one often finds out how common one's feelings are. By knowing that others, too, are feeling the same anxiety, one feels less "crazy" or "out of joint" with the world.

Sometimes talking with a friend is not adequate, and one needs the help of a professional person. In such cases, usually a few minutes with an instructor or counselor will help a person discover why he or she feels anxiety. In other instances, the treatment for anxiety is time— minutes, days, perhaps weeks. For instance, time usually reveals that the student who does not enjoy the treatment or evaluation activities of the chosen profession may enjoy research, design, teaching, administration, writing, or consulting in the same profession. Because of the many opportunities open to the health professional, it is highly likely that whether or not he or she knew it at the time, the choice of a career in the health professions was a wise one.

In all these methods, the key to decreasing anxiety, once its source is identified, is to evaluate what reasonable alternatives are present.

REFERENCES

1. Carroll, L. *Alice in Wonderland*. New York, Delacorte, 1977.
2. Greenfield, M.: Creating a 'learning society.' *Newsweek*, May 16, 1983, p. 100.
3. Scully, R. and Shepard, K. F.: Clinical teaching in physical therapy education. An ethnographic study. *Phys. Ther.* 63:439–355, 1983.
4. Rosarii, M.: The allied health student as a hospital employee. *J.A.M.A.* 213:2055–2057, 1970.

Chapter 2

FOCUS: CLINICIAN

Clinical education allows persons who were classroom students to become students in the clinical setting. Here they are given their first opportunity to become practitioners in their given field and, under supervision, to assume the responsibilities, problems, and privileges of that role. At first they may spend a few hours at a time in the clinical setting while their activities are closely supervised. As they near the completion of their professional education, they will be expected to assume an increasing amount of responsibility in their role as a professional helper, or "clinician."

In the traditional use of the term, the "helping professions" were limited to those in which there was prolonged, one-to-one contact with the patient. For the purposes of this book, however, it is expedient to expand the meaning of this term to include all of the health professions. Indeed, all health professions *are* helping professions in the sense that they benefit individuals in society. The health professional does have some contact with the patient, at least to the extent that the patient's life is affected by the health professional's activities, whether directly or indirectly.

Whether viewed in the traditional or the expanded sense, "helping" in the health professions is a complex, many-faceted phenomenon, possibly quite different from the student's anticipations. Students may discover that they like to work with and even help people, but not in the therapeutic helping relationship, or that they wanted to help in a one-to-one relationship with the patient, but their present choice of profession does not provide this opportunity. Each of these concerns will be considered.

Working with People

Occasionally a student gets as far as the clinical setting before discovering that the amount of time spent in actual patient contact is not what he or she anticipated. A profession that demands many hours of contact each day may reveal to the student that he or she really does not enjoy working with people.

It is difficult for a student who has already entered a program in the health professions to concede that he or she does not like working with people. Such a student needs to be reminded that he or she may not necessarily be in the wrong profession but rather may become one of those professionals who pursue careers in areas where little contact with other people is required; such careers include research, design (of equipment, departments, public buildings, and so forth), and writing, among others. What better way to demonstrate a concern for others than to contribute to the progress of the health professions by working in these areas! A more difficult problem faces students who want to work with people and find that this is not going to figure significantly in their jobs. Such persons may need to consider switching into a related field.

Characteristics of Helping Relationships

Most students conclude that they like to *be with* people. Some discover, however, that they do not enjoy *helping* people. The difference is that they like to have friends, peers, and colleagues around them, working beside them in a shoulder-to-shoulder relationship, but they do not like to have people dependent on them. A common example is the student who insists she wants to work with children until she undergoes a clinical experience in pediatrics. She then concludes that playing with children is enjoyable but that working with them, especially when they are ill and in pain, is quite another thing!

Helping ranges from performing highly intimate acts to performing simple personal ones. Intimate help is that which is offered to someone whom you love deeply, for whom you are willing to do a big favor. The offer of intimate help in its most extreme form means that you are willing to risk even your life for this person. In contrast, personal help is that which one offers acquaintances or strangers when giving directions, assisting a person physically, or donating money to a good cause. Personal help demands personal involvement in the act but should be distinguished from intimate involvement, which is reserved for families and the closest of friends.

THE SOCIAL HELPING RELATIONSHIP

Another way to view helping concentrates on the tools and activities utilized rather than on the degree of involvement with the other person. Any help in which the tools for helping are not specific, well-defined, professional skills can be called social helping. Therapeutic helping, discussed below, is limited to specific professional skills. Contrary to this, social helping takes many forms, because the number of tools for helping are as infinite as one's own resources. One helps a child across the street, one helps allay an old man's loneliness by paying him a visit, one helps the woman upstairs by lending her five dollars (again!). Sometimes this type of helping stems from an unselfish or "altruistic" motive of wanting to benefit someone else, and other times from a subconscious desire to fulfill one's own neurotic needs.[1] Physically disabled persons are often victims of the latter motive.

A brilliant example of this was related by a health professions student. On weekends, the student cared for a 13-year-old paraplegic lad. One Saturday, they were shopping in a large department store and paused at a vending machine for a Coke. First the student bought a Coke for his young friend and then turned to buy one for himself. The lad had just taken the first sip and was resting his Coke can on the arm of his wheelchair when a small woman laden with bundles rushed up and dropped a dime into the hole in the can. She patted the astounded boy on the head and exclaimed, "Poor, poor boy. I hope that helps you get better." She then gathered up her packages and scurried away. Did the woman help? If so, *whom* did she help?

Beatrice Wright, in her excellent book, *Physical Disability: A Psychological Approach*, discusses the patient's interpretations of social helping:

> The act of helping may be disturbing to the recipient because it is not simply an act that may be more or less useful to him; it is primarily a social relationship that expresses a variety of attitudes on the part of the participants. . . .
> Disparaging aspects of receiving help have a variety of contents. Sometimes the proffered help is interpreted by a person with a

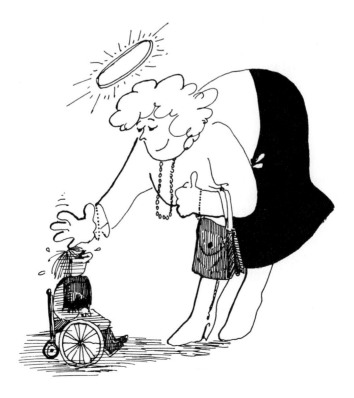

disability as meaning that he is considered more helpless than he actually is, and therefore not only is the help unnecessary but it also questions his status. Sometimes the help is felt to be motivated by hypocritical self-aggrandizement; the helper, being intent on inflating his own ego, is completely insensitive to the wishes of the recipient. Sometimes the act of helping is resented because it calls attention to the person's disability or is felt to set him apart against his wishes. Underlying this unwillingness to be noticed is the fear of being devaluated as a disabled person. Not only does he feel that his social standing is jeopardized, but also his defenses against feelings of self-devaluation become threatened. Sometimes the help is seen as oozing pity, in which it is generally rejected with bitter condemnation.[2]

The helper in the social relationship uses any available tools rather than special skills, and the help may or may not be appreciated. It is especially important to note that a physically disabled person is victimized by unwanted help, and sometimes it is viewed as an act that jeopardizes his or her feelings of worth and independence. Clearly, the health professional does not want to do this, as there is another kind of help available; it can be termed "therapeutic help" and takes place within the "therapeutic helping relationship."

THE THERAPEUTIC HELPING RELATIONSHIP

Therapeutic helping is of a personal but not intimate type, in which the primary tools are specific, well-defined professional skills. It can be administered by the health professional who meets a patient only once. For instance, the prosthetist may measure the stump of a patient's amputation, then return to the shop to develop a prosthesis; a dietician may interview the patient only once, then return to the dietetics office to evaluate nutritional status and plan the diet; or a medical technologist may collect a blood specimen and return to the laboratory to perform extensive laboratory analyses. Each of these health professionals is helping in a therapeutic manner because they are all performing professionally competent acts that will benefit the patient. Another facet of their therapeutic helping took place during the one short visit with the patient. If they could maintain or enhance the patient's self-worth during the interaction, they benefited that patient.

Therapeutic helping can also exist in a relationship that extends over a period of time. In these extended relationships, trust develops between patient and health professional. In a later chapter, this is referred to as "professional closeness." Dependence between the two also develops in extended relationships. If dependence allows the patient to realize more fully his or her personal health goals, dependence can be called "constructive dependence." If it hinders the patient in realizing legitimate health goals, it can be called "detrimental dependence." In Chapter 7, these two types of dependence are described.

Carl Rogers, a leading psychologist today, defines the helping relationship in the following manner:

... By this term I mean a relationship in which at least one of the parties has the intent of promoting the growth, development, maturity, improved functioning, improved coping with life of the other. The other, in this sense, may be one individual or a group. To put it another way, a helping relationship might be defined as one in which one of the participants intends that there should come about, in one or both parties, more appreciation of, more expression of, more functional use of the latent inner resources of the individual.[3]

Helping in a therapeutic relationship, then, takes place between a person who has a special problem and another person skilled in techniques that can alleviate or diminish that problem. The relationship can be established at the first meeting and is therefore as pertinent to health professionals who see a patient only once as it is to those who see a patient over a prolonged period of time. Specific limits are imposed by the relation between the individual's problem and the health professional's skills; for example, a speech therapist cannot enter into a therapeutic helping relationship with a patient who has no speech problems. The differences between helping as a social relationship and helping as a therapeutic relationship are reviewed in the following chart.

COMPARISON BETWEEN HELPING AS A SOCIAL AND AS A THERAPEUTIC RELATIONSHIP

Helping as a Social Relationship	Helping as a Therapeutic Relationship
May be an intimate or personal act.	Is a personal but not intimate act.
Helper utilizes a wide variety of resources.	Helper primarily utilizes well-defined, specialized professional skills.
Relationship does not necessarily allow participants to realize personal goals. (Can foster either constructive or destructive dependence.) *Further discussed in Chapter 7*	Relationship should always allow participants to realize personal goals. (Should foster constructive dependence.)
Can result in continued interdependence or self-dependence. *Further discussed in Chapter 13*	Should result in self-dependence; dignity is maintained through professional closeness.

Within the therapeutic helping relationship, an important point sometimes overlooked by helpers is that their own desire to help is only one factor in the situation. The patient's personality, motives, and other characteristics are equally decisive. A physician recalls one type of difficult patient he and his colleagues encountered:

A 51-year-old attorney specializing in medical negligence was enraged when his many complaints were ultimately diagnosed as multiple sclerosis. Known for his flashy wardrobe and courtroom pyrotechnics, he roamed from doctor to doctor, refusing to understand the nature of his illness, and threatening to sue the previous "bastard" who had tried to help him. He was like Job (xiii:4), who raged, "Ye are forgers of lies, ye are all physicians of no value." He adamantly refused treatment and demanded more and more tests and consultations. Eventually his doctors did not return his calls for appointments and were frightened and depressed about him . . .[4]*

*Excerpted by permission of the New England Journal of Medicine, 298:8813, 1978.

This dramatic instance is not the only type of barrier one encounters. For example, some patients have a problem responding to any kind of help, even though the services offered will seemingly benefit them. For these patients, receiving help may be seen as a sign of weakness. Other types of patients also create challenges to the person who wants to help. In an article entitled "Taking Care of the Hateful Patient," the author reports four types of patients that health professionals dread: demanders, dependent clingers, manipulative help-rejecters, and self-destructive deniers.[5] The issue of patient types is examined in more detail in Chapter 6. The reader is reminded of them here only to highlight the fact that helping as an ideal is not always easily executed! When barriers arise, the health professional feels frustrated and may even engage in behavior that is less than beneficial to the patient.

New Dimensions of Helping

In the opening paragraph of this chapter, it was explained that helping traditionally connoted one-to-one contact with a patient over a period of time; this can now be expanded to include limited contact with a patient or, in some instances, indirect contact through reports, specimens, and so forth. There are two other ways in which the definition of helping can be expanded: One is possible as a result of the introduction of the assistant, while the other is found in the practice of referrals. Each of these will be presented briefly.

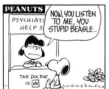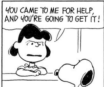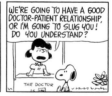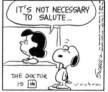

© 1952, 1958, 1968 United Feature Syndicate, Inc.

THE ASSISTANT

Many health professionals are experiencing a rather dramatic change in their professional roles with the introduction into health care of a growing number of "assistants." The term itself is confusing because some assistants, such as the physician's assistant, engage in a program equal in length and rigor to many programs now considered to be for health professionals. At any rate, almost every health field at present consists of at least two groups of people distinguished primarily by the amount and type of formal preparation required to practice in their fields. One consequence of this is that some who entered a health profession with the understanding that they would help in some particular manner (i.e., one-to-one patient care) are experiencing anger and disillusionment. Although it is understandable how they feel, they should be reminded that this narrow definition of helping may not, in fact, be in the patient's best interest. Helping a patient should be more broadly defined as providing the best possible service (both quantitative and qualitative) at the least possible cost.

Professional assistant programs were introduced in recent years to help provide low-cost quality care, to create employment opportunity for people who did not want to or could not pursue a professional program, and to alleviate serious manpower shortages in many health fields. The extent to which these particular goals have actually been met to date is widely disputed. However, it should be emphasized that the possibility of better quality health care may well still be an important consequence of having introduced assistants into the system of health care delivery. This rests less on the idea of decreased costs to patients and more on the idea that a specialization of services enables each person in the system to most effectively apply those skills for which he or she is best trained. Ideally, with time the mutual dependence of professional and assistant will become more apparent. When this happens, assistants will be considered less as supportive persons and will be acknowledged more fully for the unique contribution their presence makes to the quality of health care. Unfortunately, some health professionals still interpret a division of skills to mean that the assistant will completely take over evaluation and treatment procedures, leaving the hapless professional with administrative tasks.

This need not be the case. The health professional will find that there are areas of direct evaluation and treatment for which he or she must, on the basis of unique professional skills, continue to assume responsibility. The patient benefits from receiving from each person what he or she is most highly qualified to give. In the case in which diagnostic, evaluation, and treatment techniques are partially administered by an assistant, the helping relationship operates in a slightly different manner: The professional (acting now as supervisor) applies specific skills (administrative and supervisory) to the assistant, who in turn applies other specific skills (evaluation and treatment) to the patient.

In short, the health professional who asserts that he or she is interested only in helping the patient must be willing to apply professional skills in the direction that will most fully benefit that patient. In some cases, this will mean being a competent supervisor to the person performing diagnostic procedures previously performed by the health professional, or now providing part of the direct patient care.

REFERRING PATIENTS

Sometimes it is hard for the health professional to refer a patient to someone else who can do the job more effectively, even though it may be in the patient's best interest. The reason is that health professionals do not take their jobs lightly and therefore find it painful to admit failure. Perhaps weeks or months have already gone into trying to help that patient, either through direct patient care or through attempts at analyzing results from diagnostic tests.

There are at least three situations in which steps should be taken to implement referral. Patients should be referred in the following cases: (1) when progress is hindered by personality conflicts between the health professional and patient; (2) when progress is hindered because of a detrimental amount of dependency between patient and health professional; and (3) when progress is hindered because the health professional is not experienced in, or does not have, adequate techniques or equipment for providing proper services to that particular patient.

The last is common today when the generalist is disappearing from the health professions. The likelihood is slim that one individual health professional will have all the necessary information.

Helping, then, does not always entail simply using one's own resources. Rather, in some cases it may mean knowing where to refer the patient for further evaluation or treatment. In this manner, the health professional's integrity as a helper can be maintained in the most inclusive sense of the word.

THE CLINICIAN AND HEALTH POLICY

A chapter on the health professional as helper would not be complete without some mention of the health professional's responsibility in regard to the institution of health care itself. Today's policies favor some racial and age groups over others. A greater emphasis on acute care of the sick rather than on preventive measures for maintaining health raises important questions about where the health care dollar is being spent and how reasonable priorities can be set.

Distributive justice is the principle that concerns the comparative treatment of individuals in the allotment of benefits and burdens. The goal of distributive justice is to limit "arbitrary" distinctions and assure a "proper" share to each party with a legitimate claim to the thing being distributed. It is easy to see that health policy and practice depend to a great extent on the interpretation of distributive justice that is accepted by a society. It has bearing, for example, on who should have access to the health care system and the types of qualifications required for receiving services within it. It helps to determine the proportion of total benefits one should receive and the price to be exacted for those benefits. Therefore, justice is not the only value related to health care, but it certainly is one important value.

In the United States, as in many parts of the world today, distributive justice considerations are based on the assumption that persons are "fundamentally equal." For example, the Bill of Rights and Amendments of the United States Constitution spell out the particulars of each person's "inalienable right" to "life, liberty, and the pursuit of happiness." This assumption of fundamental equality supports the idea that each patient should be treated as *inherently worthy* of the health professional's consideration.

If everyone is "fundamentally equal," should treatment then be identical for all? Common sense tells us that this is not what justice based on "equality" calls for. Justice, as an eliminator of "arbitrary" distinctions, must provide the basis for justifying an unequal distribution. In short, what we really seek is not a radically equal distribution, but one that is "fair" or "equitable."

Commonly accepted criteria for achieving an equitable distribution are special merits of some persons and special needs of some persons. A merit notion supports allocating resources in accord either with how hard a person tries or with the kind of results he or she achieves. Distribution according to need is quite a different approach. Here the explicit goal is to help diminish the difference in well-being among persons, and the means of achieving this is to compensate the person who has the deprivation. Medical care is more appropriately distributed according to need.[6]

However, even if one agrees that medical need is an appropriate criterion for the distribution of health care resources, the problem of *costs* that are incurred in trying to respond to the need remains an issue.

This brief discussion highlights that the health professional who becomes involved in health policy must make a commitment to understanding the trade-offs and gains that various positions will yield.

The health care provider is perceived by society not only as a person who provides a specific technical service but also as one who is able to interpret important health-related issues and help effect needed change. He or she is consulted by legal and consumer-interest agencies for aid in matters of law, practice, and public policy.

This social responsibility role of the helper is increasingly being acknowledged in the health professions. Students are being introduced to basic legal and ethical concepts and advised of health-related policies. Individual health professionals are acknowledging this role by involving themselves in government and lay organizations designed to face key issues and effect change.

Becoming involved in improving the health care system does not require that one hold a federal office or receive an appointment to a post in the Department of Health and Human Services. These positions are vital, but the task cannot be done at top administrative levels alone. Equally important is the health professional's involvement in local organizations, church groups, neighborhood health centers, and the policy-making body of his or her institution of employment.

REFERENCES

1. Toi, M., and Batson, C. D.: More evidence that empathy is a source of altruistic motivation. *J. Pers. Soc. Psychol.* 43:281–292, 1982.
2. Wright, B.: *Physical Disability: A Psychological Approach.* New York, Harper & Row, 1960, p. 224.
3. Rogers, C. R.: On Becoming a Person. Boston, Houghton Mifflin and Company, 1961, pp. 39–40.
4. Groves, J. E.: Taking care of the hateful patient. *N. Engl. J. Med.* 298:883–887, 1978.
5. *Ibid.*, pp. 884–887.
6. Purtilo, R.: *Justice, Liberty, Compassion: Humane Health Care and Rehabilitation in the U.S.* New York, World Rehabilitation Fund, Inc., 1981, pp. 13–16.

Chapter 3

FOCUS: PERSON

The final chapter in Part I focuses on the health professional as a person. In what kind of activity should a health professional engage in order to stay healthy and job-satisfied? What guidelines are there to follow? What are the main pitfalls that the health professional should watch out for? The chapter progresses along three lines of thought: (1) taking care of oneself; (2) building strong working relationships with colleagues; and (3) assuring high-quality performance in oneself and others.

Taking Care of Oneself

Everyone would agree that one is ultimately responsible for one's own health. One feels better, looks better, and is able to function more fully when taking care of one's own health. Furthermore, there is much evidence to suggest that health professionals who are healthy physically and psychologically are more satisfied with their jobs than those who are not. There is a positive correlation between satisfaction in one's work experience and one's level of healthiness.[1] Much is to be gained personally and professionally from taking good care of oneself. However, many health professionals have serious health problems that are obviously related to lifestyle. Clearly, knowing the benefits of staying healthy and actually staying healthy are not the same! Why do health professionals fail to take care of their health?

THE ILLUSION OF INVULNERABILITY

Many health professionals are so used to being helpers that they believe themselves somehow invulnerable to illness or debilitation and therefore fail to take the same kinds of precautions to safeguard their health that they instruct their patients to take. Goethe, in his "Elective Affinities," illustrates that everyone has a potential for organizing a world that fits his or her illusions:

> And so they all, each in his own way, reflectingly or unreflectingly, go on with their daily lives; everything seems to have its accustomed course, for indeed, even in desperate situations where everything hangs in the balance, one goes on living as though nothing were wrong.[2]

For a health professional, ill health is fundamentally "wrong" insofar as the helper believes he or she should not be vulnerable to the same weaknesses as persons who need help from the professional. It is easy to deny that one is fully vulnerable to the particular fates and misfortunes that strike down others in the natural lottery of life. One person, reflecting on his own sudden onset of severe illness and its long convalescence reflects:

> I have come to the conclusion that the psychology of my experiences has a constant theme, which I have referred to loosely and generically as a feeling of invulnerability—a feeling that affects attitudes, moods, and thoughts. Within 13 weeks I had, in effect, condensed three states of life: childhood, adolescence, and a kind of skittish maturity. Each of these stages has its own delusion of invulnerability—invincibility in childhood, independence in adolescence, and safety in maturity—and accompanying each of these delusions is a whole way of acting and responding to the world.[3]*

Ethical codes and oaths in the health professions do not provide assistance to persons who wish to take good care of themselves. Indeed, throughout history all of the major ones have emphasized the health professional's responsibility to *others*, with striking negligence in talking about responsibility to one's own self. Not one of the major oaths or codes makes reference to a moral obligation to take care of oneself. It appears that neither the professional associations nor the public are very much concerned with the health professional's struggle to combat the illusion of invulnerability.

There are at least two ways in which the tendency to believing oneself invulnerable—and thereby neglecting to make sensible decisions about one's own health—can be constructively overcome. The first is to adopt good work habits. The second is to make constructive time for oneself. Although apparently obvious, the particulars of how to go about each of these deserves attention.

STYLES OF APPROACHING PROFESSIONAL TASKS

Popular bookstands are filled with prescriptions for more effectively managing one's time, stresses, and responsibilities in the workplace. Unfortunately, many of them do not take into account personal strengths and habits as reasonable starting points. Therefore, rather than suggesting a particular course of action, the following paragraphs outline two styles that one can use as models in trying to cope with the many tasks and responsibilities related to professional life. While neither, taken alone, is adequate, some aspects of the two models taken together can create a balanced approach to stresses and problems in the workplace.

Two characters from Greek mythology, Sisyphus and Pandora, pro-

---

*Reprinted by permission of the New England Journal of Medicine, 308:1268, 1983.

vide contrasting models for consideration.* There is much to be learned from each, as well as some illustrations of what to avoid when organizing one's priorities and approaching one's tasks.

One model is Sisyphus.[4] He is portrayed as possessing competence, single-mindedness, perseverance. As a king, being "held responsible" required that Sisyphus willingly place himself in a position of decision-making and accept as an integral aspect of the role the consequences (sanctions) that would follow if the task was not completed well. In the Sisyphus approach one has a task to perform and pursues it with undying diligence.

The Sisyphus type of health professional is decisive, acts autonomously, competes with vigor, accepts complaints, guards territory, and sees little need for input from others. Things are "in control." When colleagues offer assistance, noting that his shoulders seem weighted down by the burden of the office, he responds, "It's not heavy, it's my duty!"

The person who adopts this approach fosters and values *efficient* decision-making within our highly bureaucratized and fragmented structures of health care. The Sisyphus-type health professional also places a high value on *competence*. One can see that Sisyphus traits support specialization in the professions, where each contributor has more highly competent but narrowly defined roles to play—an important quality because specialization is being discussed by many health professions today.

The Sisyphus-model emphasis on holding oneself accountable for one's activities makes this type of health professional supportive of accountability-oriented procedures such as informed consent, institutional review mechanisms for clinical research, quality assurance policies, continuing education requirements, and peer review practices.

With so many positive values fostered by the Sisyphus approach, one may not be surprised that the entire social work code of ethics is organized around the concept and language of this type of "responsibility,"[5] and that the codes of numerous associations of the health professions place it centrally in their ethical guidelines. In fact, one might ask, has this approach any shortcomings at all?

The major shortcoming is revealed in the plight of Sisyphus himself. Sisyphus was not a well-liked fellow, though that did not create the major problem for him. However, his activities were such that during his tenure as king of Corinth he incurred the wrath of the gods, who doomed him to Hades. As the administrators of this efficiently run institution tended to do, they drew on his strengths in deciding what his eternal task would be. Sisyphus has to forever roll uphill a heavy stone, which

---

*The following comments on the two styles were first presented by the author as the Commencement address at the MGH Institute of Health Professions, Boston, Massachusetts, August 5, 1983. Used with permission.

forever rolls down again. He keeps pushing, never reflecting, never trying an alternative route, never attempting to renegotiate the terms—always pushing up the same path again and again and again. . .*ad infinitum.*

His accountability is awesome; the fastidious persistence with which he exercises his task, exhausting. He is rigorously responsible, *but he never quite succeeds.*

If only once, just once, Sisyphus would break away to try the alternative route up the backside of the mountain, or better yet, around it! If only once he'd say, "Phooey, this isn't going to work, I'm going to bed!" While his dogged persistence generates much useful activity, the tragedy of Sisyphus is his inability to reach his goal—and to recognize that it may be attainable by some other route.

There is another problem with the Sisyphus model. Modern-day Sisyphus-type health professionals are becoming immortalized too—in the literature of "burnout." The demands of professional life can be exhausting, and most leaders today are not placed in immortal bodies and spirits. In the literature of burnout, one sees such a mortal less as "smiling competence," strolling coolly down the corridors with chart in hand, and more as a closet alcohol or drug abuser;[6] more as divorcée;[7] or more as an ugly autotron harboring chronic rage and depression. This "burnout" phenomenon destroys some of the most committed leaders.[8] The strains are so exhausting that eventually the morning sun is robbed of anticipation; joy is bleached into boredom; meaninglessness—like the morning fog in Carl Sandburg's poem—comes "on little cat feet," obscuring the promise of the horizon.

Because there is such a high price to pay for many who adopt a Sisyphus approach only, it is worthwhile to consider alternative or additional modes of functioning as a professional.

It seems that some of the serious difficulties accompanying a strictly Sisyphus approach can be mitigated by lacing them liberally with Pandoran traits. Therefore, let us consider this model.

Pandora was a leader in her own right, being the first mortal woman. Pandora was playful, imaginative, mischievous. Her inquisitiveness was unbridled. Her spirit of optimism and ingenuity was a delight to behold.[9]

Virtues required for operating within this model include the acknowledgment of surprise, the ability to embrace rather than oversimplify ambiguities, willingness to accommodate uncertainty, courage to act in the face of the unknown, optimism, risk-taking, love of the lyrical, a propensity for dancing rather than marching, and an "at homeness" with improvisation.

One can readily see the contrast with the model of Sisyphus and begin to see its strengths. Imaginative exploration is required in order to overcome the uselessness, in some situations, of trying old—even time-tested—routes for today's changing health care system demands. The weakest link in the chain of the Sisyphus approach is its inability to cope with what is new and uncertain.

In *Medical Choices, Medical Chances*, the authors address head-on the issue of *uncertainty* in health care:

> We are all, to some degree . . . afraid of uncertainty. Because our conception of rationality has no place for uncertainty, we find it difficult to be rational about uncertainty. Instead, when faced with uncertainty we become anxious—[and] are tempted to retreat into a false sense of certainty, which affects our capacity to make decisions . . . but we cannot make wise decisions when we deny ourselves the benefits of conscious awareness of uncertainty.[10]

Today the health care system that most of us have grown familiar with rapidly is skidding off the edges of this society's peripheral vision, and in its place is a largely undefined horizon.

An example of uncertainty is how health care costs are going to be kept—or brought—down without severely compromising the values of equitable access and high quality of care. For example, "diagnosis-related groups" is an attempt to rethink the mechanism of third-party reimbursements. The incentives built into this approach create an emphasis on doing *less* for patients rather than more. The history of how this new practice will affect access, costs, and quality is almost completely unwritten.[11]

How are health professionals, whose ethos traditionally has included the bidding to "do the best (most) possible for the patient" going to accommodate to these new federal directives? McCue has shown that health professionals who are faced with uncertainty about patient care decisions tend to order more tests, do more treatments, rather than less. The new directives fly in the face of this type of logic.[12] The old paths up the mountain, however deeply trodden by those before us, are not assured routes to success in this uncertain moment.

Other practices, long believed invulnerable to change, are being called into question. An example is confidentiality. The advent of computers, for example, is raising doubts about whether this—a persistent concept in health care oaths and codes—has become an outdated concept. A recent article in a health care journal was entitled "Confidentiality: A Decrepit Concept."[13]

In an article adressing confidentiality issues in social work practice, the author reflects:

> Confidentiality has become a highly complex ethical and legal issue. Those professionals uninitiated to its complexities generally function with a few simple guidelines such as, "don't talk about clients outside work" and "when a subpoena arrives, you have to answer it." Unfortunately, numerous sticky situations arise in daily practice, and clinicians, administrators, and those concerned with personnel matters often find the standard guidelines inadequate. There may be no single, definitive answer to tell the confused practitioner what should be done. Various sources can be consulted for guidance, but in the end, the individual must often exercise professional discretion, con-

sult his malpractice policy to determine the extent of coverage, and stick his ethical neck out and do what he thinks best under the circumstances. If the troublesome problem is researched intensively, conflicting guidelines and mandates often emerge.[14]

In short—given the uncertainty that characterizes large areas of health professions policy and practice, health professionals necessarily must be risk-takers, innovators, probability seekers.

However, most readers know that Pandora is not remembered mostly for her vitality, optimism, and ingeniousness, but rather for her mistake. Impulsively she opened a box—the wrong box—and let escape and be lost all human blessings, leaving only hope. Clearly, the Pandoran mode needs "tempering." Aristotle based his theory of excellence on seeking the mean between two extremes of character traits. . .a principle well applied to the health professional's search for excellence and balance. Only in trying out various traits and approaches can each person finally find a set of options that combine the correct amount of each characteristic for optimizing professional success while avoiding burnout or diffuse lack of directiveness. Pandora and Sisyphus present two extremes of approach. Ideally, the reader will avoid the detrimental effects of each while capitalizing on the considerable strengths of both.

THE NEED FOR SOLITUDE

No matter how wisely one picks and chooses to develop a lifestyle that allows ample doses of both Sisyphean and Pandoran traits, the health professional still needs to claim time to be alone. In other words, a vital strategy for survival is solitude.

What *is* solitude? In its most fundamental sense, it's one expression of one's state of being alone in the world. Solitude is a positive, active state of being: Although the experience of solitude is not identical to happiness and may even be "bittersweet" (accompanied by sorrow or anger), nonetheless it is *sought out* as a need in itself, not foisted upon one as a result of feeling rejected or "out of contact."[15] In general, it can be thought of as the "positive dimension" of aloneness, in contrast to loneliness, which is also an expression of being ultimately alone in the world but is a form of suffering.[16]

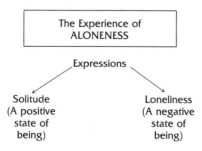

Pooh Bear, the most philosophical and reflective member of the community at Pooh Corner, sought solitude often. It was said of him by his neighbors:

> And He sits and thinks of the things they know: He and the Forest, alone together . . .[17]

Other philosophers have emphasized that seeking solitude is an activity directly related to community with others. Tillich maintains that it is the necessary (and perhaps sufficient) criterion for relationship.[18] Bugbee suggests that it is necessary for bringing to consciousness who we are in the world and how we are related to other people.[19] In short, it's a time to be *with oneself* only, not with others, and to engage in activities that can better prepare one for relationship. Therefore, its importance for the health professional is obvious.

Yet, many health professionals do not in fact find their lifestyle and work conducive to considered reflection. Both the structure of institutions themselves and the psychological demand of this "inward-looking" activity create barriers.

Health care institutions, like other bureaucratic systems, have efficiency as an overriding value. In order for efficiency to be realized, schedules, policies, and routines must be implemented and followed. Therefore, former routines of work and play are replaced by the new, usually more rigorous demands of the hospital schedules and operations, and there is little encouragement from one's employer to engage in solitude-seeking behavior!

From a psychological viewpoint, the inward-looking process of solitude activity itself is taxing. Solitude work can lead one into aspects of one's existence that have been carefully kept hidden for years. The process can be excruciating and, for some, too painful to pursue. Furthermore, when a health professional sees a colleague who is seeking solitude, very often he or she sees someone who is acting aloof from the very projects that help to create the health professional's *raison d'être*. The solitude-seeking person's need to withdraw from, move away from, the colleague is easily interpreted as personal rejection. When the concerned person asks, "What can I do to help?," the response all too often is, "Leave me alone!"

Insight into one factor underlying the experience of rejection by would-be "helpers" in such situations is provided by considering the discrediting or stigmatizing quality of not being needed. Nowhere is the plight of the "not needed" or "no longer useful" more vividly portrayed than in Eliot's "Choruses" from *The Rock*:

> No man has hired us
> with pocketed hands
> and lowered faces
> We stand about in open places
> And shiver in unlit rocms.
> Only the wind moves

Over empty fields, untilled
Where the plough rests, at an angle
to the furrow. In this land
There shall be one cigarette to two men
To two women one half pint of bitter
Ale.[20]*

The health professional, whose identity is laden with "helping" skills, easily experiences it as a *personal* rejection when a colleague prefers to just "be alone"!

And so one begins to get a fuller picture: Neither the social structure, nor one's own energies, nor even one's closest colleagues and friends are likely to support an activity that is life-supporting but that *also* requires that one be left alone.

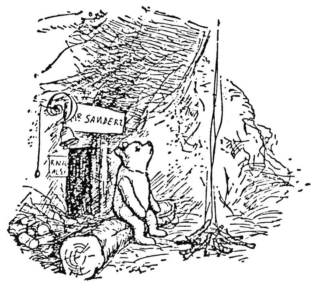

From *Winnie-The-Pooh* by A. A. Milne, Copyright 1926 by E. P. Dutton & Co., Inc.; renewed, 1954 by A. A. Milne. Reproduced by permission of the publisher.

Some ideas to try in fostering time for oneself include the following:
1. Set a conscious time and place to be alone.
2. Become bold in identifying to others what you are doing.
3. Take notes on your reflections.
4. Remind yourself often that the basic minimum requirement upon which most or all other health-supporting activity depends is to take time to be with oneself.

In addition, one can help others to have their own time alone by learning to recognize this need in others and encouraging it.

Taking Care of Each Other

It is not enough to cultivate character traits for survival in one's work or to make time for oneself. Also needed for success and satisfaction

*From "Choruses from 'The Rock'" in *Collected Poems 1909–1962* by T. S. Eliot. Copyright 1936 by Harcourt Brace Jovanovich, Inc., Copyright © 1963, 1964 by T. S. Eliot. Reprinted by permission of the publisher.

in one's career are colleagues with whom one can share the joys, dreams, and frustrations of everyday practice. Broski and Cook surveyed medical dieticians, medical technicians, physical therapists, and occupational therapists to determine levels of job satisfaction.[21] Each of the groups expressed the highest level of satisfaction in their relationships with colleagues, suggesting that persons in a wide range of health professions are fortunate to have competent, reliable, and enjoyable people with whom to work.

SUPPORT GROUPS

The persons working in a health care situation have several forms of common language, all of which help to establish bonds among themselves and create a type of supportive network when the going gets rough.

The Language of Caring. Health professionals speak the language of caring—about the patient's problems, prognosis, and progress; about the department; about what is happening in their field; and about health services in general. They voluntarily place themselves in the mainstream of human suffering, thereby showing that they care. No neon lights beckon them in. No one commits them to this role. There are no locked doors preventing their departure. They choose to be there because they care enough about human suffering to want to effect certain changes by the use of professional skills.

But having made themselves available to those who need their skills, all health professionals assume commitments that extend beyond themselves and each other, beyond friends and relatives, into the heart of society. The common dilemma into which they are plunged by continuous technological progress is expressed well by Kenneth Vaux:

> An initial question we face is that of the meaning of human value under the impact of technology. Decisions that need to be made day by day in hospitals and clinics of a medical center are always both particularly immediate and profoundly universal. . . . In the clinical settings of modern teaching hospitals the constant weight of human anguish, combined with the ever-present fact of death which is the refutation of not only our life urge but the biomedical commitment as well, conspires to create an insensitivity toward persons and a devaluation of human dignity.[22]

When faced with such momentous issues, the bond of caring extends across external barriers.

Technical Language. Another language shared by health professionals is the technical language of each specific profession. While this may seem irrelevant at first glance, it should not be overlooked entirely as a means whereby potential differences can begin to be resolved. For example, an older graduate who feels she has nothing in common with the young student may see him in a much different light after discussing with him newer approaches to treatment of amyotrophic lateral sclerosis or a better method of analyzing cholesterol levels. Similarly, the student may gain new respect for the older person who has taken time to explain a new piece of equipment or to demonstrate an interesting technique.

The Language of Gratitude. Gratitude or appreciation is expressed too seldom by persons working together. A simple word of thanks can create more good will than many months of competent work together.

The three kinds of language—the language of caring, technical language, and the language of gratitude—can help to reduce tensions among co-workers and foster a sense of "belongingness" among them. Together they can realize mutually shared goals and values.

To help assure maximal support, when looking for a position in a new setting it is advisable to identify persons in that setting who will make potentially good sources of support. At least one person who appears to be a potential source of support should be recognizable if one is going to accept the position. If no one person promises to be such a resource, it is better to look elsewhere. In addition, one should try to gain some understanding of how support is expressed within the department and larger institution. To make an assessment, the following guidelines may be useful:

1. Inquire of your future employer whether there are meetings or other sessions where problems associated with the everyday stresses of health care delivery are discussed.

2. Ask some of the people you will be working with what they believe to be the sources of the most intense stress in that environment.

3. Ask some of the people you will be working with how each as an individual deals with the stress of his or her position, and whether, as a whole, the environment is a supportive or divisive one.

4. Make a mental note of those who appear to be potential sources of support, or if no one appears to be. A setting in which everyone denies that problems exist or becomes defensive about such questions when they are tactfully posed, probably signals that stresses are dealt with alone, without the support of one's colleagues.[23]

Fortunately, only in rare situations are no supports available. In fact, being a support to others often is the key to finding support from them when it is needed. The old adage, "To have a friend is to be one," holds true in the workplace.

THE HEALTH CARE TEAM

Many institutions today incorporate a "teamwork" approach to health care. The health care team enables individuals to work together cooperatively with the goal of more effective patient or client management. Individuals in the health professions function within the context of the health care system. This system is made up of two broad categories of actions, actions flowing from hierarchical decisions and those flowing from community-derived decisions.

Within the *hierarchy*, the power to make decisions flows from very few persons to affect very many. Power differentials are necessary and accepted. The power and the responsibility weigh heaviest at the top. A value realized by this mode of functioning is efficiency.

In contrast, within the *community* framework the power to make decisions is more equally diffused throughout the institution, or at least among the members of a health care "team." Power differentials are less obvious. Professionals with different skills function together as mutual support and task sharers. Values realized by this mode of functioning are equality and mutuality.

Therefore, two important values are realized in the two forms of activity—efficiency and mutuality.

The idea of the health care team is that all team members are more equal. All are working together cooperatively and efficiently toward the institutional goal of patient management. Therefore, the two sources of action (hierarchy and community) are brought into closer approximation—with an emphasis on community-directed rather than hierarchical decision-making.[24]

One of the most striking aspects of the health care team is its accommodation to personal and professional differences among the team members. Writing on the health care team, Brill notes:

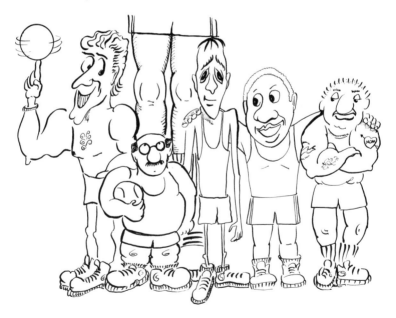

Team members bring their own personal and professional values and norms to the team, and in the process of either building a new team or becoming part of an already formed team, there must be an accommodation among the various norms and values involved. Achievement of this accommodation is a necessary step in team formation, and once it has been achieved, it is a major factor in holding a team together and enabling it to work. It is important to remember that there will be significant differences in values among team members, and this diversity can be a source of strength, in that it promotes a critical attitude and examination of the principles involved.

The three fundamental values, cited earlier, that underlie human services—the worth of human life, the capacity of people for change, and the ability of an outsider to facilitate that change—should be held in common by all team members in human service. Beyond that, there is room for great variation. The manner in which variations are accommodated and the norms that develop will be indicative of the health and strength of the team and whether maximum use can be made of its potential.[25]

The potential for accommodating personal differences while improving patient care has been voiced in numerous articles. Most emphasize with Thomasma that two important functions of the team are to create a common language and encourage a common process of decision-making.[26]

The team itself should become a means of support, growth, and increased effectiveness for the health professional who wants to maximize his or her strengths as a person while performing the necessary professional tasks.

Taking Care to Do Well

A chapter on the how's and wherefore's of maximizing one's personal-professional functioning would not be complete without giving at least brief attention to the importance of maintaining high professional standards of practice for oneself and others. Two mechanisms for maintaining the high quality of a group are (1) peer review and (2) whistle-blowing.

Peer Review. This procedure involves evaluating each other's work in a formal, usually written, way. It serves several purposes: It provides constructive criticism and a means of increased self-awareness for the person being reviewed; it provides protection to patients or clients should the person being reviewed be incompetent to perform his or her professional tasks; and it is a means of assuring society that a health professional is fulfilling the conditions of his or her "contract." All of these taken together help to ensure a high quality of health care while providing support and reassurance to the various members of the health care team.

Whistle-Blowing. Sometimes the situation arises in which a colleague is not functioning in a manner that is acceptable, because he or she seems to be a danger to good patient care or in other ways in acting unethically or incompetently. As a result, many professional ethical codes today include a statement about the moral responsibility of a health professional to report such conduct, or "blow the whistle."

Consider the following two stories. Would you "blow the whistle" in either instance? Why or why not?

The first concerns a health professional who is faced with a question regarding the activity of her superiors in an institution:

Judy Morris is a dietician at a small community hospital. She is a single parent with two children, and she provides for their needs totally. Her present job allows her to earn a nice salary and live comfortably. She likes her position and does a good job.

Part of the function of the Dietary Department is to provide catering services for hospital affairs. Lately, several members of the hospital's administrative staff have been holding personal parties that are being catered by the Dietary Department and charged to the hospital's operating budget. The dietary staff are aware of these events and resent the fact that they must provide these services on top of their regular work. Judy is also afraid that the patient meal service may suffer as a result of the catering. She has approached the Director of Dietary Services about the matter and he promptly told Judy that "if she liked her job, she would overlook these events."

At the same time, Judy has noted that several employees have been pilfering food items from the storeroom. It is part of Judy's job to report people who are stealing. One evening, Judy caught David, a cook's assistant, stealing a roast beef. According to policy, David should be reported and would probably be fired for stealing.

Can Judy justifiably report David and yet continue to provide— and thus condone—the catering services without reporting them?

The second story involves two health professionals working in surgery:

Henry Arnold, a 44-year-old electrician, was married and the father of four children. At age 14 he had had rheumatic fever, and shortly thereafter a heart murmur was noted during a routine physical examination. He was without symptoms until five years prior to admission, when he began to notice fatigue and shortness of breath with only slight exertion. He was referred to a cardiologist who diagnosed rheumatic heart disease with a damaged heart valve. His symptoms became progressively more serious as he developed severe congestive heart failure. The decision was made to replace the damaged valve with an artificial valve.

A week later he underwent open heart surgery. Early in the procedure, Jack Carstens, one of the pump technicians, noted that there was a large pool of blood on the floor of the operating room; the tubing connecting the pipe to the patient either had failed to be connected or had been insecurely fastened at the locking connector. Judging from the volume of blood on the floor and the rate of flow of the pump, Jack estimated the length of time Mr. Arnold's brain was without blood (and therefore without oxygen) was six minutes. The surgeon decided to reconnect the pump, complete the operation, and "hope for the best," since the actual time of cerebral anoxia was unknown.

Postoperatively, Mr. Arnold was transferred to the intensive care unit, which was routine procedure for the post–open heart surgery patients. The rumor of the "accident" in the operating room spread quickly through the nursing and professional staff of the intensive care unit and soon after through the rest of the hospital. Mr. Arnold never regained consciousness, although his surgery itself was successful. His family had been prepared before the surgery for the possibility of death or disablement as a result of the "unavoidable consequences of high-risk surgery" and never thought to question the possibility of an accident.

At two weeks postoperatively, Mr. Arnold died.

Mrs. Arnold received a bill from her insurance company for $5500, the portion of the hospital bill not covered by her husband's health insurance.

Should Jack Carstens have "blown the whistle"?*

These and similar cases will present themselves to health professionals. Although there often is conflict because of the individual involved, there is a responsibility to help maintain high standards. Failing to "blow the whistle" in instances of obvious misbehavior hurts the health professions as a whole. One's own professional growth and personal integrity are at stake in such situations.

REFERENCES

1. Lacy, W. B., Houghland, J. G., and Shepard, J. M.: Relationship between work and non-work satisfaction: is it changing and does occupational prestige make a difference? *Sociol. Spectrum* 2:157–171, 1982.
2. Goethe, J. W.: *Elective Affinities*. New York, Penguin Books, 1978.
3. Frank, J.: Illness and invulnerability. *N. Engl. J. Med.* 308:1268–1274, 1983.
4. Pinsent, J.: *Greek Mythology*. London, Hamlyn Publishers Group, Ltd., 1969, pp. 69 ff.
5. National Association of Social Workers, Inc.: *Code of Ethics of the National Association of Social Workers*. Washington, D.C., 1979. (Adopted by the 1979 NASW Delegate Assembly, effective July 1, 1980.)
6. Schnurr, S.: The alcoholic professional. *Fam. Commun. Health* 2(1):33–59, 1979.
7. Kaplan, S. R.: Medical school and women over 30. *J. Am. Med. Wom. Assoc.* 37(2):39–50, 1982.
8. Halenar, J. F.: Doctors don't have to burn out. *Med. Econ.* 58(21):148–161, 1981.
9. Pinset, J.: *Op. cit.* pp. 48 ff.
10. Bursztajn, H., Feinbloom, R. I., Hamm, R. M., et al.: *Medical Choices, Medical Chances*. New York, Delacorte Press/Seymour Lawrence, 1981, p. xiv.
11. Association of American Medical Colleges: The "DRG" system of prospective payment. *Medical Care Prospective Payment: A Staff Report* (Revised April 1983). Washington, D.C., pp. 2–4.
12. McCue, J. D.: The effects of stress on physicians and their medical practice. *N. Engl. J. Med.* 306:458–463, 1982.
13. Siegler, M.: Confidentiality in medicine: a decrepit concept. *N. Engl. J. Med.* 307:1518–1521, 1982.
14. Wilson, S. J.: Confidentiality. In Shankar, Y. (ed.): *Ethical Issues in Social Work*. Springfield, Ill., Charles C Thomas, 1982, pp. 338–356.
15. Purtilo, R. B.: Loneliness, the need for solitude and compliance. In Withersty, D. J. (ed.): *Communication and Compliance in a Hospital Setting*. Springfield, Ill., Charles C Thomas, 1981, pp. 91–115.
16. Rubenstein, C. M., and Shaver, P.: The experience of loneliness. In Peplau, L. A., and Perlman, D. (eds.): *Loneliness: A Sourcebook of Current Theory, Research and Therapy*. New York, John Wiley & Sons, 1982, pp. 206–224.
17. Milne, A. A.: *Now We Are Six*. New York, E. P. Dutton and Company, 1927.
18. Tillich, P.: *Systematic Theology*. Vol. 1. Chicago, University of Chicago Press, 1957.
19. Bugbee, H. G.: Loneliness, solitude and the twofold way in which concern seems to be claimed. *Humanitas* 10:313–328, 1974.

*Adapted from Veatch, R. M.: *Case Studies in Medical Ethics*. Cambridge, Harvard University Press, 1977, p. 157. Used with permission.

20. Eliot, T. S.: Choruses from "The Rock." *The Complete Poems and Plays 1909–1950*. New York, Harcourt Brace and World, 1962, p. 99.
21. Broski, D. C., and Cook, S.: The job satisfaction of allied health professionals. *J. Allied Health* 7:281–287, 1978.
22. Vaux, K.: *Biomedical Ethics*. New York, Harper & Row, 1976, p. xi.
23. Purtilo, R. B., and Cassel, C. K: *Ethical Dimensions in the Health Professions*. Philadelphia, W. B. Saunders Company, 1981, p. 142.
24. Purtilo, R. B.: Responsibility and health care teams. In Agich, G. (ed.): *Responsibility in Health Care*. Dordrecht, Holland, D. Reidel Publishing Company, 1982, pp. 215–226.
25. Brill, N.: *Teamwork: Working Toegether in the Human Servies*. Philadelphia, J.B. Lippincott Company, 1976, p. 64.
26. Thomasma, D.: Moral education in interdisciplinary teams. *Surg. Technol.* Jan./Feb. 1982, pp. 15–19.

Part I Summary

The person who enters the health professions brings to the job many personal qualities, expectations, and abilities. Each individual must take these personal characteristics into consideration when deciding what kind of health professional he or she wants to be. The first step to success in the health professions, then, is to gain an understanding of one's own needs, desires, and capabilities.

Three kinds of learning constitute the formal education of a student in the allied health professions. Knowledge deals primarily with intellectual abilities. Skills deal primarily with those activities that demand application of theoretical concepts to practical situations, often requiring fine coordination of mind and body. Attitudes are those feelings that reflect how a person will (or would like to) respond in a given situation. The two environments in which professional preparation takes place are the classroom and the health facility. Each setting is highly suitable for particular kinds of learning, but both are equally important in professional education.

The notion of helping has always been associated with the health professions. However, helping is a complex human interaction that can be either beneficial or highly detrimental to the person receiving help. Helping can be illustrative of either a social or a therapeutic relationship. The health professional helps within the limits of the therapeutic relationship primarily by utilizing professional skills to obtain a specific desirable result.

Certain problems arise as a result of the helping component of the health professions. Some students discover that (1) they did not understand the extent to which their chosen profession would demand that they work with people; (2) they do not enjoy working with other people; (3) they enjoy working with people, but not helping them within the therapeutic relationship; or (4) they did not understand the many facets of helping, such as supervisory competence and patient referral.

Part I carefully considers the *person* who becomes a health professional. The themes addressed here will recur throughout the course of one's professional career.

Several suggestions for establishing good work habits and making adequate time to reflect on one's goals are offered in Chapter 3. The health professional as an individual also must learn to work effectively with colleagues, establishing strong support groups and functioning as a full contributor to the health care team. Several new mechanisms for assuring high standards of professional practice and fostering professional growth have become a part of the health professional's experience. Among them are the peer review process and admonition to report unethical or incompetent colleagues.

Part II directs the reader's attention to the *person* who, because of particular circumstances, becomes a patient.

Part I Questions for Thought and Discussion

1. In what important ways is professional education different from other types of formal education?
2. What are some skills that are important to all health professionals?
3. What are some skills that are more important to your particular profession than to the health professions as a group?
4. You go to a patient's bedside to perform a procedure. Before entering his room you read his chart. Then you go in, greet the patient, ask how he feels, explain the procedure, make certain he is comfortable, carry out the procedure, get him a drink of water that he requests, bid him good-bye, and make notations in his chart.
   (a) What components of this interaction could be classified as social helping? Why?
   (b) What components could be classified as therapeutic helping? Why?
5. Barbara S. and Joan B. are two health professionals who work together in a large hospital. Both are in their late twenties and have worked together for the last three years. While they enjoy a friendship at work, their personal lives are so different they do not often socialize outside the hospital.

   During the month of March, Barbara notices an aloofness in Joan. Whereas they used to share coffee breaks and lunch, Joan now makes excuses. Joan now seems "too busy" to talk to Barbara. Barbara is upset and approaches Joan regarding the matter. During the conversation, Joan begins to cry. She confides to Barbara that her husband has been fired from his job. Joan is embarrassed and very worried. The bills are mounting fast, and the tension in her married life is increasing. Joan is terrified that the others will find out and asks Barbara not to tell. Barbara reassures her. She tells her that her secret is safe and offers to help in any way she can.

During the first two weeks in April, things get worse. Joan calls in sick several times and Barbara covers. Several times Joan is late, and, on two occasions, she left immediately after lunch. Joan's work is being left undone, and others are bearing the brunt of her errors. Barbara feels she is being taken advantage of. She has done Joan's work and even lied to the director regarding Joan's whereabouts.

One day over lunch, two of the others in their unit start complaining about Joan. They say they are tired of her getting away with things. One has recently had to cover Joan's work on a sick day and says that things were a mess. They tell Barbara that they are going that afternoon to talk to the director.

Barbara's upset. What should she do?

Part II
THE PATIENT

Part II

It is not enough for us to do what we can do;
   The patient
      and his environment
         and external conditions
   Must contribute to achieve the cure.

HIPPOCRATES

In Part I, it was shown that the health professional's personality, interests, and expectations all help to determine his or her effectiveness as a professional person. Part II examines closely the person who seeks professional help—the patient. Almost every person becomes a patient at some time, and the reader can undoubtedly recall some of the fears and problems he or she experienced as a patient, as well as the sympathy and special attention accompanying that experience.

In most cases, the person's role in society during a period of illness or incapacity differs significantly from the role he or she held before becoming sick.* Part II examines how sickness affects people and how the health professional is significant in their recovery. Chapter 4 discusses patients' problems, while Chapter 5 deals with privileges associated with being sick. Chapter 6 examines an individual's values and their possible modification. Chapter 7 discusses the several interactions patients have to engage in because of their current situation.

The health professional should ask the following questions as he or she reads about the patient as a person: (1) How does my professional help affect a patient? (2) Toward what attainable goals should a patient strive? (3) What should I look for in a patient's responses to give me a clue to his or her own set of values?

---

*"Sick" here denotes the presence of disabling symptoms caused by disease or injury.

Chapter 4

PROBLEMS OF THE PATIENT

Most of the patients' problems are related to the altered role of sick persons in society, and to the resulting changes in self-worth experienced in the company of those with whom they have previously had meaningful relationships. Fortunately, these problems have received considerable attention in recent years, and the reader will likely have one or more courses in which they are discussed. Some common problems are presented here.

Losses

A central problem associated with becoming ill or sustaining an injury is that the experience entails losses. The loss may be in the form of decreased physical or mental function. A physician who suffered a stroke and thus became a patient himself reflected:

> The depression I refer to comes from a sense of loss of a cherished possession. It may be the death of a loved one, an object stolen, or a fantasy dispelled—such as not getting a job one wanted, a date, or a publisher for a book. In my case the loss was a significant part of my body's ability to function . . .
> . . . Since depression is a sense of loss, I'm mostly set off by some disappointment in my physical improvement. There are many. Either some symptom reappears after I thought I was over it or I'm aware of another physical limitation, such as the inability to repair items needing delicate hand control . . .[1]

Persons who becomes blind, deaf, or paralyzed, those who lose control of movement or vital body functions, and those who through illness become incapable of making judgments experience similar loss. The loss may also involve a change in physical appearance, such as in the case of the person who must have teeth extracted, must undergo an amputation, or is badly scarred following a severe burn.

The significance of these losses for each person is determined by a complex interweaving of several factors, including the pathological process itself, the change in environment or societal role necessitated by the condition, and the coping mechanisms the patient has developed throughout his or her life. Thus it is understandable that actual physical loss will be more disabling for some persons than for others.

Patients react to health professionals in ways that express their concern about their losses. The medical technologist's blood tray, for example, often evokes a response of hostility or joke-making. On entering a patient's room, the medical technologist may be called a vampire, a robber of one's lifeblood. "Are you people selling my blood?" or "Do you have a license to take my blood?" is a common inquiry. The x-ray technologist is sometimes accused of destroying cells with the x-ray equipment. Professional persons who require physical or emotional exertion of a patient are said to be sapping the strength of the latter. All these comments reflect the patient's need to preserve his or her body from further loss.

LOSS OF FORMER SELF-IMAGE

A natural extension of loss of function or previous physical appearance is the overwhelming fear that one has literally lost oneself. Some patients feel that they have actually died, and almost all go through a stage of profound denial if the loss promises to be extended or permanent. So powerful is denial that it can be significantly detrimental to the patient's recovery or adjustment.[2] All people have feelings from time to time that they just aren't themselves that day, or that what they did in a particular situation was not typical of the "real them." For most people, this sense of self-alienation is temporary; however, it may become more lasting for a person experiencing illness, and is an especially serious problem for those who are chronically ill or permanently physically impaired.[3]

The feeling that one has lost oneself results from the patient's conviction that what he or she is closely relates to a preconceived body image. That is, for most people, *self-image* (what one is) depends to a large extent on body image (what one perceives onself to look like). The idea of body image was first described by Head[4] in the 1920's and Schilder[5] in the 1950's. They felt that a person's body image is represented neurologically in the brain. Today there is less emphasis on neurological representation, and body image is conceived as a psychosocial concept concerning a person's frame of reference about himself or herself. That is, body image is now regarded as a *social* creation. In spite of the proverb's bidding, most of us still do "judge a book by its cover." Painful sanctions are imposed on those whose appearance deviates from some societally determined standard of normality. Approval and acceptance are given for normal appearance only. There is a very close relationship between appearance, accompanying body image, and sense of self-worth.[6]

This concept is particularly valuable because it emphasizes that the body image is a result not only of how one actually looks but also of how one thinks one looks. There are some people, of course, who have exaggerated notions about their beauty and charm. Recall the vain, ugly witch in the story of Snow White, who stood proudly in front of her

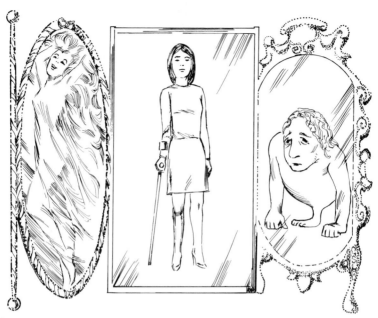

The patient's fantasies about the distortion of her former appearance may override what she sees in the mirror.

mirror each morning asking, "Mirror, mirror on the wall, who's the fairest of them all?"

A person who becomes sick or injured often has as exaggerated an idea of his or her undesirability as did the witch about her charm and beauty. This self-depreciation is undoubtedly increased by today's emphasis on physical attractiveness. It cannot be denied that some physical deformities and odors are repugnant to just about everyone. Affected individuals suffer from having to watch the unguarded reactions of others. However, in many instances the person's perception of the degree of deformity far exceeds what a mirror objectively reveals or what others see.

It is important to realize that whether or not a physical change is visible to others, the patient has, in one sense, lost his or her old self. Such a person will distrust the health professional who tries to offer encouragement by implying that things are going to be just as they were. It is more important, however, to realize that the patient need not have lost himself or herself completely as the result of the trauma and is still the worthwhile being that he or she was prior to illness or injury. As one might expect, part of the health professional's success depends upon an adeptness at helping the patient either reclaim his or her old image as recovery occurs or, when necessary, discover a realistic and satisfactory new body image.

In an article entitled "Reestablishing a Child's Body Image," the nurses conducting the study concluded:

The children quickly perceived our attitudes in the way we looked at, touched and moved them, as well as in our willingness to talk to them about their condition. More than anything else, perhaps, the nurse needs to give the patient permission to explore the changes in his body image.[7]

They also emphasized that touching the patient may be a most important factor in conveying acceptance as well as in offering comfort and support. In general, this approach is equally effective with adults, although their body images are more established.

The challenge of assisting in the process of establishing a new body image is nowhere illustrated more clearly than by the following situation related by Roy Campanella, former catcher for the Brooklyn Dodgers, who became a quadriplegic as the result of an automobile accident:

It didn't hit me at first. I didn't get the full meaning of it all at once. But then it came through to me . . . she (the therapist) was gonna teach me—Roy Campanella—how to catch a ball. . . . There I was, a guy whose claim to fame—such as it's been—had been built on my ability to catch a ball. Cripes, Roy Campanella, Campy—Number 39 with the Brooklyn Dodgers. . . . She lobbed the ball to me—gentle-like from only seven or eight feet away. . . . Gee, the way I used to catch standing up and now I can't even catch sitting down. Not only that, but when I would try to catch it I would topple over. Not once, but several times. . . "That wasn't fair, nurse," I managed to stammer. "You're cheating. You caught me off guard!" We both knew it wasn't so. . . .[8]

Part IV is devoted to describing ways in which health professionals can help patients to realize their sense of worth in the face of such difficult truths as Roy Campanella was confronting in the scene just described.

LOSSES ASSOCIATED WITH HOSPITALIZATION—HOME AND PRIVACY

Although not all people who become ill or who are injured must be confined to a hospital or similar institution, the large number that must be hospitalized warrants the reader's consideration of some of the problems associated with it. In the following discussion, the word "hospitalization" will be used to denote confinement to any health care institution.

Hospitalization is a traumatic experience for almost everyone. First, it usually significantly disrupts an individual's personal life as well as the lives of family, occupational associates, and friends. The problems associated with the disruption may be primarily social, but it is likely that they will also be economic owing to loss of work, hospital expenses, or both. The economic burden is especially acute for one who is the breadwinner in a family. A single parent has the burden of finding and paying for suitable guardians for the children. A child, teenager, or other student loses valuable instruction and may have to drop out of school. A professional person may have to forgo participation in an important project. Whatever the individual's personal responsibilities, he or she is likely to be affected both socially and economically by necessary hospitalization.

In addition to the disruption, the patient is often aware that entering the hospital signals that the battle of coping with an illness has been lost. This psychological defeat can be as deleterious to the patient's welfare as the physical manifestations of the illness itself. A psychiatrist who has worked extensively with people hospitalized with myocardial infarction suggests that the accompanying "ego-infarct" occasioned by the heart attack is often more of a barrier blocking the patient's recovery than the heart damage itself.[9] In submitting to hospitalization, the person is finally admitting openly that the problem is out of his or her control and that people professionally qualified to render certain services are needed. The patient is understandably anxious about leaving his or her health, perhaps life, in the hands of strangers but feels there are no other alternatives.

The disruption and sense of defeat that usually accompany the patient's admission are made greater by the fact that the person is placed in the middle of the mysterious hospital world. In the strangeness of this other-world that is vaguely associated with sickness and dying, he or she is robbed of both home and privacy.

Loss of Home. Not every patient experiences the loss of home negatively. Some people associate home with strife or boredom and try to escape it at all costs. Occasionally, a person will feign illness in order to be admitted to the hospital, thereby escaping the unpleasantness of home life. These patients present special problems for the health professional and are discussed in Chapter 5.

Most people do not associate home with strife or boredom. On the contrary, most see it as a haven in a complex, fast-paced world. What makes home so desirable for most people when they are away from it, and so much taken for granted when they are there? Two qualities of home, among others, missed by most hospital patients are (1) comfort and (2) security.

Comfort can be interpreted in a number of ways. The reader has undoubtedly entered a home where there was incredible chaos and disarray. In the midst of the pandemonium, the family members appeared perfectly at ease; this was their idea of living. Undoubtedly, the reader has also entered a home where even the teacups seemed to sit primly on shelves, where dust *dared* not settle and curtains never ruffled. In the midst of this porcelain perfection, these family members also appeared perfectly at ease!

The comfort of home might best be described as freedom to extend oneself naturally and completely into one's immediate environment: to do (or not do) what one wishes, when one wishes, how one wishes. The environment within the home, whether there be 1 or 40 rooms, can be changed to conform to one's own needs, habits, and desires.

The bed is a good example of how hospitals disregard the sleeping needs and habits of a person. Almost anyone would agree that a good night's rest greatly determines one's outlook on life the next day, and most people acknowledge that their bed is one of the important comforts of home. The standard hospital bed is of a given height, width, length, and firmness. Although the hospital personnel stop short of treating patients in the manner of Procrustes, the hospital murderer-robber in Greek mythology who invited his guests to sleep in his guest bed and rewarded them by chopping off their legs if they were too long, hospitals make little effort to ensure proper bed size, mattress firmness, and other personalized comforts for their patients.

The obvious difficulties in totally personalizing health care are readily apparent to all those in the health professions. Nevertheless, the difficulties should not signal complete resignation on the part of health professionals. The more that can be done to minimize discomfort for the patient who is away from home, the more readily he or she will be able to direct energies toward healing, adjustment to disability, or rehabilitation.

The security of home is also lost by the hospital patient. Security is characterized in large part by familiarity—knowing where things are and what to expect. The familiarity of home may be symbolized by objects in the home. A favorite chair for relaxation, a magnifying mirror for applying make-up, a reading lamp, a family picture, or a ragged toy may all be real but subconscious symbols of security to the person. The mere arrangement of furniture in a particular room or the sight of a tree or birdbath in the yard may give a person a sense of belonging. These familiar objects all too often are left behind when the person goes to the hospital.

Familiarity may be expressed in a routine. Many persons have one or two favorite television programs that they must see each week, or they put aside one afternoon a week for a favorite hobby or activity. Often these familiar, orienting activities are absent. It is not at all unusual for a person to become confused about what day of week it is because these landmarks are missing. The person who likes to start the day with a cup of coffee and the morning paper will be unsettled when, in the hospital, the coffee is served with breakfast and the morning paper arrives during the bath, just before he or she is scheduled to go to the first treatment session of the day.

Familiarity is most significantly embodied by the people and pets in the home. The grandmother may literally live for the companionship of the small granddaughter. A single person looks forward to a weekly visitor, or finds companionship in a pet. Children have the familiarity of family and playmates. The loss of security imposed by restrictions on the nearness and companionship of loved ones or pets is acutely felt by the hospitalized patient and is increased by harsh restrictions regarding visiting hours, numbers of guests admitted, and, most of all, the exclusion of children from the bedside of sick or dying loved ones.

That most patients do try to retrieve a little of the security and familiarity of home is revealed in the contents of their bedside stands. A stand tells one as much about the patient as the contents of a small boy's pocket does about him. Generally, the table top is cluttered with get-well cards, flowers, candy, and stuffed animals. In the top drawer are stamps, writing paper, rosaries, or religious books, yesterday's newspaper, assorted ointments, Kleenex, a transistor radio, and more! The author once found a smoked herring after a roommate complained that the patient in the next bed was sneaking fish into his bland diet. Hidden caches of forbidden cigarettes and nonprescription drugs (especially sleeping pills, tranquilizers, and laxatives) are common finds, and a patient who imbibes liquor regularly will go to all lengths to maintain a supply. A health professional who wishes to learn about his or her patient should check the contents of an open drawer with the speed and diligence of Sherlock Holmes. The bedside stand thus will reveal untold mysteries about the patient's personality.

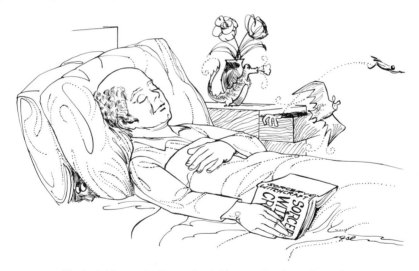

The bedside stand will reveal untold mysteries about the patient.

The reader should note, however, that patients are sometimes understandably sensitive about having a health professional snoop around the hospital room, even if only to read a card attached to a bowl of roses or to hang up a bathrobe in the closet. Their sensitivity about these seemingly innocent gestures is due to the fact that, in addition to losing the comfort and security of home, the patient is also robbed of privacy.

Loss of Privacy. Some investigators contend that living creatures need a space to call their own. They need to have a territory that is exclusively theirs.* While admittedly there are pitfalls in generalizing from animal to human behavior, there is some experimental evidence to support the idea that humans do need private space.

A fascinating example of what might be interpreted as a need for private space is recounted in Langdon Gilkey's *Shantung Compounds*, a classic account of the behavior of Westerners in a Japanese internment camp during World War II. For example, he relates how in one woman's dormitory some of the occupants were caught in the middle of the night edging their beds a fraction of an inch into the other women's space in order to increase their own space (each was allotted 18 inches). The problem was solved only when the housing committee intervened and marked lines on the floor, defining each person's rightful space. Gilkey speculates that a very basic need for private space in Western society is not often considered, because most people are not in situations that threaten their private space.[10] Only in institutions or under unusual circumstances such as a disaster shelter does space become a phenomenon with which to contend.

The experience of women thrown together in an internment camp dormitory may not appear to bear much resemblance to today's hospitalized patient. Nevertheless, the parallels should not be wholly excluded from the health professional's consideration. The patient who is uprooted from his or her home and placed in a hospital room (usually with at least one other person, a stranger) may, for the first time, feel a loss of private space. The door to this room has no lock. The "walls" are curtains through which health professionals and others can intrude without warning. There is no opportunity for holding a confidential conversation, for having a good cry without others hearing, for engaging in lovemaking with one's spouse. The light switches either are out of reach or have outlets that can be controlled by persons entering the room. Except in rare circumstances, all the usual privacy "props" are uprooted.

This lack of privacy increases the irritation of some patients. Little annoyances become major issues over a period of time; it can be devastating for the person who always has an afternoon rest to have a hard-of-hearing roommate who always watches two hours of soap operas at that time, or for the nonsmoker to be in a ward with a person who lights up one stogie after another.

The lack of privacy is also a source of frustration to the person who wishes to withdraw from others for a while in order to organize his or her thoughts and try to ascertain how the illness or injury will affect the future. This withdrawal is a natural reaction, one that we all experience during times of crisis or change.

---

*Two now classic books supporting this theory are Konrad Lorenz' *On Aggression*, New York, Harcourt, Brace and World, 1966; and Robert Ardrey's *The Territorial Imperative*, New York, Atheneum, 1966. Following their publication there was a rash of books supporting or discounting their claims, the most controversial of which is E. O. Wilson's *Sociobiology: The New Synthesis*, Cambridge, Harvard University Press, 1975.

Health professionals, fearful that the patient's withdrawal may develop into an escape from dealing with some important aspects of reality, often do not allow patients this time for withdrawal and stillness. A friend now 55 years old, who is severely afflicted with cerebral palsy, and who for the first time since his youth is living in a private home, told me that the most difficult aspect of the many years of institutionalization was that people never left him alone to think.

Thus, in Western society every person has come to expect and need a measure of privacy. The patient, when robbed of privacy through hospitalization, is likely to feel deep-seated, intense frustration.

LOSS OF INDEPENDENCE

The loss of home and privacy is rooted in the far more basic loss of independence. Hospitalized patients' reactions to this loss are easily discernible if one considers the structure of an institution. Total institutions can be defined as a place of residence and work where a large number of similarly situated individuals, cut off from society for an appreciable period of time, together lead an enclosed, formally administered life. An institution is a place where (1) the inhabitants work, sleep, and play in the same place rather than perform these three functions in separate places, as one does in the outside world; (2) many daily activities are carried out in the immediate company of other people; (3) there are two levels of persons—the inmates, patients, and the like, and the staff, officers, or guards; and (4) contact with people outside the institution is controlled by the staff.[11]

Most health facilities are not as tightly organized as total institutions such as a prison, but one can nevertheless draw striking parallels between the restrictions imposed by both. For instance, patients have almost every minute of the day scheduled for them, and they are limited as to how and where the unscheduled time can be spent. They are herded from place to place for therapy, x-ray, and other activities. Visiting hours are fixed, and the switchboard operator may choose not to put calls through after a certain hour at night. In every way, the dependent state of the patient is reinforced.

The hallmark of this dependent state is the hospital gown. Presidents and kings dare not defy the potential danger or indignity of walking down the hall in that gaping garment!

The patient outside the hospital setting also experiences a loss of independence. He or she may be too weak to carry on simple daily activities. Charles Clay Dahlberg, the physician mentioned at the beginning of this chapter, who at the age of 55 suffered a stroke, claimed that the period immediately following his release from the hospital was one of the most difficult of the entire ordeal for this very reason:

> I started planning all the things I could do with the incredible amount of free time I was going to have. Chores I had put off, museums and

galleries to visit, friends I had wanted to meet for lunch. It was not until several days later that I realized I simply couldn't do them. I didn't have the mental or physical strength, and I sank into a depression.[12]

In some cases, the patient may be on a restricted diet, may not be allowed to smoke or drink, may be asked to exercise (or to rest) at given intervals, and may be required to keep appointments for tests or treatment. For the acutely ill, this is a temporary frustration. For the chronically ill and permanently disabled, it is a way of life. Such impingements on one's freedom undoubtedly interfere with the happiness of many individuals.

Stigma and Support Systems

A brief look at the issue of stigma and lack of support systems for sick or disabled persons may help to explain further why all of the losses associated with sickness or disability take on such importance for the patient. Taken alone, each loss is difficult to accept. However, when combined with stigma and an awareness of being alone (without supports), these losses can become overwhelming. The next chapter addresses itself to the fact that becoming sick in this society does not result only in "problems." There are some "privileges" associated with sickness as well. Indeed, in some ways the terms "sick" and "disabled" act as labels that may benefit such persons in need of special attention by establishing their eligibility for special treatment.

Carlson suggests that accepting a label of "disabled" has beneficial consequences for many physically limited persons, because it may enable them to seek mechanisms for alternative methods for coping with their limitations.[13] Most of us assume that being sick is going to help us achieve the means for regaining health, and so we go through the necessary process of demonstrating that we belong to the category of persons labeled "sick."

However, the privilege deriving from the label carries with it the negative assumption that the person is more vulnerable or weak than those who do not bear the label.[14] And in a society that highly values autonomy and independent functioning, this weakness can, paradoxically, tend to decrease the labeled person's claim on the scarce resources of society. Labels, in general, tend to place a person in a "sigmatized" position in society. A stigma is an attribute that makes a person possessing it different from others in a negative way. It is, therefore, a deeply discrediting feature.[15] The person who is sick or disabled often buys the idea of being less worthwhile, or not fully human, at least initially, because the losses mean giving up part of his or her *essence*. That is, as discussed earlier in this chapter, a person may feel as though he or she has really died.

When the losses are permanent, and especially if visible disability results, the feeling of being less than human engulfs some persons. Staring at the person can only promote such a feeling. In this society we stare when we see something that is incredibly curious or bizarre or when we wish to show our disapproval. Thus, the person who is the constant recipient of amazed, bold stares is bound to feel like a freak in a side show. Further, Beatrice Wright lists ten fears within people themselves that support the erroneous idea that disability is a sign of inferiority:

1. My disability is a punishment.
2. It is important to conform, not to be different.
3. Most people are physically normal.
4. Normal physique is one of the most important values.
5. Physique is important for personal evaluation.
6. A deformed body leads to a deformed mind.
7. No one will marry me.
8. I will be a burden to my family.
9. My deformity is revolting.
10. I am less valuable because I can't get around (or see or hear) as others can.[16]

Bruce Hillam, a professor of mathematics who became a quadriplegic at the age of 16, wrote a letter to me after reading an earlier edition of this book. Commenting on the list of fears, he says,

> I had never seen Beatrice Wright's list on why some people feel they are inferior. [Among physically limited persons] there is a tremendous concern over body image, particularly of a sexual nature. Sort of the "who would want to go out with me" thing. You relate this to the fact that over 80 per cent of marriages where one partner suffers a spinal cord injury end in divorce and you wonder. . . .[17]

He goes on to explain the difficulty he and his friends in the rehabilitation center had in trying to get some sense of what kind of sexual function he, as a 16-year-old quadriplegic, could expect for the rest of his life:

> I think it was a frank and honest concern, but no one either knew, or would tell me who to ask. I found out later that my parents had asked several people the same question, including a doctor, who said it would depend on me and my prospective mate's inhibitions, and stopped there.[18]

Such responses to a person's questions are bound to leave him or her feeling radically different from other people.

One of the most damaging elements of being a stigmatized person in society is that the *shame* some members of the stigmatized group feel about their condition works against their finding others in the same situation with whom they can share their feelings. This is a dominant theme in a recent book composed of interviews with women who talk about their disabilities.[19] Fortunately, with the rise of "grass roots" support groups this is less true than it has been in times past, but it remains a problem for many who are unnecessarily made to feel utterly alone in their experience. Patients make significantly better adaptations to catastrophic illness when placed with other similarly affected persons. A method of peer counseling can be used, whereby a "veteran" patient introduces a new person with the same problem into the group. The whole procedure often is coordinated by a member of the health care team.

Families are more systematically being called on to act as a support network for such a person; they are becoming more actively involved in a person's recovery or adjustment. Although this involvement has always been one source of support, new and more formal means of including the family are being proposed. One health professional writing about issues related to successful rehabilitation of patients goes so far as to suggest establishing a contract with the whole family rather than with the patient alone.[20] This seems a particularly viable idea when the recovery and adjustment process is going to be lengthy and difficult, if the family wishes to be integrally involved.

Some church and lay groups, too, are providing means of support for people in times of crisis. A Quaker meeting in the city where I live has a system that ensures that no one is ever left alone in a time of sickness or at the death of a loved one. By dividing their time, the members of the group are able to give around-the-clock support if necessary.

However it is provided, one of the most important elements in a patient's successful return to society is the support of significant others *besides* the health professionals,[21] and the accompanying knowledge that he or she is not alone and rejected. A man who learned he was suffering from motor neuron disease and was told there was no treatment or cure reflected some months later in an article entitled "Where There's Hope, There's Life,"

> . . . Care and support and the encouragement of my friends is helping me to live a reasonably full and meaningful life despite my severe disabilities. More than anything else they help me to be positive and to keep a ray of hope alive. . . .[22]

Special Problems of the Outpatient

The outpatient is in a special position within the health care setting. Therefore, a brief discussion of this person's position is in order.

The outpatient has the difficult position of sitting on the fence between two worlds. He or she may appear completely well and therefore not be stigmatized by the label of "sick" or "disabled." But he or she is definitely a *patient* for the following reasons: Physical or mental function is impaired enough to produce discomfort in the person or result in his or her inability to proceed with some activities formerly taken for granted;

the symptoms are severe enough to have been openly acknowledged by the person and confirmed by a physician; the person has agreed to participate in a treatment or ongoing diagnostic regimen that requires regular trips to the health facility; and the visit takes high enough priority in the patient's life so that other competing activities must be sacrificed.

From the health professional's perspective, outpatients are in many regards indistinguishable from inpatients. But there are notable differences too. For instance, outpatients may feel the loss of self-image even more keenly than other patients. That is, the person in hospital is continually surrounded by others in a similar predicament and is allowed to look and act sick. The outpatient does not have this license. He or she comes into the treatment setting for a brief period of time and then returns to the world of the well and able-bodied. In some instances the person may have to fight for time off work, or may lose pay or vacation time. A parent with young children may have to go to extreme measures to find someone to care for the children. The trip to and from the health facility can be so arduous as to make the person question the worth of a treatment. Even just the process of going for treatment can be discouragingly complicated and may help to explain some of the patient's reactions to health professionals and others in the health facility.

The outpatient is not threatened with the losses associated with hospitalization mentioned in Chapter 4. Those outpatients who were previously hospitalized are often grateful that they can remain in familiar surroundings this time. But they find that there is a price to pay for being at home, and this is more disturbing to some than to others. For instance, the realization that being at home may not represent a complete recovery of independence can be devastating. Recall Charles Clay Dahlberg's description of this experience after returning home following hospitalization for a stroke. If he had continued as an outpatient, he would have probably brought these concerns to the treatment situation.

More troubling for some is that the camaraderie existing among patients and staff in a hospital setting cannot be found in the home situation. If the outpatient was previously hospitalized, he or she can feel the difference and mourns it as a loss. The outpatient who has never been hospitalized sometimes continually feels excluded from the "action" that appears to be taking place in the health facility. Such a person feels like a spectator at a game he or she wanted to play and play well. Everyone else knows each other, understands the rules, and has a better chance of "winning." Consequently, the outpatient may feel jealous of those who are in closer contact with the healers and worry that he or she is not getting adequate attention.

Underlying this situation is the feeling in society that one goes to the hospital to be healed or to die. Patients believe this, and so does everyone else. The outpatient may thus regard himself or herself as a person cut adrift and may experience periods of intense loneliness. Society expects the person to be a picture of health and vitality because he or she spends the majority of time among the well and living. But friends, family, and associates know that the person penetrates, and in some intrinsic way also belongs to, that mysterious other-world of the sick and dying. On the other hand, hospitalized patients may envy the outpatient, who, to them, is identified more with well people than with themselves.

Further, the term "outpatient" usually implies that one is still "on the way" to some other physical or mental condition. In this regard, most outpatients are distinguishable from the chronically ill and permanently physically limited, and their expectations will be different. Specifically, they will still be envisioning recovery rather than working toward adjustment. In fact, even if they know that they will experience progressive debilitation and that they are being treated in an attempt to maintain function or relieve pain, the rest of society may well harbor the belief that they should be getting better at any time. Therefore, the hapless outpatient, because he or she occupies a tenuous position, may experience hostility from, and be stigmatized by, both sick and healthy people.

Finally, it should be noted that the outpatient may be carrying a financial burden not shared by the inpatient. Many insurance policies and other types of third-party payments do not include outpatient services or else pay for only a small portion of them.

The health professional who is mindful of these special problems attending the outpatient will be better able to respond to the outpatient's questions and to deal with any difficult behavior appropriately.

Uncertainty About the Future

At some time in every recovery or adjustment process, a patient's uncertainties about the future loom menacingly before him or her. These uncertainties are based on both fact and fantasy, the seriousness of the possibilities for the future usually at least partially determined by the length and severity of the limitations imposed by the event.

Of course, even patients whose conditions will not leave them with a visible disability or permanent loss are also filled with anxiety about the future. They do not have to contend with the stigma of a deformed body, but they do share many questions with those whose deformities are visible. Some patients are especially anxious about their ability to provide economically for themselves or their families. Young people often express concern (as, to a lesser extent, do older patients) that their condition will inhibit normal sexual or childbearing functions. Others may be equally anxious about resuming a former social role or being able to engage in an activity that gave them satisfaction.

The effects of uncertainty are manifested in many ways during the time the patient is receiving health care. Anxiety causes some patients to be overly fearful of a particular testing or treatment procedure. He or

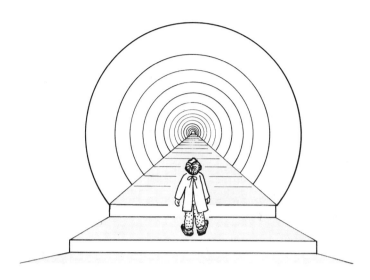

she may doubt the health professional's competence when there is no rational basis to do so, and may refuse care. It is easier for the health professional to understand such reactions if it is realized that they are irrational responses arising from anxiety about the patient's uncertain future.

Anxiety causes some patients to become extremely rigid or conservative in their outlook. Psychiatrists state that this increased rigidity naturally accompanies anxiety, and that the fearful patient is more likely to cling to any familiar solution, even an inadequate one, than to experiment with other alternatives.[23] The unfortunate result is that such a patient prolongs his or her problems rather than finding simple and available solutions. This patient wants desperately to hear the health professional say, "You are going to get right out of that wheelchair and run across the room someday"; "after this, you will again know what it means to go a full day without pain"; or "your biopsy shows that you do not have cancer."

For this reason, it is often the experience of a student that a patient asks, "do you think I'm improving?" The student, in a sincere effort to console a distressed patient, must exercise the greatest care not to give false information or instill false hope in him or her. The wise health professional does not try to "play God" or use supernatural powers to see into the future. However, among the many questions the patient may have is one not often asked: "Will you be present to see me through this situation, whatever the outcome?" To this the health professional can respond by assuming that everything possible will be done for the patient and that he or she will not be carelessly abandoned in this time of crisis. This one certainty must be just what is needed to stimulate the patient to work toward recovery or adjustment.

REFERENCES

1. Dahlberg, C. C., and Jaffe, J.: *Stroke*. New York, W. W. Norton, 1977, pp. 62–63.
2. Bergsma, J., and Thomasma, D: *Health Care: Its Psychosocial Dimensions*. Pittsburgh, Duquesne University Press, 1982, pp. 99–100.
3. Meenan, R. F., Yelin, E., Narett, M., et al.: The impact of chronic disease. *Arthritis Rheum*. 24:544–549, 1981.
4. Head, Sir Henry: *Studies of Neurology*. Vol. 1. London, Hodder & Stoughton, 1920.
5. Schilder, P.: *The Image and Appearance of the Human Body: Studies in the Constructive Energies of the Psyche*. New York, International Universities Press, 1950.
6. Kellerman, J. M., and Laird, J.: The effect of appearance on self-perceptions. *J. Pers*. 50:296–315, 1982.
7. Smith, E. C., et al.: Reestablishing a child's body image. *Am. J. Nurs*. 77:445–447, 1977.
8. Campanella, R.: *It's Good to be Alive*. Boston, Little, Brown & Co., 1959, pp. 207–209.
9. Cassem, N.: *Psychological Aspects of Cardiac Disease*. Lecture presented at University of Massachusetts Medical Center, Worcester, June 2, 1977.
10. Gilkey, L.: *Shantung Compound*. New York, Harper & Row, 1966, pp. 80–81.
11. Goffman, E.: *Asylums*. New York, Doubleday & Company, 1961, pp. xiii, 5–8.
12. Dahlberg, C. C., and Jaffe, J.: *Op. cit.*
13. Carlson, C.: Psychosocial aspects of neurological disability. *Nurs. Clin. North Am*. 15:309–320, 1980.
14. Purtilo, R. B., Sonnabend, J. S., and Purtilo, D. T.: Confidentiality, informed consent and untoward social consequences in research on a "new killer disease" (AIDS). *Clin. Res*. 31(4):464–472, 1983.
15. Eisenberg, M. G.: Disability as stigma. In Eisenberg, M. G., Griggins, C., and Duval, R. G. (eds.): *Disabled People as Second Class Citizens*. New York, Springer, 1982.
16. Wright, Beatrice: *Physical Disability: A Psychological Approach*. New York, Harper & Row, 1960, p. 172.
17. Hillam, B.: *Personal communication*, April 9, 1977.
18. *Ibid.*
19. Campling, D. O. (ed.): *Images of Ourselves: Women with Disabilities Talking*. London, Routledge and Keegan Paul, 1981.
20. Epstein, Nathan B., et al.: The family as a social unit. *Can. Family Phys*. 22:1411–1413, 1976.
21. Carlson, C.: *Op. cit.*
22. Griffiths, G.: Where there's hope, there's life. *Practitioner* 226:1365–1366, 1982.
23. Bursztajn, H., Feinbloom, R. I., Hamm, R. M., et al.: *Medical Choices, Medical Chances*. New York, Delacorte Press, 1981, p. xiv.

Chapter 5

PRIVILEGES OF THE PATIENT

Special Privileges Given to the Patient

That there are particular privileges reserved for those who temporarily are struck down by physical or mental impairment can probably most easily be recognized by recalling the privileges you had as a child when you were sick. What did your mother do for you then that she otherwise would not do? Common answers from students include the following:

Meals were brought to me in bed.

I didn't have to go to school.

I had first choice of the toys.

I was exempt from doing the dishes.

I had the television (or radio or stereo) brought to my room.

I was given a cold washcloth for my forehead.

I had fresh orange juice or chicken soup (or some other special food or home remedy).

Sympathy for the sick person is part of the message being conveyed by the privileges extended to him or her. However, inherent in the granting of the privileges is a message that the privileges are also an encouragement to keep up the good fight back to health. The second message was well conveyed by the design of this get-well card.

Parsons, a sociologist who provided a classic description of the role a person assumes when he or she becomes ill, emphasized both the privileges and the accompanying expectation of society that the person will try to return to health. He outlines four characteristics of the person: First, the person becomes exempt from the usual social responsibilities. For example, a student may be excused from taking an exam because of the "excuse" (viewed as a justifiable excuse) of illness; second, the person cannot be expected to take care of himself. In other words, the person is allowed to regress to a dependent state, and society as a whole assumes the role of a nurturing parent. However, the person may lose these privileges if he or she does not take some responsibility for getting well. Indeed, Parsons' third and fourth characteristics of the sick role are (3) the patient's desire to get well and (4) proof that he or she is trying to get better by seeking professional help.[1]

Increasingly, the emphasis on the patient's role as active agent in the healing process, and not just as a passive recipient of the health professional's ministrations, is being emphasized.[2] Curiously, the healing touch of E. T. came not from the others who tried to take care of him

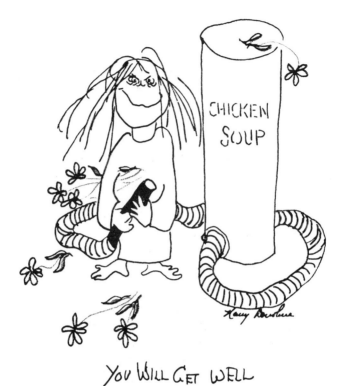

You Will Get Well

Crocus Card by Nancy Donahue, the Forers. Used with permission.

during his lonesome sojourn on the planet Earth; rather, he himself had the power for his own healing. Similarly, many patients are reckoning with their responsibility for their own health, or their part in the restoration of it. They are believing that some of the "help" they need is to seek professional help, as Parsons suggests, but that they have information about their own lives that can assist in the process of healing as well.

Part of this "taking responsibility for their own illness" is crucial to patients' healing. However, the author has observed a kind of "braveness" in many patients in recent years that at first appears to be an example of "taking the bull by the horns" and assuming full responsibility for the course of treatment; at some juncture in the course of the illness, however, the braveness dissipates and leaves the patient feeling fully out of control and frightened. A woman who was diagnosed as having an adenocarcinoma of the lung, treated with immunotherapy and chemotherapy, lends insight into the dynamics of "bravery" among patients in the following excerpt:

> The need to exert some kind of control over the irrational forces that we imagine are loose in our bodies also results in what I have come to recognize as the "brave act" put on by people who have cancer. We all do it. The blood-count line at Memorial Hospital can

be one of the cheeriest places in New York on certain mornings. It was on this line, during my first visit to Memorial, that a young leukemia patient in remission told me, "They treat lung cancer like the common cold around here." (Believe me, that was the cheeriest thing anyone had said to me in months.) While waiting for blood counts, I have heard stories from people with lymphoma who were given up for dead in other hospitals and who are feeling terrific. The atmosphere in that line suggests a gathering of knights who have just slain a bunch of dragons. But there are always people in the line who don't say anything at all, and I always wonder if they have at other times felt the exhilaration felt by those of us who are well. We all know, at least, that the dragons are never quite dead and might at any time be aroused, ready for another fight. But our brave act is important. It is one of the ways we stay alive, and it is the way that we convince those who live in "The Land of the Well People" that we aren't all that different from them.[3]*

Surely, part of the health professional's role today is to assist the patient in maintaining as much bravado and control over the events of his or her life as possible while still being on hand to provide professional assistance and skills when they are appropriate to the healing process.

Some Advantages of Staying Sick

Society is willing to give privileges to a person who is sick, but it does expect him or her to want to recover and to resume former responsibilities. What then happens in the rare case when a person does not want to get well? Clearly, for these people the tender loving care and protection—the privileges—they receive while they are ill outweigh those granted them when they were well. One way a person stays sick is to feign symptoms long after they are gone, or to fabricate them if they never existed at all. Such a person is called a malingerer.

Sometimes the problem is more complex. The patient may have symptoms of organic illness in the absence of organic pathology. This patient is said to have a hysterical symptom, or to have undergone a conversion reaction—i.e., a psychological problem has been converted into an organic (physical) symptom. A third kind of person may refuse to take the necessary measures to relieve the symptoms, thus destroying his or her chances of ever returning to society as a healthy, responsible person.

ESCAPE AND FINANCIAL GAIN

One may wonder what such patients gain by their behavior, considering the advantages of a healthy, independent, and active life. They see protection from the threatening outside world as one advantage of staying sick. This is especially true of a patient who has been hospitalized or institutionalized and is suddenly faced with discharge. The uncertainty about the future that was discussed in the last chapter becomes a paralyzing fear for some. Their response to the fear is to stay sick.

---

*Excerpted by permission of the New England Journal of Medicine, 304:699, 1981.

Financial gain is also an advantage. The malingerer is seen often in clinics that treat industrial injuries. Many malingerers have jobs that are boring, offering no opportunity for advancement; therefore, they welcome any means of escape from the job as long as workmen's compensation or some other form of disability insurance will subsidize them.

During the author's stay in Sweden in 1981–1982 she learned that a particularly problematical group of people for the health professionals there were laborers in the 50- to 60-year-old group who were dissatisfied with their jobs and presented with symptoms that were disabling but difficult to quantify medically. These persons felt that they had paid enough into the Social Security System and saw younger people using up the funds these older folks had worked hard to establish and maintain. The patients usually wanted to go into early retirement, rather than waiting until the customary 65-year retirement age.[5] In the United States, the question of gaining early retirement or receiving extensive disability often goes through the courts. An increasing number of people are involved in lawsuits in which they must exhibit symptoms in order to win their cases; it is often impossible to prove malingering.

SOCIAL GAIN

Social gain is a third advantage. A common social end achieved is manipulation of one's family and friends. If the results are rewarding enough, an individual may decide that it is not expedient to be restored to his or her former symptom-free life.

Argan, Molière's malingering imaginary invalid, is a perfect example of such a person. He manipulates everyone in his life by virtue of his weakened condition. When his daughter Angélique is old enough to be married, he chooses a physician as her husband. Toinnette, the maid, asks Argan why the physician has been chosen, when Angélique is obviously in love with someone else.

> Argan: My reason is that, in view of the feeble and poorly state that I'm in I want to marry my daughter into the medical profession so that I can assure myself of help in my illness and have a supply of the remedies I need within the family, and be in a position to have consultations and prescriptions whenever I want them.
>
> Toinnette, boldly: Well that's certainly a reason and it's nice to be discussing it so calmly. But master, with your hand on your heart, now, *are* you ill?
>
> Argan: What, you jade! Am I ill? You impudent creature! Am I ill?
>
> Toinnette: All right then, you *are* ill. Don't let's quarrel about that. You *are* ill. Very ill. I agree with you there. More ill than you think. That's settled. But your daughter should marry to suit herself. *She* isn't ill so there's no need to give *her* a doctor.
>
> Argan: It's for my own sake that I'm marrying her to a doctor. A daughter with any proper feeling ought to be only too pleased to marry someone who will be of service to her father's health.[6]

The world thus revolves around Argan's medicines and body functions. His emotional dependency is revealed in his continual tattling to his wife about the annoying Toinnette, who confronts him with his hypocrisy. His brother Béralde observes, ". . . One proof that there's nothing wrong with you and that your health is perfectly sound is that in spite of all your efforts you haven't managed to damage your constitution and you've survived all the medicines they've given you to swallow."

Argan quickly counters, "But don't you know, brother, that that's just what's keeping me going. Mr. Purgon [the physician] says that if he left off attending me for three days I shouldn't survive it."[7]

Audiences for 300 years have been laughing at Argan's obvious self-deluding rationalizations. They laugh, of course, because they can identify with Argan's reluctance to give up the privileges of the sick. However, most differ from Argan in that they do not enjoy these privileges enough to allow themselves and their loved ones to be imprisoned forever by their symptoms and debilitating disorders.

Responding to a Malingerer

The health professional occasionally meets an Argan in the professional working situation and should be prepared to know how to help him or her. It is understandable that most health professionals become frustrated when confronted with a patient who apparently does not want to get well but who wants the attention of treatment, often at the price of attention that the health professional judges should be given to another patient.

> Marilyn Siegler is a 19-year-old woman who has long had "family problems." Her father is a successful businessman, and her mother is very much involved in the charitable and social activities of the large city in which they live. Marilyn has felt, from the time she was a child, that her parents favored her older brother, who now has decided to become a partner in their parents' business.
>
> Marilyn has been seen by numerous counselors and psychiatrists since her teen years, when she made a suicide attempt. All agree that her feelings of rejection are the basis for her unhappiness. Several attempts have been made to bring the parents in for family counseling, but they have always been too busy.
>
> Marilyn is now a junior in college. She went from boarding school to a college dormitory, where she has been living throughout the three years. During the past six months she has developed a progressive weakness in her legs, until now she is paralyzed completely from the hips down. She is confined to a wheelchair. Extensive tests have revealed no physical basis for the disabling symptoms, though there is the possibility of a rare neurological disorder, as yet undiagnosed. Recently her parents have decided it would be best for Marilyn to return home, where they plan to employ a private tutor for her.

You are living in the dormitory where Marilyn lives. She has been a patient in the clinic where you are currently serving as a clinical affiliate as a part of your professional preparation. You know much more about Marilyn's clinical history than any of the other people in the dorm.

Early one morning, about one A.M., you go out in the hall to stretch your legs because you are burning the midnight oil in preparation for an exam. Much to your astonishment you see someone who resembles Marilyn, in Marilyn's robe, walking into Marilyn's dorm room. The door closes quickly, before you can call out to her.

What, if anything, should you do now? As a personal acquaintance of Marilyn? As a health professional?

What can be done to help such a person? Obviously he or she is in need of help. The following suggestions may assist a health professional confronted with a person believed to be malingering. First, believe the patient until all reasonable evidence that he or she is sick or debilitated has been legitimately discounted. Every member of the health professions who is in contact with the person can assist in this process. For instance, if the patient is hospitalized, a dietician or radiological technologist, who often is in briefer contact with a patient than, say, a nurse or occupational therapist, may be able to provide helpful information by sharing observations. Such persons often are not asked for their opinions because their contact is so brief. To the contrary, patients are often more relaxed and unguarded with them and may exhibit behavior not noted during a longer association. In addition, discussing the issue in staff meetings will alert a large number of people to the problem. If the patient is not hospitalized, one can sometimes tactfully employ the assistance of family and friends.

In all cases, such fact-finding must be carried out with the idea that the patient is legitimate in his or her complaints of symptoms until proven otherwise. Sometimes gathering information about a patient can take on the aura of a witch hunt, and the patient understandably grows to distrust and despise the health care providers. It is for this reason that I urge belief in the patient's report until there is well-documented evidence of malingering, to which one is willing to testify under oath in court.

Second, once a case of malingering is proved, it may occasionally be worthwhile to talk with the patient privately. In most cases, however, it is better to recommend him or her to a professional counselor. The most important thing to remember is that the patient can't be coerced into wanting to return to society until his or her underlying problems are solved. Health professionals often become involved in this problem-solving process by working closely with the psychologist or psychiatrist and by reinforcing the patient's actions that contribute to healing and subsequent independent functioning.

REFERENCES

1. Parsons, T.: *The Social System.* Glencoe, Glencoe Illinois Free Press, 1951, pp. 436–437.
2. LeShan, L.: *The Mechanic and the Gardener.* New York, Holt Rinehart and Winston, 1982.
3. Trillin, A. S.: Of dragons and garden peas. A cancer patient talks to doctors. *N. Engl. J. Med.* 304: 699–700, 1981.
4. Abramson, M.: Ethical dilemmas for social workers in discharge planning. *Social Work in Health Care* 6:33–42, 1981.
5. Purtilo, R. B.: *Justice, Liberty, Compassion—Humane Health Care and Rehabilitation.* New York, World Rehabilitation Fund, 1981, pp. 37–38.
6. Molière, J.-B.: *The Misanthrope and Other Plays.* Translated by John Wood. London, Penguin Books, 1959, p. 218.
7. *Ibid.*, p. 257.

Chapter 6

INCENTIVES FOR GETTING WELL

Chapter 5 maintained that in spite of certain privileges, most sick people to want to return to the mainstream of society. However, the losses described in Chapter 4 must first be regained or, if they are permanent, mourned,* before the patient can move toward a new sense of well-being. This process of coming to grips with one's losses is necessary because the lost capabilities, position in society, or objects were cherished by that person. The present chapter deals with those things that patients cherish in life. Taken together, they constitute what can be called a person's *value system*. Some values in that system are shared by all humans and some by the person's society or subgroup; still others are highly specific to the individual. The unique combination for each person constitutes his or her conception of "the good life." One important role of the health professional is to help a patient regain or replace old values, thereby helping him or her to realize the good life as much as possible.

Societal Values

One well-recognized characteristic of "the human condition" is that we, as human beings, organize ourselves into societies—complex interactions among individuals and groups of individuals. With their ability to communicate and reflect, humans are technological beings who build tools to assist in the completion of daily tasks; historical beings who build cultures based on the wisdom and knowledge of those before them; political beings who organize behavior into systems of laws that govern interaction; and esthetic beings who create nonfunctional objects and treasure them for their beauty alone. Humans are also religious beings, performing rituals and believing in supernatural powers; and they are ethical beings, able to distinguish between right and wrong and to adjust behavior accordingly.[1] As a result, human beings rarely can find satisfaction outside the limits of a society.

---

*Health professionals sometimes fail to consider adequately that patients must mourn many kinds of losses. Although mourning is usually associated with losing a loved one, it applies to a far wider range of losses as well. For a good account of a person in the process of mourning the loss of her former self-image, see Simone de Beauvoir's account of her mother as she is dying of cancer in A Very Easy Death. New York, G. P. Putnam's Sons, 1964. See also Ruth B. Purtilo: Similarities in Patient Response to Chronic and Terminal Illness. Phys. Ther. 56:279–284, 1976.

Since the individual identifies so strongly with his or her societal affiliation, and at times in history was identified entirely by it, it is not surprising that human values are held in common by most or all members of the human society. However, it is more difficult to find agreement on which values are universally acclaimed as the most desirable. Literary and philosophical writings are cluttered with contesting interpretations of what constitutes the good life and which values uphold it. Despite the wide range of conflicting beliefs, one does find some common threads of agreement regarding necessary components of a good life.[2]

Rawls' list of "primary goods," although not necessarily all-inclusive, provides an idea of the scope of values such a life might include. *Social* primary goods include rights, liberties, powers, opportunities, income, wealth, and self-respect. (Self-respect, or what is commonly called dignity, is necessary in order for a person to have a sure conviction that a life plan is worth carrying out or capable of being fulfilled.) The realization of these goods is at least partially determined by the structure of society itself. *Natural* primary goods, also partly determined by societal structure but not directly under its control, include health, vigor, intelligence, and imagination.[3] Together these social and natural primary goods provide a sort of "index of welfare" for any individual. Rawls' proposition that persons in Western societies would desire these goods is defensible partially because he states them so generally.

Western society seems to be organized on the principle that human life itself is a basic value and therefore ought to be sustained. However, beyond that, certain *qualities* help to give it meaning. Beginning with the idea of life itself as a basic value, one can begin to envision certain other values that are instrumental in assuring a high quality of life. Some of these instrumental values seem directed at the most basic level of existence only; examples include physical safety, a modicum of freedom to make decisions about one's own life, and the assurance that others will keep their promises. Many laws are designed to ensure that at least this most basic level is maintained and that those who try to destroy it are punished.

Other values are perceived to be necessary for life-in-community and for the realization of some qualities characteristic of life above the bare subsistence level. Good health is an example of values in this category. Others include the attainment of some reasonable level of wealth and the assurance that institutional arrangements will be just (for instance, that offices within institutions will be filled according to a standard that preserves equality of opportunity for all, and that due process will be followed in adjudications). Rawls' notion of self-respect should be included here also, as should vigor, intelligence, and imagination.

There is an important moral aspect to the idea that upholding certain values can produce the good life in the community. This moral aspect is evidenced by the emphasis that is placed on the development of certain

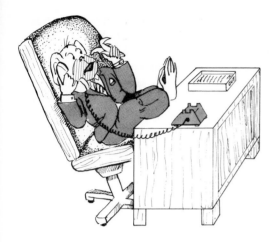

"Please, Miss Baxter, no more human applicants—they're just too darned conscientious."

desirable character traits, or *virtues*. Many would maintain that high moral character is conducive to the achievement of being a better person. But there is dispute over which character traits and practices are the most central to this life. For instance, in ancient Greek thought the virtues of temperance, prudence, justice, and fortitude were considered central. But early Christian thinkers, particularly those in the Middle Ages, argued that these alone were not sufficient and that to be a "good person" one also had to have faith in God, maintain hope, and be loving or compassionate. Other world religions and schools of philosophical thought contribute their lists. On one thing they all, except for the most extreme positions, agree: Character traits alone are not enough to assure maintenance of the good life. They tend to further it, but human experience shows that the positive relationship between the good person one is and the types of actions one engages in are not always consistent. For example, the Apostle Paul lamented, "For the good that I would, I do not; but the evil which I would not, that I do" (Romans 7:19).

In addition to those previously mentioned values that are believed to support human life and sustain it at a level above a minimal quality of existence, some other societal values appear to arise from the peculiar habits and practices of a given community or era. A good example in modern Western society is the value placed on individual autonomy. At no time in history has there been such an emphasis on the importance of having control over one's own life, of independent functioning and radical self-reliance. Failure to succeed is often interpreted as not trying hard enough, the underlying belief being that individuals can pull themselves up by their bootstraps.

The value placed on individual autonomy understandably lays an immense burden on the person whose independence has been diminished by illness or injury.

Somewhat paradoxically, this value of autonomous independence is juxtaposed beside the value of conformity to societally established norms of behavior, dress, and general appearance. There is a "catch 22" built into the concept that one must be an autonomous individual but must not be different, or at least not *too* different! And what is acceptable (attractive, desirable) is based on arbitrary standards arrived at by exclusivistic types of reasoning. The discussions of self-image and stigma in Chapter 4 explain how society punishes those who fail to conform to its notion of normality by making such persons feel less than human. Thus, this societal value, like the value of independence, causes great consternation to a patient who, naturally enough, needs acceptance by others.

Of course, there are values other than those of autonomy and conformity that spring from the idiosyncrasies of a given society, although these are two of the most important ones.

When a person is placed in a position in which it is impossible to live up to society's expectations and the values it dictates, he or she may experience tremendous anxiety and discomfort.

The importance of proving that he is still an integral part of his social group is exemplified by the sick or injured teenage boy. The lengths to which he goes to maintain his teenage identity become apparent when one walks into his hospital room: The evidence is plastered on the walls, tied to the bedposts, and hanging from the ceiling. In his appearance, manner and language, the teenage patient declares, "I'm still 'in'."

The teenager is by no means the only one to try to preserve peer-group identity. The man whose role in society is that of the rough-and-ready laborer will overtly show how disdainful he is toward the ridiculous hospital; his buddies may tease him unmercifully about being bedridden, about the nurses, and about having to use the bedpan. Their jibes and his responses are efforts to reassure themselves that he is still one of them and is not to be identified with the world of either the sick or the educated.

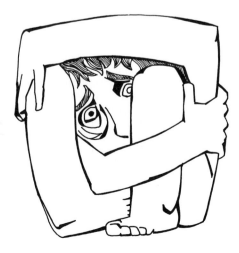

When a person is placed in a position in which it is impossible to live up to society's expectations, he or she may experience tremendous anxiety and discomfort.

Personal Values

It has been suggested that most people have some values that are based on those of society (or a subgroup of society). I have called these societal values. In addition to societal values, individuals have *personal* values that are not derived from societal norms. Realization of these values does not necessarily depend on interaction with other members of society; they are strictly one's own thing.

Most people cherish more than one personal good, or value. Literature provides striking examples of the exception: Ahab braved the high seas believing the good life consisted of getting revenge on the great white whale, Moby Dick; Sir Lancelot suffered the gravest adversities in his relentless quest for the Holy Grail; and the hobbit, Bilbo, defended his ring against the terrifying schemes of Gollum. The lifestyles of Ahabs, Sir Lancelots, and Bilbos are not the same as those of most individuals. Most people have many personal values, some more clearly defined than others, and go through life trying to realize several values simultaneously.

The health professional should be mindful of this multiplicity of personal values when working with patients, as most of them tend to feel, at one time or another, that all is lost. Professional persons often provide the bridge between despair and new meaning in life by simply making the patient aware that although some of the values he or she cherished may be out of reach now, others are not. The definition of goals that will lead to the adoption of new values is the responsibility of the health professional who works with a patient over a period of time, rather than of one who sees the patient only once or occasionally. However, any health professional can help in this process, sometimes in the most unexpected ways. The story of Mr. Mason clearly illustrates this.

Mr. Mason entered the hospital with a severe headache on May 14. That evening, he sank into a coma and was rushed to surgery, where a small brain tumor was removed. This procedure relieved the headaches but left his left arm and leg partially paralyzed.

In the following weeks, he was examined by almost every kind of health professional in the hospital. He was chronically depressed and lethargic and refused to talk to anyone. His progress was thought to be hindered by his apathy, but repeated attempts by his family and health professionals to spark his interest were largely unsuccessful.

One day, a new dietician stopped by to see Mr. Mason. She had never met him before and did not know how unresponsive he was. She greeted him with enthusiasm (which the others found it increasingly difficult to do), asking him how he was. Mr. Mason retorted, "It doesn't matter how I am now. All that matters is that I can be home by the seventeenth of July to give my daughter away. She is being married. My only child."

The dietician wrote on Mr. Mason's chart: Mr. Mason wants to be home by July 17 because his daughter is being married. On second thought, she telephoned the head nurse, giving the message; the

nurse, in turn, mentioned it to several of the other health professionals. The entire staff then began to direct Mr. Mason's energies toward
returning home to walk down the aisle on July 17.

Mr. Mason immediately began to work feverishly and was able
eventually to realize his dream. To be able to perform what he felt
was his fatherly duty and to be present at this marriage were important
components of Mr. Mason's idea of the good life. The astute dietician
who stopped by just once was instrumental in identifying for the
other health professionals one key to Mr. Mason's cooperation and
subsequent recovery.

This is one example of how astute health professionals can coordi-
nate their efforts to help a patient realize a goal that is important to her
or him.

In some instances an individual's personal values will conflict with
each other. An example is the case of the person who is excessively
obese. Although there are many factors contributing to obesity, it is
generally thought that many such people find security in consuming
food. Unfortunately, their habitual eating eventually causes breakdown
of their body and shortening of their lifespan. Therefore, the basic value
of *life itself* is endangered by the competing personal value of *feeling
secure*. Because both of these values are essential to good health, treatment is often directed toward helping the person derive security from
aspects of life other than eating. Similar examples can be made in regard
to other life-endangering practices, such as smoking, excessive use of
alcohol, and lack of good sleeping habits.

The "Good Life" of the Individual

Two sets of values have been presented so far, societal and personal.
They have been discussed separately to emphasize their differences. In
a health professional's attempt to help steer patients' efforts towards
goals consistent with the patient's own idea of the good life, it is
important to gain an understanding of how the two sets of values are
interrelated.

HARMONY WITH SOCIETY

Usually a person adopts a set of personal values that overlap in part
with societal values and are harmonious with them. A schematic representation of this person's value system follows:

Area A	Area B	Area C

Area A represents values developed by society to assure its continued functioning. The individual accepts these values, but does so simply because he or she wishes to live harmoniously in society. Examples of such societal values include obedience to traffic and other laws, adherence to practices of etiquette, and willingness to pay taxes.

Area B also represents societal values, but the person *internalizes* them so that they are perceived as one's personal values. His or her motivations for accepting them, then, are those of wishing to live harmoniously in society *and* experiencing personal benefits from them. Examples of these values include friendship, economic independence, and the cultivation of certain virtues such as courage and compassion.

Area C represents personal values that are important not to the continued functioning of society but to the individual. Motivation for protecting them is centered entirely on the personal benefits they render to him or her. Examples of individual values include the cultivation of enjoyable hobbies and the accumulation of personal possessions. As we saw earlier, the value might be in the form of a function, like Mr. Mason's function as father of the bride.

Most people find fulfillment only if they have some values in each of these areas and are able to integrate them into a workable and satisfactory lifestyle. They need the personal values to individualize themselves. They need the societal values represented in areas A and B in order to feel like an accepted part of their society and of humankind. Frankena makes a distinction that may be helpful here. I have been maintaining that everyone has some conception of what a good life involves. Frankena suggests that it is possible to say of anyone who lives according to his or her system of values, "That person has a good life." However, when a person's value system includes values that help to uphold and further society as well, we say that such a person *leads* a good life.[4] Frankena is pointing out that moral approval and acceptance are afforded to the person who is concerned with societal well-being as well as his or her own and who tries to live in harmony with societal standards. One can conclude that the person with many values in area B will receive the most support from society during recovery or adjustment following illness: Such an individual is perceived to be a sound citizen and a good individual with a sense of personal identity.

CONFLICT WITH SOCIETY

Not everyone adopts a set of personal values compatible with societal values or even with those of his or her own social or cultural subgroup. A schematic representation of this person's value system is as follows:

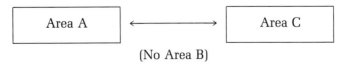

(No Area B)

Area A, societal values, is in conflict with area C, personal values. In the extreme form, as shown, there is no area B because the person has not internalized any societal values. Such a person either desires not to live in harmony with society or, more likely, believes that there are no benefits to be derived from doing so. Some examples of people whose values clash with societal values are the hermit, the outlaw, and the saint or martyr. The hermit or outlaw rejects societal values and replaces them with his own; the saint or martyr rejects societal values and replaces them with some "higher" set of values. There are varying degrees to which such persons divorce themselves from societal values: The woman who goes through a red light in order to make it to her tennis match on time is replacing a societal value of obedience to traffic rules with the personal value of reaching her destination to play that game of tennis; similarly, the conscientious objector who does alternative service is refusing to accept a societal value in the name of a higher law. Most people experience some such conflict from time to time, but seldom is it as lasting or profound as that experienced by the outlaw or martyr.

Such people are a source of anxiety to the majority of people who live in harmony with society by accepting the status quo no matter how unsatisfactory their existence may be. A good example is provided by the chorus of peasants in T. S. Eliot's *Murder in the Cathedral*. Here Archbishop Thomas Becket comes to the city to indict those who have been oppressing the peasants. But rather than welcoming him, the peasants are afraid of this man with a vision. When they hear that he is coming from France, they gather outside the cathedral, chanting:

> We do not wish anything to happen.
> Seven years we have lived quietly,
> Succeeded in avoiding notice,
> Living and partly living . . .
> O Thomas, return, Archbishop; return, return to France.
> Return. Quickly, quietly. Leave us to perish in quiet. . .[5]

But it is not only peasants who are threatened by the person living outside the scope of societal values. The health professional, too, is sometimes wary of such a person. The author experienced this when treating a person who had been convicted of murder and released on parole but who kept talking about regaining the use of his arm so that he could do "another job." Such experiences challenge the widely accepted dictum in health care that to maintain the patient's dignity and uphold the personal values at all costs is vital. The extent to which the patient's personal values and those of society must each be attended to is one of the most difficult quandaries for the thoughtful practitioner.

CONFLICT WITH HEALTH PROFESSIONALS

Are the values of the health professions generally compatible with those of society? Do they uphold personal values of patients? It is maintained by some that the values of the health professions as a whole are not drawn from universal concerns, and therefore may not be in harmony with the values of society and of many individuals in it. The claim is made that the health professions constitute a select, elitist in-group of like-minded people whose value system reflects their allegiance to each other. It follows that even the patient whose personal values are compatible with widely held societal values may run into difficulty when faced with the values imposed by the health professions. This view of the interaction between patient and health professional as one marked by conflict is being articulately expressed by a number of contemporary writers, among them Eliot Friedson. In one book he proposes that there is no such thing as the health professional-patient relationship and that instead one must regard the interaction as the health professional-patient conflict. When the two come together, a power struggle ensues. In his opinion, all too often the health professional "wins," to the detriment of the patient's well-being and, one can infer, of society's well being.[6]

The idea that health professionals are not in tune with societal values probably is overstated. Health professionals do, after all, function in society not only as health professionals but also as citizens, as parents, as friends, and even as patients.

However, undoubtedly the health professional sometimes errs on the side of thinking he or she knows what is best for the patient, and rushes headlong into a plan of action inconsistent with the patient's needs and wishes. A fine example of this is portrayed in the dialogue between a patient Oblomov, and his physician in the nineteenth century Russian novel by Goncharov:

> "If you go on living in this climate for another two or three years, lying around, and eating rich, heavy food . . . you're going to die of a stroke."
> Oblomov was startled. "What am I to do? Tell me, for God's sake."
> "Do what other people do—go abroad."

Oblomov replies that his financial situation won't allow that. The physician replies:

> "Never mind, never mind, that's no affair of mine; my duty is to tell you that you must change your way of life, the place, the air, occupation, everything—everything. . . . Go to Kissingen, or to Ems," the doctor said. "Spend June and July there, drink the waters; then go to Switzerland or the Tyrol, take the grape cure. . . ."
> "The Tyrol! How awful! . . . But what about my plan for the reorganization of my estate? Good heavens, Doctor, ..."
> "Well, it's up to you. My business is simply to warn you. You must be on your guard against passions, too. They hinder the cure. You should try to amuse yourself by riding, dancing, moderate exercise in the fresh air, pleasant conversation, especially with ladies, so that your heart is only moderately stimulated and by pleasant sensations." . . .
> "Anything more?"

"As for reading or writing—God forbid! Rent a villa facing south, with plenty of flowers; have lots of music and ladies around you . . ."

"What sort of food?"

"Avoid meats, all fish or fowl, also starchy foods and fat. You may have light bouillon, vegetables, but be on your guard: there is cholera almost everywhere now, so you must be very cautious. You may walk eight hours a day. . . ."

"Good Lord," Oblomov groaned. . . .[7]

Clearly the health professional who unwittingly foists his or her own notions regarding what is best for the patient onto the patient may as well be talking to a wall. A balance must be struck between what is possible and desirable from the patient's perspective and what the health professional judges best.

Discovering a Meaningful Value System

In recognizing the complexities involved in acquiring and maintaining a value system, the health professional gains an idea of how great a challenge it is to help a patient discover a new and meaningful value system following injury or illness.

To illustrate the process, we can take Mr. Mason's case a bit further and speculate what might have happened if Mr. Mason's condition was such that he could not be home by July 17 to walk his daughter down the aisle on her wedding day. The dietician's information would have still been very important for the following reasons: (1) It would provide the other health professionals with valuable insight into Mr. Mason's reactions to them; he undoubtedly would become increasingly hostile and depressed as July 17 drew near. (2) It would alert the health professionals to explore alternative values and goals to offset the disappointment of not being able to attend his daughter's wedding. (3) It would give them an opportunity to express their sympathy at his having missed such an important event in his life. The second point is particularly important here. The health professionals have been able to identify some of Mr. Mason's goals and are intent on now discovering some acceptable substitutes for those he cannot realize.

VALUES CLARIFICATION

Such a process is usually referred to as "values clarification." There are several useful means of learning what a patient's values are and thereby enabling him or her to understand them more clearly.

One obvious source of information is the patient himself or herself. Not all patients are reluctant to tell the health professional what they consider to be important. On the contrary, most patients are eager to talk about their values. Conversations about the patient's job, family, pets, hobbies, travels, past achievements, or material possessions reveal much information.

Family and friends, when available, are also good sources. They are usually eager to assist, and an alert health professional will detect clues from casual conversation (e.g., "I'll tell you one thing; the fishing trip just wasn't the same this year without Joe.").

Finally, the patient's chart and other medical records offer information about ethnic and family background, religion, occupation, age, birthday, and medical history. All this information can lead to conversations that will uncover personal values.

What else can you do to discover the patient's values?

DISCOVERING AND RECLAIMING VALUES

In addition to being able to identify a patient's values from the numerous sources, a health professional must work on the premise that everyone's values change from time to time. Circumstances, unexpected opportunities, tragedy, and new insights all act as controls in one's notion of what should be considered valuable in one's life. However, the circumstances that force or enable most people to change their values usually evolve slowly, while those that force a patient to do so may appear in a matter of minutes or hours!

> Daniel Janowski was the star football player on his hometown team in a small South Dakota town. On homecoming night he ran the winning touchdown for his team.
>
> Following the game, he, his buddies, and their girlfriends went to celebrate at a cottage at a nearby lake. They had a few beers and were grilling steaks when Jack said he would race Daniel across the lake. Loving the dare, Daniel ran to the water's edge, dived into 3 feet of water, and broke his neck.
>
> He was carried from the water, unconscious. A hospital helicopter took him to the emergency room of the large hospital 40 miles away, where a diagnosis of fractured cervical vertebra at the level of C5 was made.
>
> It is nine months later. He is totally paralyzed from the neck down. His weight is down to 125 pounds from his previous 165.
>
> He works diligently in the rehabilitation program, although he suffered one period of deep depression. He says now that he has "much to live for."

What types of values might Daniel have that would allow him to feel as if there is 'much to live for' when so much has radically changed?

The process of replacing some of the patient's old values may take weeks or months. For one thing, the person must learn what the illness or injury really means in terms of long-term impairment. A woman who had multiple sclerosis once told me that it took her years to stop doing silly things that overstressed her. She said, "It was because I didn't know my disease; now I know it, like a friend, strange as that may sound. Not knowing was the hardest part. . . ." The process of adjustment is also based on the joint support of family, friends, and health professionals. The entire staff of health professionals can be instrumental in identifying possible new interests for the patient. Further, some studies suggest that the richness of the person's financial and emotional resources and the job satisfaction, prior to the illness or injury, help to determine the patient's ability to identify new values afterwards.[8] The following are some general guidelines for determining when a patient should change a value or alter a goal:

1. Enlargement of the scope of values is indicated in the case of all-inclusive suffering, when the problem is to be able to see as valuable those aspects of life not closed to the person.

2. Subordination of values is indicated when the importance of the value has been overrated.

3. Containment of the negative effects of disability is needed. A person may believe that he or she can't do many things after the illness. For example, a man with a leg amputation may think he can no longer go to his bridge game, believing the amputation to have somehow affected not only his mobility but also his ability as a bridge player.

4. When a value retains substantial importance, as in the case of physique, the patient must not compare what can be done now with what could be done before; rather he or she must concentrate on what can still be done.[9]

Helping a patient to identify new values when such conditions are operant is not always an easy task for the health professional, and, as was discussed previously, it is obviously more difficult to set meaningful goals for persons whose lifestyles, beliefs, and behaviors vastly differ from one's own. A common error by the health professional is the use of his or her own values as a standard for others. Especially in the case of a patient whose illness or injury will keep him or her from not being able to quite measure up to what he or she was before, seeing the "healthy" health professional may make the patient forever feel inadequate.

A patient's chances for a satisfactory adjustment today are far more promising than in any other period in history. To understand why, one must compare the structure of past societies (as well as some tribal societies today) with that of modern Western society.

In the past, the individual was considered almost entirely in terms of his or her societal functions. Because he or she existed for society, societal values were naturally much more highly regarded than personal values. Health care was aimed at alleviating disabling symptoms so that a person could return to a productive position in society. This, of course, resulted in a drastic loss of status for the person with a chronic condition or permanently disabling symptoms. At best one became a beggar or a burden to the community. At worst one was thrown to the lions or ostracized and left to starve. In most ancient societies, children born with deformities were killed or allowed to die.

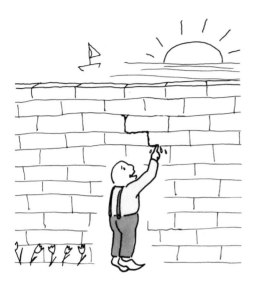

In modern Western society, the individual is more highly valued than anywhere else or ever before in history. One might go so far as to say that society exists for the individual.

The increased emphasis on the importance of the individual influences the modern interpretation of sickness and health as well as the direction of health care. A chronically sick person is often no longer able to contribute to the continued functioning of society, and a physically limited one may not be able to contribute to society in the same way as before. However, health care is aimed not only at restoring a person to a productive position in society but also at individual satisfaction and fulfillment.

The health professional today understandably is faced with a greater challenge than were any of his or her predecessors, who could direct a patient's values exclusively toward resuming societal productivity. Goals were based on societal values (area A). The health professional, as another cog in the wheel of society, was responsible for the health care of a society rather than that of the individual. Today, however, goals are set so that the patient can find a value system based on both societal and personal values. The health professional is responsible for the health care not only of society but also of the individual in society.

The health professional examines the patient who is about to be discharged from professional health care. Is the patient still "sick" or is the patient restored to health? The answer is intrinsically related to how successful the patient has been in defining a value system compatible with the new limitations and opportunities created by the illness or injury. The health professional may have been instrumental in defining this value system, but it is now up to the patient to transform the new values into functioning realities.

REFERENCES

1. Adler, M. J.: *The Difference of Man and the Difference It Makes*. Cleveland, Meridian Books, World Publishing Company, 1967, p. 91.
2. MacIntyre, A.: The nature of virtues. *Hastings Cent. Rep.* 11:27–34, 1981.
3. Rawls, J.: *A Theory of Justice*. Cambridge, Harvard University Press, 1971, p. 62.
4. Frankena, W. K.: *Ethics*. 2nd ed. Englewood Cliffs, N.J., Prentice-Hall, 1973, p. 62.
5. Eliot, T. S.: *Murder in the Cathedral*. In *T. S. Eliot: The Complete Poems and Plays 1909–1950*. New York, Harcourt, Brace, and World, 1952, p. 180.
6. Friedson, E.: *Patient's View of Medical Practice*. New York, Russell Sage Foundation, 1961.
7. Goncharov, I.: *Oblomov*. Translated by Ann Dunnigan. New York, New American Library, 1963, pp. 104–105.
8. Honig-Parnass, T.: The relative impact of status and health variables upon sick-role expectations. *Med. Care* 21:62–68, 1983.
9. Wright, B.: *Physical Disability: A Psychological Approach*. New York, Harper & Row, 1960, p. 137.

Chapter 7

INTERACTIONS OF THE PATIENT

The last chapter explained that both societal and personal values are important components of a patient's value system. The extent to which an individual is able to realize these values determines his or her happiness and self-fulfillment. This chapter is concerned less directly with the patient's values as such, discussing instead some key aspects of the patient's interaction. The first section discusses dependence, an important component of interaction between a patient and an individual health professional; the second treats the patient's interaction with health professionals as a group; and the third concerns the patient's interaction with society during and immediately following recovery, or, if there is permanent limitation, during the process of adjustment.

Interaction Within a Dependence Relationship

Some people who become ill or injured need more support than others, but all experience some confusion in the face of such disruption and need to be reassured.

Although there has been much discussion in recent years regarding possible new models of the health professional–patient interaction, the relationship is still primarily one of authority-dependence, with the health professional being turned to for some measure of reassurance. The authoritative healer is expected to evoke healing forces, apply appropriate technology, be a mentor, clarify values, and be a role model as well as mediate between the sufferer and society. Patients have different responses to the authority of the healer, depending on their own needs and on the way in which they have learned to respond to other authority figures in their lives. Therefore, the interaction with the health professional can be either a comfort, enabling interaction, or a further source of suffering. To illustrate, consider the following patient:

> A 35-year-old sculptor with metastatic disease of the breast was treated by competent physicians employing advanced knowledge and technology and acting out of kindness and true concern. At every state, the treatment as well as the disease was a source of suffering to her. She was uncertain and frightened about her future, but she could get little information from her physicians, and what she was told was not always the truth. She had been unaware, for example,

the irradiated breast would be so disfigured. After an oophorectomy and a regimen of medications, she became hirsute, obese, and devoid of libido. With tumor in the supraclavicular fossa, she lost strength in the hand that she had used in sculpturing, and she became profoundly depressed. She had a pathologic fracture of the femur, and treatment was delayed while her physicians openly disagreed about pinning her hip.

Each time her disease responded to therapy and her hope was rekindled, a new manifestation would appear. Thus, when a new course of chemotherapy was started, she was torn between a desire to live and the fear that allowing hope to emerge again would merely expose her to misery if the treatment failed. The nausea and vomiting from the chemotherapy were distressing, but no more so than the anticipation of hair loss. She feared the future. Each tomorrow was seen as heralding increased sickness, pain, or disability, never as the beginning of better times. She felt isolated because she was no longer like other people and could not do what other people did. She feared that her friends would stop visiting her. She was sure that she would die.

This young woman had severe pain and other physical symptoms that caused her suffering. But she also suffered from some threats that were social and from others that were personal and private. She suffered from the effects of the disease and its treatment on her appearance and abilities. She also suffered unremittingly from her perception of the future.[1]*

What could the health professionals have done to further mitigate this woman's suffering?

It is of prime importance to understand that dependence is established as soon as the patient enters into relationship with a health professional. Any of three types of dependence (see next page) can be exhibited by the outpatient as well as by the inpatient; by the patient who has a short, acute illness that will lead to complete recovery as well as by the permanently limited patient who needs long-term care. Moreover, a patient can manifest any of these types of dependence in a relationship with any health professional; it is incorrect to presume that the type of dependence a patient shows is determined solely by the amount of time the two are in contact.

Dependence reflects the patient's attitude toward the health professional as an authority figure who has control over some important aspects of the patient's life. The patient probably does not fully understand these feelings toward the health professional; they may be interpreted as awe or respect, as vague admiration, as infatuation, or even as intense hostility. The patient is somehow aware both that the health professional's support is intrinsically related to his or her progress and that such support is needed. To some extent, the health professional can alter the patient's attitude.

---

*Excerpted by permission of the New England Journal of Medicine, 306:639, 1982.

TYPES OF DEPENDENCE

Three types of dependence can be differentiated in any discussion of dependent relationships: detrimental or overdependence, constructive dependence, and self-dependence. These three types of dependence will be referred to many times in the rest of this book, so they should be noted carefully.

Detrimental Dependence. Detrimental or overdependence is based on an excessive insecurity, an intense sense of self-depreciation, and the desire to find personal identity in relation to someone else. It develops when one person has a neurotic need to cling to another, who either does not know how to control the amount of involvement between them or needs the possessive aspect of the relationship, or both. They consequently become intimately entangled in each other's problems to the point where they are no longer helpful to each other but are unable to terminate the relationship gracefully.

The classic example of this relationship is that of wives who lose themselves in their husbands' work. They claim no greatness for themselves and may feel they do not even *exist* apart from who they are in relation to their husbands. Concomitantly, the husband is made to feel entirely responsible for his wife's well-being and for her continued existence. She takes no responsibility for what happens. Although one may despise the other or there may be mutual hatred between them, they continue to control each other's lives. This dependence handcuffs both people to the relationship while each blames the other for their mutual imprisonment. They cannot express what they really feel about each other because the fate worse than their present imprisonment is rejection by the other person. The result is continuing mutual dependence.

Detrimental dependence as it applies to the patient–health professional relationship will be discussed at length in later chapters. However, it will be briefly described here. The patient may have a neurotic need to cling to the health professional, and the health professional may desperately need to be liked either to prove his or her competence or to control another person. Detrimental dependence may possibly result if only one of them has these neurotic needs, but it will undoubtedly result should they both have them; it is especially devastating in a long-term relationship. Once the health professional and patient become overly dependent on each other, they will hesitate to discontinue treatment or evaluation procedures even after it becomes apparent that the patient no longer needs treatment. They may arrange to see each other outside the clinical setting. If the patient does not improve, he or she may begin to blame the health professional; by the same token, the health professional may accuse the patient of not wanting to improve. Such is the double bind of detrimental dependence. To illustrate, consider the story of Arthur Cranston.

At first everyone thought Arthur Cranston was a delightful person. He was never late for his appointment, with you or others, cooperated thoroughly, and maintained a cheerful attitude in spite of his symptoms.

Naturally, everyone was concerned when after several treatments he received no relief from the symptoms. A meeting of the health care team was called, and the members tried to outline another approach with the hope that he might find some relief. In the meanwhile he has begun to telephone you between treatments, usually to ask a question in regard to the home aspects of his treatment regime, but also to chat. You learn at the meeting that he also has begun calling the other members of the team, exhibiting the same behavior. Furthermore, you learn that he has been bringing small gifts to the others. You recall that last week he brought in some donuts for you and your staff, . . . a gesture that you appreciated and thought nothing more about at the time.

Another couple of weeks pass, and his calls are becoming more frequent. He also has begun calling you at home, and you learn that the others have been receiving similar calls.

Yesterday he telephoned while you were with another patient. You ask the secretary to tell him you will call him back. The secretary does so. Later the secretary says, "Mr. Cranston said to tell you that he knows you are lying and just don't want to talk to him. He says he is coming over this afternoon and will wait in our receiving area until you have a few minutes. I told him you were pretty tied up this afternoon and asked if it was urgent. He swore at me and said, 'Of course it is'."

At noontime Mr. Cranston's primary physician meets you in the cafeteria line and takes you aside to say that her colleague across town identified Mr. Cranston as the person now threatening a lawsuit against him because he finally began to refuse Mr. Cranston's frequent visits to the clinic for what were essentially social calls. You relate your present predicament to the physician.

What should you do to affirm Mr. Cranston as a person worthy of your respect while assuring that the other patients and you are not victimized by his dependent behavior?

How can the team members assist each other in this situation?

A patient who enters the health care world with an attitude of total dependence becomes a problem for everyone. Health professionals find that the feeling of dependence is easily transferred from one person to another. It is the health professional's *role* that creates the initial dependence; the individual health professional at any given time can only increase or diminish it.

Constructive Dependence. Constructive dependence is based on respect. At some level the patient acknowledges that he or she has a need, and that fulfillment of the need means establishing some dependence on the health professional. It is, however, not a neurotic desire to cling to the other person. It does not entail loss of one's own identity in a relationship with another person. Both come together genuinely concerned, become personally though not intimately involved, and are able to terminate their relationship when it ceases to be mutually beneficial. This sense of trust and involvement can be established at their first meeting, benefiting both if it is their only encounter. However, if they continue to interact, mutual trust grows.

Constructive dependence enhances each individual's potential and is characterized by each accepting full responsibility for his or her own progress in the relationship. Because the limits of the relationship are understood by both, there is no fear of rejection. But at the core of constructive dependence is a paradox. The two people who trust and respect each other find that in their closeness they are able to allow each other freedom. The result, then, is independence; they have been, all along, primarily dependent not on each other *but on themselves.*

Constructive dependence as it applies to the patient–health professional relationship is discussed at length in later chapters. However, it will be briefly described here. Both people come together because of mutual need; the health professional needs to find satisfaction in applying professional skills, and the patient needs the services of these skills. Both people exhibit normal needs rather than the neurotic desires that lead to detrimental dependence. Their involvement is personal and not merely a business transaction; they express to each other those feelings and opinions that can be shared within the limited professional setting. When the patient no longer needs the services of the health professional, there will be no regret about ending their relationship because each one has benefited from it, whether it lasted for ten minutes or ten months. To illustrate, consider the story of Hilda Minier.

> Mrs. Minier is a retired schoolteacher who was severely burned on her face and arms when a campstove exploded during a camping trip with her husband. She was treated on the burn unit for three months and now returns three times a week as an outpatient.
>
> She is cheerful and cooperative in spite of the obvious physical discomfort and the cosmetic difficulties she experiences as a result of her accident.
>
> On several occasions she has telephoned you to confirm that she is carrying out the home treatment procedures correctly. She speaks to the point and does not linger or make small talk. Sometimes you have asked to call her back because you are with another patient. She does not mind waiting. You think she deserves the reassurance and is reasonable in her extra demands on your time, though you know that she is quite capable of carrying out the home procedures accurately.
>
> On your birthday she sent you a birthday card at your home. Once she and her husband sent a fruit basket to the department, and you learned that a basket has been sent to other departments as well.

What are the key differences between this interaction and the one involving you and Arthur Cranston?

COMPARISON OF DETRIMENTAL AND CONSTRUCTIVE DEPENDENCE

	Detrimental Dependence	Constructive Dependence
Basis	Insecurity, lack of self-worth	Mutual respect, feeling of self-worth
Stimulus	Overwhelming need	Genuine concern
Behavior	Mutual blame for failures	Acceptance of responsibility for oneself and for direction of relationship
Result	Continued interdependence	Reciprocal freedom, self-dependence for both individuals

Before proceeding to the discussion of self-dependence, consider the following chart, which reviews the differences between detrimental and constructive dependence. These two types of dependence involve *relationships* with other people, while self-dependence is a characteristic that an individual may or may not have.

Self-Dependence. Self-dependence simply refers to the extent to which a person depends on his or her own resources. The amount of self-dependence experienced by a person will be determined by three factors: (1) the extent to which a person was encouraged to realize his or her potential prior to illness or injury; (2) the support from health professionals and outside groups given during the recovery or adjustment process; and (3) the success of the person in daring to seek creative resolutions to prior difficulties.

A person's feeling of self-worth is too complex a matter to discuss fully here, but these three factors are central. The person who has much self-dependence will be able to function more independently of others' opinions than will the person with little self-confidence. The self-dependent person does not separate himself or herself from others; rather, he or she willingly interacts with them but still finds the main source of strength within.[2]

Self-dependence has been included in the discussion because it is important in determining the type of dependent *relationships* the self-confident person will develop. A patient with much confidence in his or her own potential will not need to cling to the other and will not become entangled in a detrimentally dependent relationship. On the other hand, if self-dependence is absent, the person will hope to find the dignity he or she lacks by overidentifying with another person. Therefore, the self-dependent patient is far more likely to realize maximal benefit from interaction with health professionals than is one who must seek himself or herself in someone else.

Interaction with the Health Professionals

In the preceding section two types of dependent relationships—detrimental and constructive—were discussed, both of which are influenced largely by the amount of *self*-dependence a patient brings to the interaction and both of which can be somewhat altered by the responses of the health professional.

The term "self-dependent" was employed rather than the more common term "independent" because the idea of self-worth was being emphasized. The previous discussion of dependent relationships dealt with a particular *attitude* that a patient brings to the relationship, one that can be manifested as easily by a woman who has just learned she is dying of cancer as by one with a splinter in her finger. The fundamental difference in attitudes depends primarily on how deeply ingrained the person's sense of intrinsic dignity, or selfhood, is; on how worthwhile he or she feels. In short, the difference is determined by the degree of self-dependence experienced.

The following section shifts the emphasis somewhat without discounting the importance of self-dependence and its role in dependent relationships. The focus is on *independence* and on the patient's progression from needing much attention to becoming able to do more and more practical things for himself or herself. The rather different situation for a patient who is dying is so important that it is discussed separately in Part VI. This section, then, deals more directly with patients who experience recovery from illness or face adjustment to permanent limitation.

The patient comes into contact with three types of health services in the health professions: (1) those concerned with preventive care and follow-up; (2) those concerned with acute care; and (3) those concerned with chronic and convalescent care.

How does the patient interpret the service provided him or her during the acute stage of illness or injury? An insight can be gained by studying the cartoon on the opposite page that is similar to hundreds of others about health services: The patient is pictured as being at the mercy of the health professional.

The health services directed primarily toward the acute phase of illness involve maintenance of body function and relief of unpleasant or life-threatening symptoms. The health professional must administer tests and treatments that are sometimes painful. "Nurturing" is a term that may describe the composite of health services in this phase. Obviously, the person who has no sense of personal worth and tends to form detrimental dependence with any authority figure will quickly assume a totally passive role in this situation. Unfortunately, too many health professionals quickly accept it. On a rare occasion an extremely insecure patient will react just the opposite way and become overly aggressive. Such patients resist all professional care because their already tenuous feelings of self-worth are further threatened by having anyone help. By declining help, they may be endangering their lives. They may even discharge themselves from the hospital or refuse medication. Such

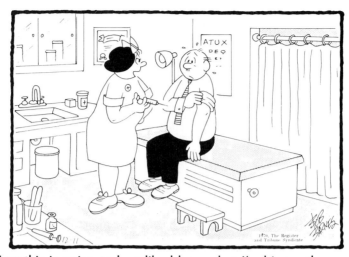

"Now this is going to hurt like blazes, but I'm bigger than you!"

Acute care: the health professional does something *to* the patient.
From Bob Barnes, "The Better Half." Reprinted by courtesy of the Register and Tribune Syndicate.

persons are not reacting to an individual health professional but to a kind of service. On the other hand, a person with a strong sense of self-dependence will neither roll over and play dead nor aggressively react against the treatment. He or she will, to be sure, enter into more negotiation about possible treatments and ask more questions. But this interest shows that the person has continued to assume responsibility for his or her own life, and it should be encouraged by the health professional.

Following the acute phase of the illness, unless the patient dies, one of three things happens next: (1) The patient recovers and goes home; (2) the patient continues as an outpatient; or (3) the patient moves into the convalescent or chronic stage as an inpatient. Both (2) and (3) will be considered next, assuming that the outpatient, in spite of the special problems associated with his position (see Chapter 4), usually continues to seek improvement or adjustment.

How does the patient interpret the services provided during the chronic or convalescent stage of illness or injury? An insight can be gained by studying the cartoon on the following page. Again the patient is pictured as being at the mercy of the health professional, but with a subtle shift. The health professional is no longer doing something *to* this person, but is instead making Mr. Decker do something for himself.

The health services provided during the chronic phase of illness or injury encourage the patient to become increasingly independent. Although the health professional is still in the authoritative role and assigns the patient activities that are sometimes unpleasant, the patient increas-

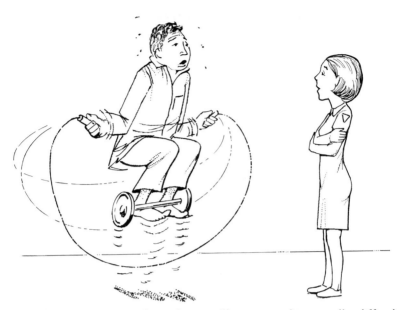

"Just 10 more, Mr. Decker, then we'll try something really difficult."

Chronic care: the health professional makes the patient do something for himself.

ingly is made aware that full recovery is ultimately up to him or her. No longer does the health professional promise, "Don't worry, we'll take care of everything"; rather, he or she says, "We're here to support you. We'll show you how, but it's up to you to take care of yourself."

Again, the success of a patient's response depends in large part on the sense of self-worth (and therefore on whether the patient trusts his or her own judgment). The fear of the unknown, discussed in Chapter 4, is a problem. But persons with a strong feeling of self-dependence will be increasingly able to move beyond that fear.

Predictably, the person given to forming detrimental dependencies will fare poorly in this process. An extreme example of the reluctance to become independent is the person who becomes a malingerer with the hope of continuing the relationship longer. Usually there are awkward moments during the transition, but both health professional and patient are finally successful in disengaging.

In summary, the patient is expected to interact with the health professionals as a group and to respond to the services they provide. The division of care into acute and chronic phases presented here is accurate but somewhat oversimplified. In most actual situations some nurturing continues throughout both phases, and from the earliest encounter the patient is encouraged to do some things for himself or herself. Nonetheless, it is hoped that by differentiating between them the reader will better understand some key processes that take place during each phase.

In addition, it may now be clearer why the patient will gain maximal benefits from interaction with health professionals if (1) help is sought when it is needed; (2) helpers are wise in nurturing and guiding the patient toward independence; and (3) the patient is willing to be partly responsible for his or her own recovery.

Interaction with Technology

Almost all health care in the United States today requires that the patient "interact" with one or more forms of technology. Technology is nothing more than "applied science," but the range of devices developed from scientific findings is immense and has radically changed the form of health care procedures offered to patients.

THE COMPUTER IN HEALTH CARE

When a patient is entering the hospital, probably the first type of technology he or she encounters is the computer. Recently I developed a rash that became so irritable and untreatable with over-the-counter ointments that I went to the emergency room in the health care institution where I work. I identified myself as an employee of the institution. The receptionist, who had been standing behind the counter and looking at me, invited me into a small side room. I sat down in the chair. She sat down too, her back almost completely to me, and faced a small screen.

"Your number," she said.

"What number?" I replied.

"Your registration number, please," she said in a kind voice.

"I don't have a registration number," I answered.

She made no attempt to look at me, but rather sat with her fingers poised at the keys and continued to stare at the screen, which, aside from four bright green spots in the corners, was totally blank.

"If you work here you have a registration number," she continued.

I asked if she knew where I would have gotten it and what kind of card it was on. She offered that I received it when I signed up at the payroll office and that the card was red. For two or three minutes I dug through my wallet, stopping only to scratch, searching for the card I was sure I had never seen. My anxiety was rising. I was feeling more and more like a failure, though I knew that was ridiculous.

After an interminably long pause she said in a resigned voice, "Well, do you know your Social Security number?"

Feeling quite confident, I gave it to her. She responded with enthusiasm, earnestly typing it onto the screen.

"Date of birth."

I gave that to her, and it, too, went onto the screen. She clicked away at the keys for several seconds.

"Ruth Purtilo?"

"Yes," I almost shouted, feeling that once again I had been brought back onto the stage of my own personal drama. Once that bit of information had been entered she was able to find my registration number, which the machine knew all the time, and we proceeded with giving the computer many more secrets about my personal history, my parents' illnesses, and a great many details about my present itching state of affairs. When she and it were satisfied, she swung her chair around and looked at me.

"It will be just a minute," she said, "and the nurse will be in to take your blood pressure."

I didn't say good-bye to the computer, but it seemed that of the first ten minutes of my entrance into the health care system, approximately eight had been devoted to interacting with this creation of technology.

Later I would learn that the information was carried by the computer so quickly that it preceded me to the pharmacy, to the nursing floor where I was admitted when the reaction worsened, and to the insurance company. But only when I received my bill from the hospital did I learn my registration number.

Much is being discussed in health care today about the effects of computers on the treatment and care of patients. At the level of health professions education, sutdents like yourself probably will use a computer for part of your learning. Many areas of professional preparation

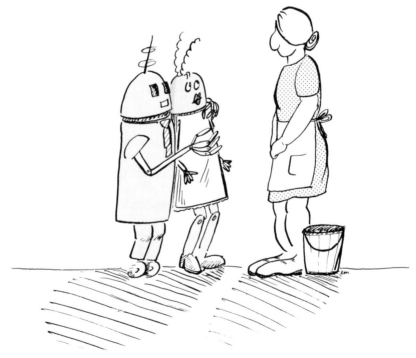

"One more "human error" and we'll be forced to seek more competent help!"

can efficiently and effectively be taught with the use of programs designed to teach various aspects of the discipline. The "silicon chip" may replace the classroom instructor in many areas of information-giving.

Within the health care system one positive outcome believed to be credited to computerized technology is the coordination of a patient's treatment and diagnostic program within an institution and across several institutions. Another positive outcome is the savings realized, once initial costs of the equipment are covered. Such savings theoretically should be passed on to patients, decreasing the overall cost of care. A third outcome is the physicians' and other health professionals' ability to use the computer for receiving information about the type of illness a patient has, thereby utilizing it as a giant storeroom of knowledge.

Some potentially negative outcomes of computerized approaches also have been suggested. One is the potential for further dehumanization of individuals in the health care system, and a second is the potential for breakdown in confidentiality as a result of extensive information-gathering and retrieval properties.

Worry about subtle dehumanizing effects is illustrated in part by the story of my admission to the health care institution. Another was related by a friend who underwent an angioplasty recently, the procedure in which a catheter is inserted into the coronary artery and a balloon is inflated to enlarge the lumen of the narrowed artery. Dye injected into the artery illuminates it and indicates when the expansion has occurred. The entire procedure is done under local anesthesia, with the patient awake.

During this patient's procedure the two nurses and two physicians never looked at him. They could "see" where the catheter was going and what was happening by looking at a screen above the patient's head. The patient said afterward that he felt very insecure during the procedure, with no one looking at him. Instead, everyone's eyes were glued to the surgical screen, the electrocardiograph print-out screen, the light flashing to indicate pulse rate, or the screen showing blood pressure. The "high tech" aspect of the procedure was working well; the patient, however, eventually grew so anxious that he began to weep, much to the shock and consternation of everyone.

Much discussion also is centered on the worry that the centralized computer information systems in health care institutions signal the end of the age-old practice of keeping patients' confidences.[3] Only the individuals involved at each step of the gathering-sharing-storing process can help to assure that confidentiality is maintained adequately. Many health professions' associations are addressing this issue today, recognizing its dangers. One group especially concerned and involved in the issue is the American Medical Record Association. In a booklet entitled *Confidentiality of Patient Health Information*, guidelines are spelled out in detail for assisting health professionals in guarding confidentiality of patient information in this new computerized era.[4]

OTHER FORMS OF TECHNOLOGY

The computer is by no means the only type of technology applied to the process of delivering health care today. Every step of the way through "the system," from receiving an immunization for travel or taking a pill for back pain, to rolling up a sleeve for the sphygmomanometer to having a CT-scan, the patient "interacts" with technology.

One effect of the development of extensive technology in the health care setting has been the increasing emphasis on the pathology itself, and not on the patient. Laennec's discovery in 1816 that a coiled piece of paper applied to the chest could enhance the sounds inside signaled more than the discovery of the stethoscope. It signaled also that the final word on what was "wrong" with a patient no longer was dependent primarily on the patient's report, but rather was dependent on the character of the technologically transmitted sound. Before that, the physician looked for a "personal statement" from the patient, and may have added to that information by putting his own ear directly against the patient's chest. Once the stethoscope was invented the distance between the patient and the health professional increased, figuratively and literally.[5] As Baron, a cardiologist, puts it,

> . . . [there is an] oft-repeated interchange between my patients and me when I am asked questions while doing a cardiac exam: "Wait a moment," I say, "I can't hear you while I'm listening."[6]

The stethoscope is one simple illustration of the many interactions between patient and technology during the course of diagnosis and treatment. The patient who cares about what is happening to him or her often is found studying the monitor above the bed, or the lab sheet at the foot of the bed, or the vital signs chart clipped to the outside of the door. Unfortunately, when the patient is unable to interpret these "codes," all too often the health professional who is asked to explain also has difficulty putting the information into language the patient can understand.

The depersonalizing effect of technology in health care often is experienced by family members as well as the patient. One young woman whose husband was dying from cancer stated how she, too, felt unneeded and unwanted amidst all of the technological equipment but, strangely, was grateful afterwards that it had bought them a bit more time before his death:

> This wasn't the way we'd planned it at all. Mark hadn't wanted to go back into the hospital, ever; he'd so clearly wished to die at home. We'd expected to have all the necessary equipment on hand there: the aspirator, the oxygen unit—everything to make the ending as comfortable as possible—but none of it had been delivered yet. It all happened so quickly—the pain, the sudden weakness, the frightening struggle for breath. We knew that lymphatic cancer often meant death

by suffocation. Was this to be it now, so soon? Could one know all along and still be caught so off-guard—ready, but never really ready? Mark had said now, calling the shots as he had all along, "I've got to have some help, San. Let's get me to the hospital."

Here we were once again, this time on the seventh floor, the hospital's resuscitation unit. Mark's bed was wheeled into a stark, antiseptic room, with no pictures or curtains and only a brick-wall view—the very setting we'd been so determined to avoid. I was thrust back into a corner, and the medical staff went to work.

A nurse came with her forms and charts to ask me for Mark's medical history, all the proper admission procedure that we'd by-passed in the emergency room. "And your husband's initial symptoms, Mrs. Albertson?" Where were all the records from Mark's other hospitalizations? What earthly good were they if they weren't used at times like these? Mike, the young physician and friend who'd come with us, saw my despair, took the nurse aside and gave her whatever information she needed.

Mark was barely conscious. His face was without color; his feet were ice-cold. Fluid drawn from his chest revealed internal bleeding, and efforts were being made to hook him up to transfusions. Blood was spattered over the walls and floor. His veins and arteries were in such bad shape from all the chemotherapy injections that the doctors were having a hard time finding an adequate connection.

I stood at the end of the bed, useless, extraneous. Was there nothing anymore that I could do? Would Mark die now, surrounded by doctors and nurses, while those of us who loved him hovered silently in the background?

An anesthesiologist was finally called in, and a suitable connection was made through the jugular vein in Mark's neck. Dr. G. came by and explained that since Mark was hemorrhaging internally, they were going to use transfusions to counter the loss of blood. The internal bleeding accounted for Mark's weakness and difficulty in breathing, his inability to retain oxygen, and the chest pains of the previous night, when some artery must have broken. Unless the bleeding itself stopped, however, the pressure on his lungs would lead to suffocation.

Out of my own anguish, I asked, "What's the point in doing all this? Can't we just let him go without all the heroics and apparatus?" The last thing both Mark and I wanted was for him to be merely kept alive by mechanical means, and Dr. G. knew it.

He seemed startled by my question, and tried to assure me that the transfusions ought to at least be tried. When I asked how long we would have, G. replied only that we would know within the next twelve hours whether the transfusions had been successful. I knew by the way he said it that if the bleeding continued, there would be little time left.

When the catheter had been secured and the transfusions begun, the fervor in the room subsided. Color rushed back into Mark's body; his breathing became more regular, and he was able to talk. I know now that if we had remained at home Mark would have died within a few hours, and that, unequipped as we were to ease his suffering, it might have been a desperate encounter with death for us all."[7]

What challenge does this state of "high technology" health care pose to the health professions? While most would affirm correctly that a return to the good old days, when the patient was made comfortable for the inevitable downward course of the disease, is not to be desired, nonetheless the need for a type of health care that attends to the person with the disease is greater than ever before. Most of this book addresses ways in which the "high touch" of the human spirit and personality can be combined with the "high technology" of interventions to assure high-quality care.

Interaction with Society

In 1860, Florence Nightingale commented on certain aspects of the interaction between the patient and people outside the health professions:

> I believe there is scarcely a greater worry which invalids have to endure than the incurable hopes of their friends . . . I would appeal most seriously to all to leave off this practice of attempting to "cheer" the sick by making light of their danger and by exaggerating their probabilities of recovery.[8]

So far the reader is acquainted with three principal factors that influence how successfully a patient returns to society: (1) ability to define a meaningful new value system if limitations to opportunities were created by the illness; (2) ability to interact effectively within a dependency relationship; and (3) ability to interact well with the health professionals as a group. After succeeding in all three areas, the patient still must overcome the biggest obstacle of all by coping with the reactions of the people outside the health professions—the rest of society.

JUDGMENT BY SOCIETY

The degree of physiological or psychological impairment does not accurately indicate how society will react to a particular patient. Other factors determining the response include the patient's socioeconomic status, the religious or philosophical significance that the patient and his or her associates and family place on the illness, and the value that society puts on health.

Many factors influence society's reactions to patients, and there have been studies on how members of a given segment or subgroup are likely to respond. These studies conclude that their responses are based primarily on the following: (1) their conceptions of health, (2) their preconceived ideas of what the patient's problems are, (3) the visibility of symptoms, and (4) the extent to which a prognosis is known.

Conceptions of health and illness also vary from person to person. In one study, the respondents (201 persons with chronic illness and 262 medical students) defined health in one of the following three ways: (1) in terms of a feeling-state, health was defined as a general feeling of well-being; (2) in terms of symptoms, it was defined as the absence of general or specific symptoms; and (3) in terms of performance, it was defined as what the person should be able to do.[9]

These interpretations of health affect not only the way a patient views his or her illness but also, equally important, the way in which others respond to it. In short, then, interaction is affected. For instance, a diabetic or hypertensive person or one with a history of cancer, mental illness, or some genetically transmitted disease, may apply for a coveted position at a firm; the person has no outward manifestation of present or past illness. If the employer has a feeling-state orientation to health, he or she may hire the person as long as the person seems healthy and able to handle the job. With a symptom orientation, knowledge that the applicant has diabetes may be enough to convince the employer to give the position to someone else. An employer with a performance orientation would probably hire the person and observe whether the new employee's condition interfered with job performance. All these possible responses would be made in spite of the patient's own evaluation of how, if at all, job performance was judged to be potentially affected by the condition.

The observer's experience is important in shaping his or her responses. The professional who sees disabled people every day or the layperson who has a disabled family member usually exhibits a much better understanding of what a disabled person can do. A physical therapist was shown this difference in perspective one day while walking with a friend. She watched with pride as a former patient deftly moved toward them, maneuvering his long leg brace and crutches with ease. Her friend nudged her and exclaimed, "There's a candidate for you! He could probably benefit from physical therapy!"

Persons who have become ill often find themselves set apart from their friends and associates. Alice Trillin, when she was diagnosed as having cancer, experienced this phenomenon as follows:

> When I first realized that I might have cancer, I felt immediately that I had entered a special place, a place I came to call "The Land of the Sick People." The most disconcerting thing, however, was not that I found it so terrifying and unfamiliar, but that I found it so ordinary, so banal. I didn't feel different, didn't feel that my life had radically changed at the moment the word *cancer* became attached to it. The same rules still held. What had changed, however, was other people's perceptions of me. Unconsciously, even with a certain amount of kindness, everyone—with the single rather extraordinary exception of my husband—regarded me as someone who had been altered irrevocably. I don't want to exaggerate my feeling of alienation or to give the impression that it was in any way dramatic. I have no horror stories of the kind I read a few years ago in the *New York Times*; people didn't move their desks away from me at the office or refuse to let their children play with my children at school because they thought that cancer was catching. My friends are all too sophisticated and too sensitive for that kind of behavior. Their distance from me was marked most of all by their inability to understand the ordinari-

ness, the banality of what was happening to me. They marveled at how well I was "coping with cancer." I had become special, no longer like them. Their genuine concern for what had happened to me, and their complete separateness from it, expressed exactly what I had felt all my life about anyone I had ever known who had experienced tragedy.[10]*

The challenge facing such a patient is fast becoming apparent. Society looks at him or her from a perspective colored by interwoven preconceptions and attitudes. Its conceptions of health, its preconceived ideas of the patient's problems, the presence of disabling symptoms in some, and the nature of the prognosis together determine for the observer what the patient should be able to do. The tragedy is that the observer's society-influenced ideas about the patient's abilities are not always consistent with the patient's own assessments.

In addition to society's interwoven preconceptions, attitudes toward the patient will also be partially determined by his or her socioeconomic status and subculture. Thus a patient may successfully interact with members of one socioeconomic class or subculture in a manner wholly unacceptable to another. In fact, one criticism often leveled at health professionals is that they help patients toward recovery or adjustment in a manner that reflects the values of the middle class or mainstream of society. Patients not sharing these values cannot, therefore, be helped as readily.

In conclusion, one responsibility of the health professional is to help the patient realize his or her potential for optimal functioning by gaining some insight into the nature of the society from which the patient came and to which he or she will return. Society's response will depend on its complex interpretation of health and illness. The atmosphere in the health facility should therefore be one of friendly support in preparing the patient for renewed contact with the society to which he or she will ultimately return.

*Excerpted by permission of the New England Journal of Medicine, 304:699, 1981.

REFERENCES

1. Cassell, E. J.: The nature of suffering and the goals of medicine. N. Engl. J. Med. 306:639–645, 1982.
2. Nadler, A., and Altman, A.: Helping is not enough: Recipient's reaction to aid as a function of positive and negative information about the self. J. Pers. 47:615–628, 1979.
3. Muyskens, J. L.: Moral Problems in Nursing. Totowa, N. J., Rowman and Littlefield, 1982, p. 154–157.
4. American Medical Records Association: Confidentiality of Patient Health Information: A Position Statement of the AMRA. Chicago, 1977.
5. Reiser, S. J.: Medicine and the Reign of Technology. Cambridge, Cambridge University Press, 1978, pp. 2, 8.
6. Baron, R. J.: An empathic rediscovery of the known. J. Med. Philos. 6(1):5–23, 1981.
7. Albertson, S. H.: Endings and Beginnings. New York, Random House, 1980, pp. 3–4.

8. Nightingale, F.: Notes on Nursing: What It Is And What It Is Not. London, Harrison Press, 1860.
9. Baumann, B.: Diversities in conceptions of health and physical fitness. *J. Health Soc. Behav.* 2:39–46, 1961.
10. Trillin, A. S.: Of dragons and garden peas. A cancer patient talks to doctors. *N. Engl. J. Med.* 304:699–700, 1981.

Part II Summary

Part II examines the person who becomes a patient. In the role of patient, he or she acquires some problems and privileges that differ from those experienced before. A person stricken with illness or injury becomes free from everyday responsibilities. Some people realize gains from the dependent state and refuse to take necessary measures to get well. Most people, however, suffer losses that create both anxiety and inconvenience and are therefore eager to return to society.

Some of the most disrupting problems involve losses associated with former self-image, independence, and privacy. Uncertainty about immediate and long-range plans may cost the patient sleepless nights. The problems of stigma and lack of support systems add to the difficulties. Outpatients share many problems of hospitalized patients and have some others as well. Understanding of patients' problems is central to a health professional's effectiveness in dealing with individual patients.

A patient's sense of loss is related to what he or she values. The individual's value system, composed of societal and personal values, serves as an incentive for getting well. Some patients are confronted with the difficult realization that, as a result of their illness, their former values are no longer realizable. The health professional can be instrumental in guiding such patients toward realistic new values.

The patient is forced into several new modes of interaction by virtue of his or her position. Interaction with individual health professionals takes place within a dependent relationship. The health professional can help direct the relationship so that it is constructive rather than detrimental to the patient.

Today almost every patient is asked to interact with technology—ranging from the stethoscope on the chest to the computer in the health professional's receiving area and at the admission point of most health professions institutions.

The patient also must interact with the health professionals functioning as a societal unit. During acute care, he or she must be able to accept nurturing from those who provide health care. When he or she begins to improve, independent functioning is increasingly encouraged. The success with which patients make this seemgly difficult transition depends largely on their sense of self-dependence.

A patient's most difficult interaction is with society. This is true to some extent whether or not appearance and capabilities are altered as a result of the illness or injury. Though societal reactions differ widely, they are likely to be affected by society's conceptions and misconceptions of health. Socioeconomic classes and subcultures have definitions of health that help to determine the patient's expected behavior.

Hippocrates was right! The patient, his or her environment, and external conditions must collaborate with the health professionals to effect the patient's recovery or adjustment. In Part III, the student will examine the communication skills that act as tools for effective interaction. Equipped with these, he or she will progress, in Part IV, to some key dimensions of the patient–health professional relationship.

Part II Questions for Thought and Discussion

1. Your patient, Miss Yuker, sustained a shoulder injury while at work. She has been collecting workmen's compensation because she cannot lift her arm over her head, which her job requires her to do. One afternoon you are riding on the same elevator with Miss Yuker. She is near the panel buttons, and you are in the rear so that she does not see you. At one of the floors, a man is still entering the elevator when the doors begin to close. Instinctively, Miss Yuker reaches above her head with her "injured" arm to push the "Door Open" button.
   (a) To whom should you report this observation?
   (b) How will reporting this incident implicate you ethically or legally?
   (c) How will what you saw affect your attitude toward the patient?
   (d) How will what you saw affect the actual interaction between you and the patient?
   (e) Does this patient have a right to continue to pretend to be injured? If she values the dependent state more than her ability to work, should the health professional force his or her own values and those of society on the patient? What is the basis for your answer?
2. If you were hospitalized for seven weeks, what aspect of home do you think you would miss most? What would be your greatest frustration? What would you find to be the most difficult adjustment to make in returning to your old role and friends?
3. If you were to lose the use of your lower extremities in an automobile accident, what would be the most difficult aspects of adjusting to this permanent disfigurement and limitation?
4. What technologies employed by your profession may be depersonalizing to your patients?

DETERMINANTS OF EFFECTIVE INTERACTION BETWEEN HEALTH PROFESSIONAL AND PATIENT

Part III

In Parts I and II, the emphasis was primarily on individuals—the *person* who becomes a health professional or a patient. Part III introduces the theme that will be continued throughout the remaining chapters of the book—the effective interaction between the two.

The tools available for their interaction must first be considered; there are both verbal and nonverbal communication tools. The setting in which health professional and patient are expected to interact must be considered next. In the broadest sense, this setting is the "global village."

Because travel has become the normal way of life, many people frequently move from one time zone to another, creating a number of entirely new phenomena. For instance, people today are the first to worry about the effects of jet lag! Given this ease of mobility, the health professional will be interacting with scores of people whose basic needs are similar but whose superficial lifestyles vary widely. How can he or she communicate with such a variety of people?

Some answers are offered in the following three chapters. Chapter 8 discusses components of effective verbal communication, while Chapter 9 is concerned with the important area of nonverbal communication and its effects on interaction. Chapter 10 reveals the possible effects of some culturally or personally derived biases on the communication process and, ultimately, on effective interaction.

Chapter 8

VERBAL COMMUNICATION

Talking Together—A Bridge to Relationship

By about the age of 2 years, a child makes all possible phonetic sounds. He clucks, cooes, chirps, and gurgles, and his audience, totally captivated, encourages him. But by the age of 4 years, a child learns that only certain sounds evoke a response from adults. The child thus begins to repress some of them and to mimic adults in combining sounds to form words. In this way, the highly complex, intricate skill of language is acquired. and an important bridge to relationship is built.

At a very young age people begin to associate verbal communication with comfort or encouragement. Similarly, patients look for verbal communication as a way of establishing themselves in relationship with the health professional and subsequently deriving comfort. For example, the 8-year-old heroine of *To Kill a Mockingbird* says of her physician:

> He was one of the few men of science who never terrified me, probably because he never behaved like a doctor. Whenever he performed a minor service for Jem and me, as removing a splinter from a foot, he would tell us exactly what he was going to do, give us an estimation of how much it would hurt, and explain the use of any tongs he employed.[1]*

Compare her statement with one by a patient interviewed in Koos' now classic study of health attitudes in *Regionville*:

> Maybe things would be better if the doc understood us, and if we always knew what the hell he was driving at, and not in big words either.[2]

Patients come to the health professional looking for comfort through communication. They do not have the technical language that is employed in health care.

A man who has a ruptured vertebral disk groans that there is a searing knife in his back, while the anemic young woman can best describe her condition as "low blood." Because patients lack language for accurate clinical descriptions, the health professional must try to translate their words into technical language.

---

*From *To Kill A Mockingbird* by Harper Lee (1960). Reprinted by permission of Harper & Row, Publishers, Inc.

The greater responsibility for effective verbal interaction between patient and health professional lies with the latter, though both must assume responsibility. By examining several interdependent components of effective communication, the reader should gain insight into this important area of human interaction.

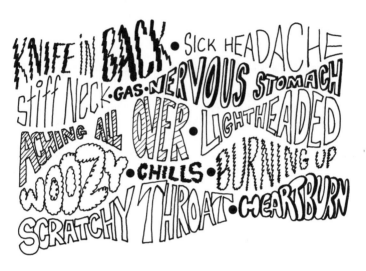

Determinants of Successful Verbal Communication

The health professional is usually required to communicate verbally with the patient in order (1) to establish rapport; (2) to obtain information concerning his or her condition and progress; (3) to relay pertinent information to another health professional or to supportive personnel; and (4) to give instructions to the patient and his or her family. Periodically, the health professional is expected to offer encouragement and support, to give rewards as incentives for further effort, to report technical data to the patient, to interpret information, to teach the patient, and to act as consultant. The health professional naturally will be more comfortable with some activities than with others, according to specific abilities and experience; nevertheless, all health professionals should be prepared to perform the entire gamut of activities.

Verbal communication is instrumental in creating better understanding between patient and health professional. This does not automatically happen. The health professional can often trace the cause of a misunderstanding to something he or she said; it was probably the wrong thing to say, or it was said in the wrong way or at the wrong time. In fact, one of the primary reasons that patients do not follow the health professional's instructions, and thus become noncompliant, is that the health professional did not utilize adequate verbal communication skills.[3]

The success of verbal communication depends on (1) the way

material is presented—the vocabulary used, the clarity of voice and the organization; (2) the attitude of the speaker; (3) the tone and volume of his or her voice; and (4) the degree to which both speaker and receiver are able to listen effectively.

PRESENTATION OF MATERIAL

Vocabulary. A health professional's failure to acquire the appropriate vocabulary leads to several problems: (1) use of the wrong word; (2) omission of important ideas; and (3) long, rambling descriptions that confuse rather than enlighten.

The descriptive vocabulary of the health professional is a two-edged sword. A student must learn to offer precise, accurate descriptions and must be able to communicate to other professionals in that mode. Some investigators suggest that when the health professional uses professional jargon in the presence of a patient, it contributes to the health professional's credibility, and may therefore increase the patient's confidence in him or her.[4]

However, highly technical professional jargon should never be used in direct conversation with the patient. It is imperative that the health professional translate technical jargon into terms understandable to the layperson when discussing the condition with the patient or the family. Even the questions asked of patients are often couched in highly technical language so that the patient has to guess at what is being asked.

> The respondent, reacting to the difficulty of language, may sense such a gap of understanding between him and the interviewer that he concludes that he is talking to a person who can never really understand and empathize with him. When this happens, one of the major motives for communication has been lost.[5]

Two problems arise when the health professional is unable to communicate with the patient in terms understandable to him or her. The first problem is obvious: The desired results cannot be obtained. The health professional attempts to receive the patient's complaints verbally. Often the descriptions are too vague, too difficult to classify. Rather than continue to work at understanding the symptoms and their significance for the patient, the health professional immediately turns to the more objective criteria of laboratory and other diagnostic findings, and bases treatment programs on experience described in the literature or derived from a large number of other patients. This "miss" in communication all too often takes as its toll the results the health professional wished to achieve, and could have, had effective communication with the patient been established.[6]

The second problem with using big technical words is that the person to whom the health professional is speaking will not be convinced that the health professional really wants to know how he or she feels.

Subsequently the health professional becomes a source of suffering for the patient rather than a means of recovery or adjustment.

Cassell has described the patient's suffering as related to the *person* who has the pain-inducing or disabling symptoms:

> Suffering occurs when an impending destruction of the person is perceived; it continues until the threat of disintegration has passed or until the integrity of the person can be restored in some other manner. It follows, then, that although suffering occurs in the presence of acute pain, shortness of breath, or other bodily symptoms, suffering extends beyond the physical. Most generally, suffering can be described as the state of severe distress associated with events that threaten the intactness of the person. . . .[7]*

The suffering of not being taken seriously as a person with serious problems is the interpretation often given to the communication gap when the health professional persists in using big words.

The complexity and impersonality of a health facility will undoubtedly be communicated to the patient if health professionals are unwilling to explain carefully to the patient, in lay terms, his or her condition and its treatment. What is *accomplished* within any allotted period of time, rather than the actual *amount* of time spent, will convince the patient that the health professional really cares. If the patient still cannot understand what is being said, all other attempts at reaching him or her will be futile.

To be sure, effective interviewing is a complex skill. Fortunately, recent studies have supported the idea that structure, organization, and formal teaching in this area are needed, and it is being widely introduced into the curricula of health professions as part of the students' formal education.[8]

The mastery of *appropriate* vocabulary, then, means knowing when and how to use professional jargon and translate it into lay terms. When this is accomplished, the patient will be able to do what is requested, will respond accurately to the health professional's questions, and will more likely be convinced that the health professional cares about him or her.

Clarity. A highly organized, technically correct, and very meaningful sentence loses its impact when poorly articulated, spoken too softly, or rushed. A patient is often preoccupied with one particular facet of a problem and, consequently, interprets everything the health professional says in light of that preoccupation.

It is surprising to some students that most patients are too embarrassed to ask the health professional to repeat an instruction, and so they try to interpret what they think they heard. Patients are sometimes hesitant because they are a bit awed by the health professions, and so

---

*Excerpted by permission of the New England Journal of Medicine, *306*:639, 1982.

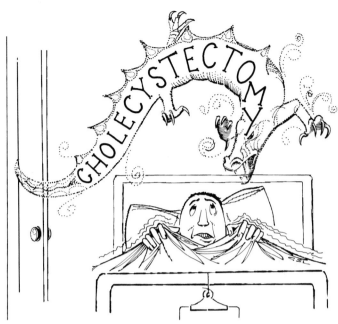

Mastery of appropriate vocabulary means knowing when and how to use professional jargon and to translate it into layman's terms.

try to act sophisticated instead of asking the health professional to repeat what was said. Patients are awed primarily because they realize that the health professional has skills that can determine their future welfare and that, regardless of their influence in the business or social world, they are completely at the mercy of the health professional in this situation. Because of this anxiety, the health professional must speak with exceptional clarity if the intended message is to get across.

Organization. A health professional often has to explain to a patient a procedure that will be done in either the presence or the absence of the former. The rambling health professional confuses a patient by jumping from one topic to the next, inserting last-minute ideas, then failing to summarize or to ask the patient to do so.

Although by no means limited to this situation, the health professional's disorganization presents a grave problem when he or she gives home instructions. Inability to progress from one step to the next, thereby reaching a logical conclusion, is usually caused by (1) a lack of understanding of the subject or of the steps in the procedure or (2) ironically, a too-thorough knowledge of the subject or procedure. The former causes the patient to grope for all the facts, while the latter causes the speaker to overlook points that are obvious to him but not to the listener. In either case, it is advisable to break down the procedure into its component parts, then practice describing it to a friend who is not familiar with the procedure. That person will readily reveal any obvious steps that have been omitted. The author recently tried this in a seminar by asking the students to make paper airplanes according to verbal instructions given them. The students cooperated all too well by doing only and precisely what they were verbally instructed to do. Some finally succeeded after 20 minutes of increasingly frustrated instruction.

The students drew two conclusions: (1) Verbal instructions alone are not always adequate; written instructions and diagrams are highly desirable adjuncts to the spoken word. (2) Verbal instruction is an art not to be taken lightly by the health professional who expects his or her instructions to be followed! (The author also drew a conclusion of her own: She will more fully familiarize herself with a procedure before trying to teach it to someone else!)

ATTITUDES

The attitude or feeling that the health professional has toward the patient will help determine the effectiveness of their spoken interaction. Most health professionals maintain a caring attitude toward the patient, and their way of speaking to the patient helps to communicate this genuine concern. However, on rare occasions the health professional may feel angry or disdainful toward the patient. The patient's understanding of why the anger or disdain is apparent can help to improve their communication. If he or she does not understand why the health professional is expressing a negative emotion, the communication between them breaks down, causing a problem.

The attitude we shall consider here, one directly concerned with spoken communication, is *fear*. When is the health professional likely to become afraid? How will this fear manifest itself during spoken communication?

The specific situations in which fear arises are numerous, and are most often connected with bad news. Such news may be that the patient has a terminal illness; the health professional knows the diagnosis but is afraid the patient will ask about the illness or whether or not it is irreversible. Consider the following example:

> Mr. Clayton Anderson, a 43-year-old contractor, fell from a scaffold, fracturing his right tibia. A month earlier he had consulted his physician of 20 years, complaining of unusual fatigue. Tests revealed no abnormal findings, and Mr. Anderson returned to work. He believes he "blacked out" prior to the fall, but this is fuzzy to him.
>
> Since the fracture is healing very slowly, Mr. Anderson has been hospitalized for three weeks. The social worker, Kim Segard, has been visiting him often, at Mr. Anderson's request. Mr. Anderson is discouraged about his slow recovery and worried about his wife and three children because he is self-employed, and every day away from work is a financial loss. Kim has been working to help Mr. Anderson arrange financial matters and provide support for the whole family.

In the fourth week of hospitalization Mr. Anderson develops a fever during the night. The symptoms persist the next day, so that all treatments must be canceled. Another series of tests is run, this time revealing a lymphosarcoma involving the bone, a type of cancer that is likely to be fatal within a year.

The physician telephones Kim to report the diagnosis and its implications for treatment. He says he is quite certain that Mr. Anderson would not want to know that he has cancer. Kim asks the physician why he has come to this conclusion, and he explains that Mr. Anderson once said of a friend who had died of cancer, "He stopped living as soon as he found out." The physician also tells Kim that he has spoken to Mrs. Anderson, who concurs with his judgment. He asks if Kim has had any discussion with Mr. or Mrs. Anderson that would provide insight into whether Mr. Anderson would want to know. Kim tries to think of something he may have said, but is unable to recall any discussions that would clarify this difficult decision. Kim believes that both the Andersons have always confronted problems directly and honestly, and says so. There is a pause. The physician says, "Well, I've pretty much decided not to tell him. I think all in all it's better for him not to know."

Kim Segard goes on seeing Clayton Anderson. About ten days later Clayton says to Kim, "You know, we have talked often, and I have come to trust your judgment. I'm grateful for the help you've given me and my family. You know I've tried to cooperate with the doctors and everyone, but I have a feeling that something funny is going on that I can't get at. My wife and the doctor are acting strange and that is scaring me. I couldn't sleep all last night and so I decided to ask you. I know you will level with me. . . . *Do I have cancer or some fatal illness?*"[9]

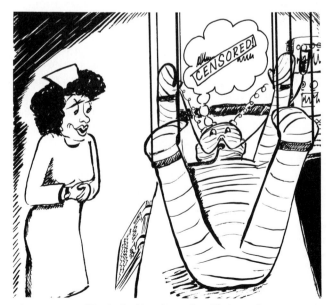

"You're looking *fine* today, Mr. Jones."

What information is it appropriate for Kim to share with Mr. Anderson?

If you were Kim, how would you handle this delicate situation?

In the professional relationship with the patient as well as in personal life, the health professional is tempted to escape a difficult situation. One means of escape is to avoid discussing a difficult situation altogether. This is often how a terminal illness is handled. A person knows he or she is dying; the doctor, the family, and the health professional also know, but they all refuse to admit it verbally and are convinced that such behavior is in the patient's best interest. This, of course, represents a total, destructive breakdown in communication.

Another means of escape is to disguise the real problem, to put confectioner's sugar on a brick and call it a cake. The bad news can also be disguised by inserting it between bits of irrelevant conversation in order to lighten its impact. A frivolous or optimistic tone of voice can serve the same purpose. This method is rarely effective but continues to be widely used. One can visualize a physician standing by a patient's bed, thumbing through the patient's chart and cheerily saying: "Well, Mr. Johnson, you are looking good today and your progress notes say that you slept well. The x-ray shows that you do have some bony changes in your spine. I see your blood tests are normal. Good! By the way, how is your wife?" The physician knows that the bony changes in Mr. Johnson's spine will mean continued pain, more absence from work, and, very likely, major surgery.

A more subtle, often effective way of disguising a problem is by using humor. The health facility is full of banter, laughter, and jokes, some of which serve useful purposes while others are destructive.

Useful Humor. Humor can be used wisely to help patients cope with stress related to their illness and accompanying problems.[10]

In communication between the patient and the health professional, joking and teasing can be used constructively to (1) allow the person to express hostility, covert exhibitionism, and anxiety; (2) permit exploration of the humor and irony of the condition in which he or she is placed by illness or injury; and (3) reduce tension when it unnecessarily exists. One device is for the health professional to poke fun at himself or herself, thus modeling for the patient that every situation has some humor in it, including his or her own.[11] Valentine Michael Smith, the Martian in Heinlein's science-fiction novel, *Stranger in a Strange Land*, suddenly realizes that in order to "grok" (fully understand) earth people, he must learn to laugh at their weaknesses, cruelties and inconsistencies. When he explains this to his friend Jill, she replies, " '. . . Apparently the pratfall is the peak of all humor. It's not a pretty picture of the human race, Mike.'

'Oh, but it is!'

'Huh?'

'I had thought—I had been told—that a "funny" thing is a thing of goodness. It isn't. Not ever is it funny to the person it happens to. . . .

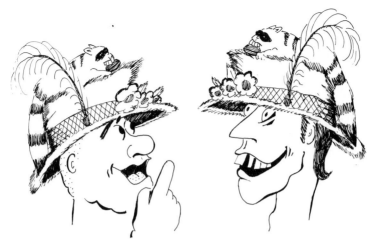

"That's the ugliest hat I've ever seen."

The goodness is in the laughing. I grok it is a bravery—and a sharing—against pain and sorrow and defeat.' ''[12]

The inexperienced health professional and the lay person are often shocked by the openness with which patients joke about themselves. For instance, patients whose legs are paralyzed often joke about rubber crutches and icy surfaces—both of which are real threats in their present situations. Persons with disfiguring injuries call themselves "freaks." Their joking helps to alleviate their anxiety about these problems. Patients with temporary or permanent sexual impotence also joke a lot about sex. It is helpful to recognize their joking as one means of expressing very difficult thoughts and emotions.

Destructive Humor. The health professional and the patient can use humor unwisely too. Continual verbal fencing to win the upper hand will likely influence other aspects of the relationship, eventually creating such a feeling of animosity that it will be impossible for them to work together.

The health professional will meet patients who use "put downs" humorously to increase their diminished feeling of self-worth. However, it is important to discourage this mode of behavior. Patients who become accustomed to buttressing their own sense of worth by insulting others soon cease to be humorous, and thus develop habits that are not acceptable to the rest of society and therefore will militate against their successful recovery or adjustment.

Besides its use as a control mechanism or as a means of boosting a faltering sense of self-worth, the patient's joking can allow verbal exploration of the limits of the relationship with the health professional. This can be beneficial to a degree. However, the joking can also serve as a way of sidestepping a real issue. To continue joking when it becomes apparent that the humor is being used as a shield can result in emotional injury to the patient or the health professional. Since it is an indirect method of coping, by itself it may not be effective over a period of time.[13]

The range of situations in which humor is used as a substitute for other verbal communication is shown in the following excerpt:

> Then there is the laugh which fills up a blank in the conversation, often associated with a thoughtful "yes, isn't it amazing?", the laugh of the older man talking to a girl, which can suggest "You are charming, but I am charming too." The laugh to attract attention, similar to that attention-attracting cough, that large confident chest-clearing, kept for a pianissimo passage, by the man who feels out of depth at a concert. The laugh, similar, which we hear in the hall from the new arrival not sure of himself, who wishes to appear sure of himself, and it makes us sure we are not sure of him. The laugh of the lone man at the theater, who wishes to show that he understands the play or understands the foreign language which is being spoken, or gets the point of the joke quickest, or has seen the play. The laugh of the creative pleasure uttered by someone who has managed to say something precise and descriptive in a conversation, whether witty or not. The laugh of relief from physical danger, or from the reprieve of the worse danger of separation. We laugh at funny hats.[14]

An equal number of variations can be found within the setting of the health facility. The use to which humor is put will determine whether it can be considered helpful to effective interaction or a poor substitute for direct confrontation.

The habit of avoiding unpleasant topics or problems either by ignoring them altogether or by disguising them does not facilitate effective communication. Later chapters deal with specific means by which the health professional can overcome the fear of discussing with a patient the latter's undesirable behavior, the former's emotional reaction to him, and any other disagreeable subjects.

VOICE TONE AND VOLUME

Sometimes a person's actions belie his or her words. This is shown in the proverbs "Do as I say, but not as I do"; and "Actions speak louder than words." Similarly, the two qualities of the voice that most influence the meanings of the words spoken are (1) voice tone and (2) volume.

Voice Tone. Give the simple question—What are you doing?—several meanings by varying the tone in which it is spoken. Compare the tones of the following people: (1) a man telephoning his wife at midday; (2) the man's wife, who has just caught their 2-year-old son writing on the living room wall with a purple crayon; and (3) the 2-year-old son trying to make up to the mother after his scolding and spanking. Each is trying to communicate more than the literal content of the spoken message.

An expression as short as "oh" can be used to express the following attitudes and emotions: anger, pity, disappointment, teasing, pleasure, gratitude, exuberance, terror, superiority, disbelief, uncertainty, compassion, insult, awe, and many more!

Tone is a voice quality that can actually reverse the meaning of the spoken word. When the patient's response is puzzling to the health professional, the latter should be alert to the tone in which the patient had communicated a message or reacted to a statement. For example, if the patient asks, "Am I going to get better?", the health professional can inadvertently confirm the patient's worst fears by answering in a not-too-convincing tone, "Yes, of course you will!"

Volume. Tone and volume are closely related voice qualities. An angry person may not only spit out the words indignantly, but may also alter the volume of the message; for instance, it is possible to communicate anger either by whispering the words through gritted teeth or by shouting them.

Voice volume controls interaction in subtle ways. For instance, if one person stands close to another and speaks in an inordinately loud voice, the listener invariably backs away. Thus, literally and symbolically, the volume of the voice does control distance between people.

On the other hand, a soft whisper automatically causes the listener to move closer. For example, a health professional may be in a crowded elevator where everyone is apparently absorbed in personal thoughts or in conversation. But if he or she turns to a colleague and begins to whisper about "an interesting case" in which a particular patient is suspected of having a rare, very contagious disease and may have infected several people before being isolated, the other people on the elevator will nearly fall over trying to lean toward the speaker in an effort to hear what is being whispered.

Inappropriately loud volume can be an irritating attention-getting device. Both health professional and patient are potential offenders, particularly if they learned at an early age to shout above everyone else to gain attention. This annoying habit is, of course, not easily broken, and the challenge seems to be to learn how to cope with the person so that he or she is offensive to the smallest number of people.

Thus, the old adage—It's not what you say but how you say it—applies to the health professions. It behooves the professional person to be sensitive to the secret messages being sent via tone and volume as well as the spoken word.

EFFECTIVE LISTENING

A considerable portion of a health professional's day is spent in listening to patients and colleagues. Elizabeth Smith lists the following levels of listening and suggests that health professionals are usually involved in the more complex levels, listed first:

1. Analytical—listening for specific kinds of information and arranging them into categories.

2. Directed—listening in order to answer specific questions.

3. Attentive—listening for general information in order to get the overall picture.

4. Exploratory—listening because of one's own interest in the subject being discussed.

5. Appreciative—listening for esthetic pleasure, such as listening to music.

6. Courteous—listening because one feels obligated to listen.

7. Passive—listening as in overhearing something; not attentive to the matter being discussed.[15]

People lack the skills to listen effectively. Thus words hit the eardrum, but the message then becomes distorted. The health professional should have two goals: (1) to improve listening acuity so that he or she hears the patient accurately and (2) to learn to ascertain how accurately a patient has heard him or her. The first step toward achieving these goals is to examine the reasons why messages get distorted. The health professional must then transfer this knowledge to his or her own experience.

Besides the often overlooked, important possibility of a hearing defect, there are at least four reasons why a health professional or patient distorts what he or she hears during verbal interaction.

The Listener's Set. A set or frame of mind often distorts meaning. It is the result of past experience. In this case, the person fails to listen to the spoken words or to note subtle individual differences among patients because he or she is very sure of what the patient will say.

Perceptual Defense. Most people tend to force an idea into a familiar context so that they can understand it quickly and ignore aspects of it that do not fit this context. This tendency is, of course, related to their mind set but is also a defense against possible change. It may be that a person's inability to accept new concepts is due to a basic lack of self-understanding. Thus, the weaker or more ill-defined a person's self-image, the greater the need to resist ideas that are more complex or ambiguous.[16]

The health professional must expect that the patient, whose self-image is jeopardized by sickness, will reject ideas that are believed to further threaten his or her world.[17]

Problem of Directives. Directive utterances are words that "direct us to do certain things with the stated or implied promise that if we do these things certain consequences will follow."[18] In the context of the health professions, instructions to patients or co-workers are directive utterances. Hayakawa warns of the obligation one assumes in promising a person that if he performs a certain act, he will recover from illness or injury: "Everyone of us, therefore, who utters directive language, with its concomitant promises, stated or implied, is morally obligated to be as certain as he can, since there is no absolute certainty, that he is arousing no false expectations. . . . It does not matter much whether such misleading directives are uttered in ignorance and error or with conscious intent to deceive, because the disappointments they cause are all similarly destructive of mutual trust among human beings. . . ."[19]

A listener often interprets directives as being more specific and concrete than the speaker intended. An interesting but frustrating phenomenon observed by the health professional is that the patient who seems to have the least cause for anxiety (that is, one who has nearly recovered) may hear more in the health professional's statements than the patient whose prognosis is far more dire. It may be that to the patient, the little failures (as interpreted by the health professional) are the hardest; near-achievement is not good enough.

Sensory Overloading. The rate at which listeners can process incoming information varies significantly. This is partially but not entirely due to differences in innate ability. Overconfidence in predicting what will be said or too little confidence in predicting what will be said also determines whether a person will cease to process informational inputs. If the person is overconfident, boredom settles in. If the person has too little confidence, he or she tends to become overly anxious and tune out the message.[20]

The rate and level of understanding at which one directs the communication will alter the listener's ability to process the information. Thus it is important that the health professional have some knowledge of the patient's basic intelligence and past experience with a subject. The listener's set, the need to defend existing precepts, the way in which directive utterances are interpreted, and the listener's innate intelligence all determine how accurately he or she will hear a message. Sometimes the health professional will be the poor listener, and at other times the patient will be. When either one or both are struggling to understand the message, it is likely to become distorted.

The health professional cannot completely control how effectively the patient listens but can, however, learn to become a more effective listener. By simply restating what the patient has said, the health professional can confirm part of a message before proceeding to the next portion of it. In addition, the following are some simple steps to more effective listening:

1. Be selective in what you listen to.
2. Realize that words are only symbols—we impose our meanings on others' words.
3. Concentrate on central themes rather than isolated statements.
4. Judge content rather than style or delivery.
5. Listen with an open mind—don't focus on emotionally charged words.
6. The average person can listen four times faster than he can speak—use extra time to summarize.[21]

The importance of becoming an effective listener is emphasized in an article from *The American Journal of Nursing*. A nurse describes how, as a patient herself, she desperately longed for a *person* who would listen to her: ". . . What I wanted was a brief, two-way relationship, an extended hand that did not hold a thermometer, a friendly face without a forced display of teeth. . . . Paralyzed by fear, in constant need of reassurance, the *asker of innumerable questions*, the patient most in need of human contact is labeled a 'pest' and shunned. . . ." [Author's italics.][22]

In Chapter 13 several ways will be presented in which the health professional can communicate that he or she is genuinely interested in the patient. All the methods require effective listening. In Chapters 15 through 20, which concern working with older people and with terminally ill patients, the importance of maintaining their dignity through effective listening is emphasized. Thus the listening skill must be acquired as carefully as other professional skills if effective interaction is to be realized.

The section on listening effectiveness completes the discussion of verbal communication. The health professional must be aware of their importance if he or she expects to obtain desirable results with patients. Verbal communication, however, is only a part of the total picture. The next chapter presents another facet of communication, one that utilizes nonverbal skills.

REFERENCES

1. Lee, H.: *To Kill A Mockingbird.* New York, J. B. Lippincott Company, 1960.
2. Koos, E.: The Health of Regionville. New York, Columbia University Press, 1954, 1977.
3. Sanson-Fisher, R., and Maguire, P.: Should skills in communicating with patients be taught? *Lancet* 1:523–526, 1980.
4. Campbell, J. H., and Helper, H. W.: Persuasion and interpersonal relationships. In Campbell, J. H., and Helper, H. W. (eds.): *Dimensions in Communications: Readings.* 2nd ed. Belmont, Calif.: Wadsworth Publishing Company, 1970, p. 132.
5. Kahn, R., and Cannel, C.: *The Dynamics of Interviewing.* New York, John Wiley & Sons, 1957, p. 113.
6. Bergsma, J., and Thomasma, D. C.: *Health Care: Its Psychosocial Dimension.* Pittsburgh, Duquesne University Press, 1982, pp. 66–67.
7. Cassell, E. J.: The nature of suffering and the goals of medicine. *N. Engl. J. Med.* 306:639–645, 1982.
8. Ivy, A. E.: *Basic Interviewing.* Monterey, Calif., Brooks-Cole Publishing, 1983.
9. Purtilo, R. B., and Cassel, C. K.: *Ethical Dimensions in the Health Professions.* Philadelphia, W. B. Saunders Company, 1981, pp. 75–76.
10. Dixon, N. F.: Humor: a cognitive alternative to stress? In Sarason, I., and Spielberger, C. D. (eds.): *Stress and Anxiety.* New York, Hemisphere, 1980.
11. King, M., Novik, L., and Citrenbaum, C.: *Irresistible Communication: Creative Skills for the Health Professional.* Philadelphia, W. B. Saunders Company, 1982, p. 16.
12. Heinlein, R. A.: *Stranger in a Strange Land.* New York, Berkley Publishing Company, 1961, p. 300.
13. Safranek, R., and Schill, T.: Coping with stress; does humor help? *Psychiatr. Rep.* 51:222, 1982.
14. Potter, S.: *Sense of Humor.* New York, Henry Holt & Company, 1955, pp. 9–10.
15. Smith, E.: Improving listening effectiveness. *Tex. Med.* 71:98–100, 1975.
16. King, M., Novik, L., and Citrenbaum, C.: *op. cit.,* pp. 5–7.
17. Kellerman, J. M., and Land, J. O.: The effect of appearance on self-perceptions. *J. Pers.* 50:296–315, 1982.
18. Hayakawa, S. I.: *Language in Thought and Action.* 2nd ed. New York, Harcourt, Brace, Jovanovich, 1964, p. 104.
19. *Ibid.,* pp. 104–105.
20. Booth, R. Z.: Conflict resolution. *Nurs. Outlook* 30:447–453, 1982.
21. Walker, R.: Effective listening. *Am. J. Med. Techn.* 35:8–10, 1969.
22. Freund, H.: Listening with any ear at all. *Am. J. Nurs.* 69:1650, 1969.

Chapter 9

NONVERBAL COMMUNICATION

Two types of nonverbal communication are utilized by the health professional to relay vital messages and facilitate effective interaction. The first is formal pantomimed demonstration, used to augment or substitute for verbal communication. The second, called "metacommunication" by communications specialists, is a type of wordless communication that alters or supplements spoken words. It includes gestures, facial expressions, physical appearance, and other such signs.

Both types of nonverbal communication can serve either to confirm and clarify or to contradict verbal communication. The allied health professional's goal should be to learn how to utilize nonverbal communication effectively.

Pantomime and Demonstration

PANTOMIME

Pantomime is the formal enactment of a particular situation. It is a professional version of charades, in which a toothy smile and round unblinking eyes express approval. To indicate the personal "I," one points to oneself or vigorously thumps one's chest. Carefully mouthed monosyllables express words whose meanings cannot be conveyed by pointing, pounding or posturing.

This type of acting out can usefully substitute for spoken or written words with the following types of patients: (1) non–English speaking, (2) aphasic, and (3) deaf.

The Non-English Speaking Patient. This patient usually comes from a cultural background different from that of the health professional, and the language difference is just one of the many causes of frustration they will encounter in working together. Chapter 10 shows how cultural bias may contribute to unexpected interpretations of the interactions between health professional and patient. The effective use of professional charades is thus a challenge in this intercultural situation.

The Aphasic Patient. The patient who is aphasic or who has other perceptual problems may come from a cultural background nearly identical to that of the health professional. His or her understanding problem, however, is the result of a brain injury that causes inability (1) to interpret

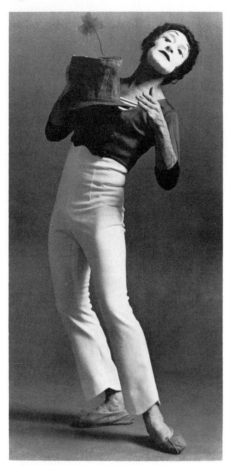

Philadelphia All Star—Forum, Inc.

incoming verbal stimuli, (2) to form words, or (3) to do both. Note that the person may be able to understand every word and know what he or she wants, but will not be able to respond verbally.

In this situation, it is advisable to begin with a simple spoken question. If the patient reacts in a manner that definitely indicates he or she understands, the health professional can proceed to more complex verbal communication. If he or she does not understand, however, pantomime actions should begin simply and be performed slowly. If the patient interprets them correctly, the health professional can proceed to more complex pantomime.

It is important to remember that the aphasic person may be able either to understand some verbal stimuli or to respond with some words. The pantomime may supplement verbal communication rather than completely substitute for it. In this way, the patient will be encouraged to communicate verbally as much as possible—a manner that is more acceptable to society.

The Deaf Patient. Deaf people can, of course, read, and some can lip-read as well, but for a few it is more effective to act out instructions than to write them down. Some health professionals who work with deaf people learn sign language as another means of communication. For instance, an intern in occupational therapy announced that she was giving a man "speech therapy" by exercising his hand. He was a deaf person who used sign language, and a crushing injury to the fingers of his right hand had "silenced" him. Besides restoring his finger motion, she was learning sign language.

Deaf people face a problem encountered by many with physical limitations: They are treated as though they are intellectually inferior. In using any method of nonverbal communication for "talking" to deaf people, the health professional must, therefore, be careful not to insult their intelligence. In pantomimed communication, it is also advisable to face the person so that he or she derives the benefit of facial expressions, lip motion, posture, and so forth.

DEMONSTRATION

Demonstration is usually used to supplement verbal instruction concerning an activity that must be repeated by the person (e.g., demonstrating how to walk with crutches or how to perform a urine test for diabetes). The health professional should perform the demonstration while standing beside and in full view of the person, because the effect of facing him or her directly is much the same as looking in the mirror—right and left are reversed. It must be kept in mind that some patients suffer from perceptual disorders and will have extensive difficulty repeating even the easiest patterns.

Pantomime and demonstration will sometimes be the only or the most effective form of communication for certain patients. In others, they will be helpful supplements to verbal interaction.

Metacommunication

Pantomime may be considered an exaggerated form of metacommunication: The goal of pantomime is to bring to the surface those postures, facial expressions, and gestures that have definite understood meanings. Pantomime more often completely substitutes for verbal messages, while metacommunication usually adds to them. Actions that accompany words modify their meaning. Since nonverbal communication or metacommunication is used during any human interaction in which two people are in each other's presence, the health professional should be aware of the effects that both have on interaction.

FACIAL EXPRESSIONS

In the last chapter, the reader was asked to consider the variety of messages conveyed by altering the tone and volume of the spoken word "oh." It is possible to omit the word altogether and, with only a facial expression, indicate anger, pity, disappointment, teasing, pleasure, gratitude, euphoria, boredom, compassion, exuberance, terror, superiority, disbelief, uncertainty, insult, or awe. In the 1960's, anthropologist Ray Birdwhistell, intrigued with the wide scope of facial expression, developed an annotation system for recording facial expressions. His system has been widely adopted and refined by others. He reported that there are 32 small units of motion (kinemes) in the face and head area. Each is seen as having a separate meaning.[1]

The subtlety with which the health professional uses facial expression in communication is illustrated by a gesture as simple as a smile. Although it is usually interpreted to mean friendliness, a smile does not always communicate that. Consider, for instance, the following five kinds of smiles:

1. The "I-know-something-you-don't-know" smile. A patient asks, "Am I going to be here very long with this injury?" The health professional smiles.

2. The "poor-poor-you" smile. The patient labors for five minutes to transfer himself from his bed to a wheelchair, but fails to complete the move and has to ask the health professional for help. The health professional smiles.

3. The "don't-tell-me!" smile. The health professional asks, "How are you today, Mr. Carlson? Is everything OK? Good!" Before Mr. Carlson can say whether or not everything is in fact OK, the health professional smiles.

4. The "I'm-smarter-than-you" smile. The patient says, "I'm sorry. I forgot again when I am supposed to return for my next test." The health professional smiles.

5. The "I-don't-like-you-either" smile. The patient shouts, "I hate you!" The health professional smiles.

These five smiles are destructive expressions used by some people in the health professions to convey an unspoken message. The fact that they are usually subconscious expressions does little to diminish their impact. The "I-know-something-you-don't-know" and "poor-poor-you" smiles are often futile attempts to disguise embarrassment or pity. The "don't-tell-me!" smile is used to hide fear of what the person may say; he or she may have a big emotional outburst! The other two, though seldom used, are means by which the insecure or hostile health professional can alienate and intimidate a patient. Fortunately, destructive smiles are rarely used. Most health professionals convey encouragement and genuine concern for the patient through a spontaneous smile.

POSITIONS, POSTURES, AND GESTURES

The way a person stands and sits in relation to another and the manner in which he or she moves communicate messages that either confirm or contradict verbal statements. For example, a threatening message is enhanced if the health professional is standing over the patient, a point not lost by satirist-cartoonist James Thurber.

It is generally agreed that eye contact communicates a positive message. If two people genuinely like each other, they will position themselves so that they can look into each other's eyes. The distance between them as they face each other further communicates how they feel about each other, but this is discussed more in the next chapter.

Even without eye contact, many things are revealed by the body. For instance, authority can be communicated by the height from which one person interacts with another. If one stands while the other sits, the former has subconsciously placed himself or herself in a position of authority. Both the angry man who jumps to his feet when making a point and the schoolteacher who stands up to see what the problem is establish their authority by their gesture. Height is unwittingly used to project a submissive role onto a patient when he or she is confined to a bed, a treatment table, or a wheelchair. In many instances, the relationship would be improved if the health professional would move down to the patient's level. In other instances, height can be used constructively to establish authority, as with an unruly child.

The extent to which the body is allowed to relax during interaction also communicates a message. The body, as a mediator of messages, uses even the tone of the muscles as a communication tool![2] The health professional who is performing a test or giving a treatment for the first time often reveals this fact by being so tense. But some investigators feel that the extent to which a person is relaxed or tense sends other messages too. For example,

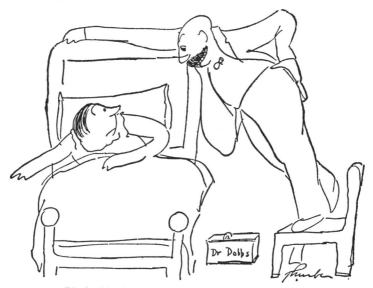

"You're Not My Patient, You're My Meat, Mrs. Quist!"

Posture is used to indicate both liking and status. The more a person leans toward his addressee, the more positively he feels about him. Relaxation of posture is a good indicator of both attitude and status, and one that we have been able to measure quite precisely. Three categories have been established for relaxation in the seated position: least relaxation is indicated by muscular tension in the hands and rigidity of posture; moderate relaxation is indicated by a forward lean of about 20 degrees and a side lean of less than 10 degrees, a curved back, and for women, an open arms position; extreme relaxation is indicated by a reclining angle greater than 20 degrees and a sideways lean of greater than 10 degrees.

Our findings suggest that a speaker relaxes very little or a great deal when he dislikes the person he is talking to, and to a moderate degree when he likes his companion. It seems that extreme tension occurs with threatening addressees, and extreme relaxation with nonthreatening, disliked addressees. In particular, men tend to become tense when talking to other men who they dislike; on the other hand, women talking to men or women and men talking to women show dislike through extreme relaxation. . . .[3]

In addition to whole-body posturing and positioning, gestures involving the extremities, even one finger, can suggest the meanings of a message. Consider the mother who folds her arms when a child begins to sputter an excuse for coming home late, the man who clenches his fist, the thumb roller, the shoulder shrugger, and the foot shuffler; what unspoken messages are they sending?

The extent to which positioning, posturing, and gesturing specifically affect the relationship between patient and health professional has not been studied extensively and is therefore open for exploration. However, one can speculate that these factors influence this relationship just as they influence all interpersonal relationships.

PHYSICAL APPEARANCE

Stereotypes are formed from outward appearances. In some instances, a person tries to adopt a stereotyped manner of dressing or speaking in the hope of being identified with a particular group.

Some health professionals adopt a stereotyped manner of dress (the uniform) in order to be identified easily within the world of health care. The "uniform" may include clothing, a patch, pin, cap, or name tag. Certain instruments also identify the person: the nurse's or physician's stethoscope dangling from the neck, the laboratory technologist's tray.

However, some health professionals today are engaged in a controversy over uniforms. One group prefers to shed the symbols of their profession and to approach each patient more on a person-to-person basis. This group bases its argument partially on studies suggesting that patients, especially children, react negatively to the white uniform. This group sees the uniform as a negative stereotype that creates unnecessary distance or gives a sense of undue authority to the health professional.

Another group defends the traditional uniform or white coat, believing it to facilitate effective interaction. This group argues that it is a quick means of identification in the entire health facility and serves as a positive stereotype in matters as simple as gaining admittance to a patient's room. Some patients actually feel more comfortable with a uniformed health professional who is about to begin a procedure that would be inappropriate in a social setting. Further, the uniform is often designed for durability and movement and may therefore be more desirable than clothing designed for less rigorous wear. Finally, it is an efficient, economical mode of dress.

Those arguing in favor of the uniform admit that these positive factors can be undermined by a health professional's actions. In fact, those on both sides agree that it is not the uniform itself but *what the person in the uniform does* that ultimately determines how the patient interprets the health professional's actions.

Besides the clothes he or she wears, there are other factors that contribute to a person's physical appearance. Grooming is often a controversial subject because hair styles, the amount and type of make-up worn by women, and the types of sideburns, moustaches, or beards worn by men are so dependent on current styles. Some professional people resist rigid rules that define physical appearance because they feel it is very important to express their individuality through their appearance. Others are less concerned that compliance with regulations governing physical appearance will damage their individuality. At any rate, the reader should be cognizant of the fact that physical appearance affects not only others' responses to one but also the way in which one perceives one's own abilities.[4]

The health professional's concern for the patient should be his or her basis for adopting a particular kind of appearance. Do body or cosmetic odors offend the patient? Does the health professional's grooming break any rules of good personal hygiene? Does it reflect the dignity of the health professional as a person? Does it present any risk of injury to the patient (long fingernails, jewelry, and so forth)? Very often, only through unpleasant experience does a health professional modify his or her appearance. A health professional should try to anticipate and avoid situations in which a particular kind of appearance will hinder professional effectiveness.

TOUCH

For a child, a touch holds great significance: Aladdin produced a genie by touching the magic lamp; Cinderella's coach appeared at the touch of her fairy godmother's wand; and a countless number of handsome princes have awakened beautiful, bewitched princesses with their kisses.

Adults give touch symbolic meaning in everyday conversation. They promise to "keep in touch," are "touched" by a tender scene in a film, and accredit the hostess with having "a special touch" for hospitality. The great religions acknowledge the power of touch; every faith has its relics and holy persons whose healing power is released if they are touched.[5] In spite of all this, most of us come from a predominantly nontouching society.

In a nontouching society, individuals do handle each other all the time, but the context is crucial. That is, they tend not to put their hands on each other except in lovemaking and well-defined rituals of greeting or celebration. (An example of the latter is a team that is joyfully celebrating its victory in a championship game.) However, the nontoucher allows himself or herself to be palpated, held, squeezed, rubbed, supported, and lifted upon entering a health facility.

These touching privileges are granted to the health professional within the patient–health professional relationship. Health professionals are actually licensed as a protection against the charge of unconsented touching (battery). Interestingly, even legitimate touching is limited. It must be recognizable as part of the diagnostic or therapeutic procedure.

Fortunately, the comforting touch is usually regarded as legitimate, and health professionals have in it a powerful tool for communicating their caring. One health professional, particularly attuned to the messages conveyed by touch, wrote:

The Language of Touch

An appendage of man—
    designed for dexterity,
        fine movement,
            adeptness.

Four fingers and a thumb—
    working in concert as
        an orchestra,
            with precision.

An instrument of function—
    directed by man's great mind,
        to create,
            to work.

But more—
The ears and tongue of the inner self—
    through the language of touch,
        listening,
            speaking.

Speaking of precious feelings—
that words cannot express,
gently,
with meaning.

Hearing the feelings of another—
never asking for clarification,
accepting,
caring.

—the hand!

SHELBY J. CLAYSON*

The health professional should be mindful that people are picking up signals conveyed by his or her manner of touching. (This is often related to the health professional's appearance and way of moving, as discussed in the section on physical appearance in this chapter.) The sensation received by the patient when his or her arm is lifted by the health professional's cold, clammy hand sends quite a different message from the gentle support of a warm, dry hand. The reassuring hand resting on a patient's shoulder sometimes speaks more loudly than the kindest words.

Patients will be much more aware of this touching than the health professional, who has become used to touching patients. The health professional probably has so firm a concept of his or her good intentions that the question of inappropriateness or improper familiarity never arises. However, touch, as one form of nonverbal communication, does involve risk. It may be a threat because it invades an otherwise private space, or it may be misunderstood. Moreover, if the health professional is not attuned to the needs of himself or herself and the patient, the touching may indeed be inappropriate.[6] But the risk, properly undertaken, likely will yield favorable results. Subjective observation by the health professional supports the idea that patients in general respond favorably to thoughtful expressions of caring conveyed through touch. Regular assessment of the amount and type of touching helps the health professional to understand a patient's reactions.

In summary, nonverbal communication is a natural, inevitable accompaniment to verbal communication. The health professional must be aware that nonverbal communication is as powerful as verbal communication. When a person's response is not what the health professional expects, the health professional's actions are probably speaking louder than his or her words.

---

*Shelby J. Clayson, School of Occupational Therapy and Physical Therapy, University of Puget Sound, Tacoma, Washington.

REFERENCES

1. Birdwhistell, R. L.: *Kinetics and Context: Essays on Body Motion Communication.* Philadelphia, University of Pennsylvania Press, 1970, p. 99.
2. Bergsma, J., and Thomasma, D. C.: Health Care: Its Psychosocial Dimensions. Pittsburgh, Duquesne University Press, 1982, p. 15.
3. Mehrabian, A.: Communication without words. *Psychol. Today,* September 1968, p. 278.
4. Wagener, J. J., and Laird, J.: The experimenter's foot in the door: self perception, body weight and volunteering. *Pers. Soc. Psychol. Bull.* 6:441–446, 1980.
5. Shriver, D. W.: Medicine and religion: some definitions and goals. In Shriver, D. W. (ed.): *Medicine and Religion.* Pittsburgh, University of Pittsburgh Press, 1980, pp. 3–20.
6. Huss, A. J.: Touch with care or a caring touch? *Am. J. Occup. Ther.* 31:11–18, 1977.

Chapter 10

CULTURAL AND PERSONAL BIASES AS DETERMINANTS OF EFFECTIVENESS

The last two chapters discussed some verbal and nonverbal tools of communication available to the health professional. It is with these tools that human interactions are achieved. But interaction also involves individual differences. Thus the health professional may discover that even with access to all the tools, effective interaction still does not result. Still to be considered is the fact that each person interprets a communication, verbal or nonverbal, according to biases derived from cultural conditioning or personal experiences.

A cultural bias is a tendency to interpret a word or action according to some culturally derived meaning assigned to it. For example, different cultures interpret the distance between persons communicating as having different levels of significance. Different cultures, then, have different kinds of distance awareness. Another example is that of different cultures which assign different levels of significance to the time in which activites are performed. Thus different cultures also have different kinds of time awareness. The culturally derived biases of distance and time awareness are discussed in this chapter.

A personal bias is a tendency to interpret a word or action in terms of some personal significance assigned to it. It is found largely in what is commonly called prejudice. It can derive from culturally defined interpretations but can also, as we shall see, originate from a number of other sources.

Cultural Bias

It used to be very easy to identify a cultural bias because one could readily distinguish between the different ways of doing things in different parts of the world. For instance, the American way differed significantly from the European way, and these two were easily distinguished from the African or Far Eastern way. But today one is suddenly faced with an infinite variety of influences within what used to be the traditional, homogenous cultures; the result is that today it is far more difficult to identify cultural biases that modify behavior.

DIFFERING CONCEPTS OF DISTANCE AWARENESS

One culturally derived bias often still evident during interaction concerns the distance between people communicating. Anthropologist Edward T. Hall, in *The Hidden Dimension*, an intriguing book that explains the difference in distance awareness among many different cultural groups, defines four distance zones maintained by healthy, adult, middle-class Americans. By examining these zones, the reader will be able to understand how they differ from those of other cultural groups. A noteworthy point is that Dr. Hall stresses that "how people are feeling toward each other at the time is a decisive factor in the distance used." The four distance zones are:

1. Intimate distance—such as that of lovemaking, comforting, protecting, and wrestling. As Dr. Hall puts it: "The presence of the other person is unmistakable and may at times be overwhelming because . . . sight (often distorted), olfaction, heat from the other person's body, sound, smell and feel of the breath all combine to signal unmistakable involvement with another body."

2. Personal distance, ranging from 1½ to 4 feet. At arm's length, subjects of personal interest can be discussed while physical contact, such as holding hands or hitting the other person in the nose, is still possible. As Dr. Hall notes: ". . . The closeness derives in part from the possibilities present in regard to what each participant can do to the other with his extremities. . . ."

3. Social distance, ranging from 4 to 12 feet. At this distance, more formal business and social discourse takes place. Dr. Hall explains: "People who work together tend to use close social distance. . .; to stand and look down at a person from this distance has a domineering effect, as when a man talks to his secretary or receptionist. . . ."

4. Public distance, ranging from 12 to 25 feet or more. No physical contact and very little direct eye contact is possible. An alert person can take evasive or defensive action if necessary. By mutual consent, both listener and speaker will remain strangers.[1]

The following two points are significant to the patient–health professional relationship. First, the health professional dealing with a person described by Hall as an adult, middle-class American performs many diagnostic or treatment procedures within the personal and intimate distance zones. The health professional invades the patient's culturally derived boundaries of interaction, sometimes with little warning. Consider, for instance, the weak or debilitated patient who comes for treatment and must be helped to a treatment table. The health professional "embraces" the person and, in some cases, actually lifts the person to the table. The significance for the patient, in terms of the touching involved, was discussed in the last chapter. The present significance lies in the distance at which it is done.

Second, and equally important, Dr. Hall's zones are restricted to a small group of people, even within one country. He is quick to point out that they do not apply to black Americans, Spanish-Americans, and Southern Europeans in the United States.[2]

When one works with an ethnic or cultural subgroup outside one's own experience or travels to other parts of the world, culturally defined zone limits readily become apparent. It is somewhat disconcerting to the average untraveled American abroad to be given hotel directions by a stranger who nearly embraces him or her; or to observe men kissing and hugging and women strolling along holding hands.

But the health professional need not travel abroad to experience uneasiness about distance zones; members of the global village, with distance zones different from the health professional's will be encountered in the health facility. The black American, Spanish-American, or Southern-European American health professional will be constantly faced with a majority of white, middle-class American patients and collegues who automatically expect *their* culturally derived boundaries to be understood and respected.

The patient who clings to the health professional or refuses to talk unless he or she is nearly in the health professional's lap may be confused or insulted if the latter unwittingly withdraws. In addition, the health professional may become aware of some things that he or she did not expect to be part of the interaction. For instance, one natural result of working within a closer range than the middle-class white American is used to is that body odors become more distinguishable. In a society where a man or woman is supposed to smell like a deodorant, a mouthwash, a hair spray, or a cologne, but *not* a body, it is not surprising that some health professionals find the patient's body odor offensive, sometimes nauseous; some admit that it so repulses them that they try to hurry through the test or treatment.

The person just beginning clinical education should be forewarned that all bodies emit odors. An x-ray technologist confided to the author that one of her biggest shocks while working in a mission hospital in India came when her assistant reluctantly admitted that patients were failing to keep their appointments because she "smelled funny," making them sick. The "funny" smell turned out to be that of the popular American soap she was using for her bath.

Bad breath is a problem. What *is* bad breath? It is *not* the smell of garlic (ask an Italian or Polish person), *nor* of onion, *nor* of tobacco, *nor* of alcohol. Its definition depends on who is asked the question. The health professional who is unable to go beyond his or her own culturally derived bias of distance awareness (with its accompanying distance zones for interaction) will have difficulty in communicating with patients. While working at close range, a reaction to body and breath odors will affect interaction. Most patients are far too ill or preoccupied with their problems to have sweet-smelling breath, and others are not aware that they are being hustled out quickly because of the salami sandwich they had at noon.

DIFFERING CONCEPTS OF TIME AWARENESS

Another culturally derived bias that affects interaction is how different people interpret time. The right time and the correct amount of time are relative, depending on the cultural perspective. One aspect of the time dimension that directly affects the patient–health professional relationship is the scheduling and maintaining of appointments with patients. Most health professionals are compulsively punctual and expect their patients to be the same. In fact, the health facility operates each day on a "schedule." Harrison points out that "punctuality communicates respect while tardiness is an insult." However, "in some other cultures . . . to arrive exactly on time is an insult (it says, 'You are such an unimportant fellow that you can arrange your affairs very easily; you really have nothing else to do.'). Rather, an appropriate amount of tardiness is expected."[3] The health professional thus may find that a patient is scheduled to arrive at "10 o'clock health-professional time" but arrives instead at "10 o'clock patient time," feeling no need at all to explain or apologize.

The amount of time spent in rendering professional service may also vary from one culture to another. How should a given amount of time (a half-hour) be spent so that the patient benefits most? By middle-class American standards, the patient is greeted briefly and the treatment or test is begun without delay. If the health professional rushes in setting up equipment, the patient may interpret it to mean he or she cares enough to hurry. When the treatment is over, the patient leaves immediately.

However, in some South American cultures, if the treatment does not begin exactly on time, it does not matter as long as it will eventually be done. Rather than rush into the procedure itself, the health professional asks about the weather, the family, and other things that may be important to the patient, sometimes spending ten minutes in this way. During the actual treatment or test, the professional person may hurry, but good-byes must not be short and rushed.

In a village in South West Africa, the health professional slowly enters the room, then greets the patient. The treatment or test may begin immediately, but at no time does the health professional rush in the least. To rush about the room while the patient remains seated is an unspeakable insult that can only mean that the health professional thinks he or she is more important than the patient.

These three examples, supplied from the author's personal experience (with the danger of overgeneralization that such references always carry), give the health professional a small idea of the variety of ways in which time must be organized within different cultural contexts.

Other problems arise for the American health professional who practices in a culture in which the ideal of "first come, first served" is not considered a just method for determining priority among patients who arrive for treatment. Who should be treated first if the patients with

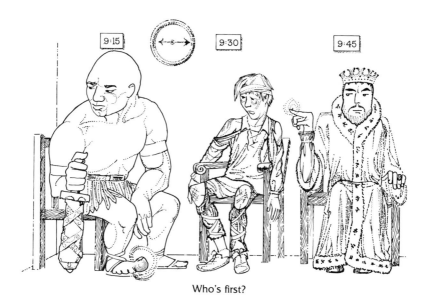

Who's first?

9:15, 10:00, and 10:15 appointments all arrive at 9:15? Should the man scheduled for 9:15 be first? Or should the oldest of the three? The man or woman? The sickest or the highest ranking official of the three in that tribe or community? The way in which the health professional handles this situation will greatly determine his or her success in the culture.

Subtle misunderstandings related to time that can arise are illustrated by an incident in Swaziland, Africa. Swazi people use their fingers to indicate numbers in quite a different manner from the Westerner who holds up two fingers to express "two," six fingers meaning "six," and so on. Each of the Swazi's fingers is assigned a number in the following way:

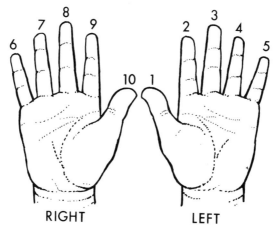

Palm view of a Swazi's hands showing that each finger represents a different number.

If asked what time he or she will return the next day, the Swazi patient will invariably hold up just one finger. If the plan is to return at 9 o'clock, he or she will hold up the index finger of the right hand; at 1 o'clock, the thumb of the left hand; at 3 o'clock, the third finger of the left hand. But the unknowing health professional will expect the whole community to arrive at 1 o'clock because just one finger was held up!

Ways of operating within and indicating time, then, are highly relative. The few examples presented only skim the surface of differences in time awareness among different cultures. The astute health professional will take this into consideration when working with people whose cultural backgrounds are different from his or her own.

Both distance and time awareness are deep-seated and culturally derived. A person usually is not consciously aware of how he or she interprets time and distance, and so neither one is easily identified as the cause of misunderstanding. Cultures help to define a person's interpretation of health and sickness. They also influence the interpretation of verbal or nonverbal communications in terms of time or distance. Cultures, then, greatly determine one's interpretation of life and must be considered when one attempts to establish effective interaction.

Personal Biases

Personal biases also contribute to the quality of communication between two people. A personal bias is an individual's feeling about a particular thing that colors his or her interpretation of it. For example, some personal biases develop from cultural biases in that an individual internalizes the cultural attitudes until he or she believes them to be entirely personal. This process is similar to that of internalizing societal values described in Chapter 6. Of course, people within cultures vary to some extent, and personal biases, as will be noted, originate from many sources.

Understanding his or her own personal biases is important to the health professional because there is no ethical or legal right to refuse care on the basis of these biases.

Race, religion, and ethnic origins are common focuses of prejudiced behavior. A fine example is the Gypsy patient. Shields observes that "the stereotype of the Gypsy is that of an unreliable, sexually immoral, or even criminal wanderer on the fringes of society." However, she adds, "beyond this view lives a centuries-old culture, distinct and strongly ritualized."[4] Non-Gypsy (Gaje) health practitioners are viewed as suspect because they so seldom recognize the basis for Gypsy behavior or are aware of Gypsy beliefs. In order to help improve understanding of the Gypsy patient, and improve interaction, Shields has developed the following chart.

REDUCING GYPSY–"GAJE" HEALTH CONFLICTS

Gypsy Beliefs and Taboos	Practitioner Response
Upper body pure, beneath waistline, polluted	Conduct physical exams from top to bottom without variation
Protective power in amulets of garlic, black pepper, etc., when worn by children	Leave on when possible, reposition rather than remove during x-rays
Lucky colors (red, green) and numbers (3, sometimes 7)	Incorporate into treatment when possible, e.g., red capsules and TID administration
Gaje (non-Gypsy) clothing and belongings unclean	Allow patients to wear own bedclothes, separate from non-Gypsies when possible
Older females have role as healers	Use older female health professionals (i.e., postmenopausal women)
Food prepared by Gaje, as is Gaje cutlery; plates unclean	Serve "unhandled" foods; use disposable plates, utensils
Special foods	When possible, allow black and red peppers, foods pickled in vinegar, garlic
Sickness from ritual pollution, relations with Gaje, supernatural beings	Allow use of religious items in hospital: amulets, votive candles, holy water
Traveling therapeutic	Encourage when possible
Extended family or clan vital to patient's well-being	Leeway in visitation restrictions; address "extraneous" visitors as immediate family
Sporadic ER visits less "immobilizing" than ongoing comprehensive care	Incorporate in treatment when possible
Social hierarchy—men over women, age over women, age over youth, unless postmenopausal, women dependent on men for health decisions	Awareness of hierarchy when seeking family opinions, decisions

From Shields, M. N.: *Hosp. Phys.,* November 1981, p. 87. Used with permission.

A similar chart could be useful for working with patients from other groups as well.

In modern society, there are additional factors besides race, religion, or ethnic origin that elicit negative responses to a person. The homosexual is one example of a person who causes anxiety. His or her sexual preferences, rather than country of origin or skin color, become the basis of discrimination.

The problem of AIDS (acquired immune deficiency syndrome), which in recent years has caused much suffering to all involved, has created a legitimate worry in the gay community that the prejudice against them would lead to restrictive policies that more closely reflected hatred of homosexuality than a reasoned approach to protecting possible vulnerable populations. An author in a medical ethics journal observed:

While confronting its internal crisis, the gay community was suddenly forced to meet the challenge produced by the first revelations of AIDS among hemophiliacs. Mindful of the history of how despised minorities had been viewed as sources of social contamination, and of the crucial symbolic significance of blood, the community attempted to forestall any efforts to link the entire gay population to the spread of AIDS through blood donations. In July 1982, Virginia Apuzzo, executive director of the Fund for Human Dignity, expressed her concern over the stigmatization that would follow the charge of "bad blood."

Without minimizing the seriousness of the problem of protecting blood recipients from AIDS, medical and lay leaders of the gay community argued for cautious, carefully circumscribed policies designed to screen donations rather than donors. Their overriding concern was the protection of the gay community from medical policies that would serve as a subterfuge for antihomosexual prejudice. "The real gravity underlying these questions—in addition to health which concerns us all—" wrote Larry Bush in the New York Native, "is that we still live in a place and time in which it is preferable to treat gays unfairly on the basis of outrageous and mistaken assumptions." Though noting that such mistreatment had not yet occurred in the blood donor controversy, Bush warned gays of the necessity to respond with extraordinary caution in public discussions.[5]

Membership in certain political or private organizations can create animosity between health professional and patient, too. Unfortunately, the biases that can work against fair treatment are many.

Discrimination based on personal bias works craftily, evasively, and with stunning certainty. Both parties involved are inevitably injured by the interaction. Gordon Allport, in his definitive work, The Nature of Prejudice (which, though written 30 years ago, is still widely considered the authoritative study and which every student in the health professions should read), warns: "It is a serious error to ascribe prejudice and discrimination to any single taproot, reaching into economic exploitation, social structure, the mores, fear, aggression, sex conflict or any other favored soil. Prejudice and discrimination . . . may draw nourishment from all these conditions and many others."[6]

Personal biases are not based entirely on another's personal characteristics. Prejudice is "an avertive or hostile attitude toward a person who belongs to a group, simply because he belongs to that group, and is therefore presumed to have the objectionable qualities ascribed to that group."[7] Actions derived only from personal biases are antithetical to those based on genuine care for an individual. Every patient–health professional relationship will undoubtedly be influenced by personal biases because a health professional will be unable to overcome all his or her own biases. In some cases, the only thing to do is to admit to a prejudice and ask another health professional to take one's place in caring for a particular patient. Though this is not an ideal means of effective interaction, in some cases it is a realistic one.

Personal bias also can be viewed from another perspective. In some cases, personal bias may produce a "halo effect" on certain individuals; that is, the health professional and patient may have common interests or characteristics, and their camaraderie is immediately apparent. This can, of course, have positive effects on the relationship, though in some such cases the extra time and energy spent on that patient are taken from the amount that should be spent on others.

One problem encountered by the health professional is that patients also have personal biases. A black health professional in a predominantly white community or a white health professional in a predominantly black community may find that patients prefer to be treated by someone who is their own color. There are obviously many other examples of personal bias, as the global village is such a complex mixture of similarities and differences. Whether the bias is culturally or personally derived, it will affect the type of communication possible between the persons involved and thus should at least be recognized as an important factor.

REFERENCES

1. Hall, E. T.: *The Hidden Dimension*. New York, Doubleday & Company, 1966, pp. 108–117.
2. *Ibid.*, p. 110.
3. Harrison, R.: Nonverbal communications: explorations into time, space, action and object. In Campbell, J. H., and Hepler, H. W. (eds.): *Dimensions in Communications: Readings*. 2nd ed. Belmont, Calif.: Wadsworth Publishing Company, 1970, pp. 260–261.
4. Shields, M. N.: Selected issues in treating gypsy patients. Hosp. Phys. November 1981, pp. 85–89.
5. Bayer, R.: Gays and the stigma of "bad blood." Hastings Cent. Rep. 13:5–7, 1983.
6. Allport, G.: *The Nature of Prejudice*. Reading, Mass., Addison-Wesley Publishing Company, 1954, p. xii.
7. *Ibid*, p. 8.

Part III Summary

The health professional is faced with many challenges, one of which is to communicate effectively with patients in the setting of a world that has been brought into physical proximity by mass transportation and into psychological proximity through the mass media. He or she is required to communicate with people who bring different levels of understanding and different needs to the situation. Six components of effective spoken communication include: (1) mastery of appropriate vocabulary, (2) clarity, (3) ability to present ideas in an orderly fashion, (4) willingness to discuss difficult situations candidly, (5) sensitivity to the effect of voice tone and volume, and (6) ability to listen effectively.

Nonverbal communication includes (1) pantomime and demonstration and (2) metacommunication (gestures, facial expressions, posturing, physical appearance, and touching). The successful health professional attends to the messages sent via these nonverbal avenues.

Cultural and personal biases affect the way in which either verbal or nonverbal messages are interpreted. One cultural bias is the use of distance; the distance maintained by individuals during interaction is a result of cultural conditioning. In the white middle-class American culture, four distance zones have been described by Hall: intimate, personal, social, and public. The distance zone within which the health professional works is often intimate or personal.

A second culturally derived bias is based on interpretation of time. In some cultures it is polite to be extremely punctual, while in others it is rude. What one does within a given period of time may differ from one culture to another.

Cuturally derived biases help to form the basis of one type of personal bias. But there are also many other bases for personal bias. Personal bias can prejudice a person against or in favor of another person. In the former case, discrimination results, while in the latter a "halo effect" is created. The health professional should be aware of the injurious effects of both. Patients, too, are influenced by their own cultural and personal biases.

Part I discussed characteristics of the health professional, and Part II, characteristics of the patient. Part III has presented the communication tools available to both for effective interaction. We will now proceed to the particulars of the health professional–patient relationship itself.

Part III Questions for Thought and Discussion

1. Dennis is a 4-year-old deaf child. His mother brings him screaming with fright to your department. You must perform some tests on him that will not hurt him but will require his attention and cooperation.
   (a) What parts of this setting may be causing his fright?
   (b) What aspects of your appearance may be causing his fright?
   (c) What steps will you take to establish communication with this child?
   (d) How may the mother be helpful in facilitating effective interactions between you and Dennis?
2. You verbally instruct an intelligent young businesswoman in the use of a home-treatment device, and ask her if she understands what you want her to do. She assures you that she does. The next week when she returns, you discover that she has done exactly the opposite! You are dumbfounded.
   (a) How will you react and what will you say when your patient glowingly reports that she did exactly what you said and you realize that she did exactly the opposite of what you said?
   (b) List the possible reasons why your patient failed to do what you asked of her.
   (c) What changes might you have made during the initial instruction period to decrease the likelihood of this happening?

3. A male intern with neatly combed long sideburns and hair down to his collar approaches a male patient and introduces himself. The patient retorts with an obscenity, exclaiming in a loud voice that he is paying for *real* treatment and is not going to be treated by a "punk." The patient's fists are clenched.

   (a) What should the male intern do in this situation?

   (b) What cultural or personal biases and past experiences may be contributing to this reaction?

4. You walk into a Brazilian teenager's hospital room to perform a procedure. She is crying softly. You have not seen her as a patient before, but you know that she is new to this country and cannot speak any English. What will you do in this situation?

Part IV

THE HEALTH PROFESSIONAL–PATIENT RELATIONSHIP

Part IV

Students are quick to observe that many experienced health professionals approach and interact with their patients in a friendly manner. Recently, after an afternoon of observation in the University Hospital, one of my students submitted a report that began: "I am a bit confused by what I saw happening between my supervisor and her patients. They seemed to almost be *friends* and yet it was somehow different too. I mean, the patient always remained patient and the health professional remained health professional. Do you know what I mean?"

This student had made a sage distinction: Although she did not quite know how to interpret it, she had observed a professional person who had mastered the art of being close to her patients while maintaining the unique health professional–patient relationship. Although it sometimes does not appear so on the surface, closeness between a health professional and a patient is significantly different from a friendship. The differentiating characteristics must be carefully defined and understood before the health professional will achieve optimal results from his or her efforts. Part IV is devoted to defining these differences. Chapter 11 provides a theoretical background for Chapters 12 and 13, which describe practical techniques of effective interaction that can be utilized by the health professional.

Chapter 11

THE PROCESS OF ESTABLISHING RELATEDNESS

The health professional–patient relationship does not just "happen." Both health professional and patient go through a process of relating to one another, each negotiating for certain conditions, carrying out agreed-upon tasks, and then disengaging from the relationship. The entire process may take place in a few minutes, such as when a patient is given a series of x-rays, or it may last through months of testing or treatment.

Enter, The Patient

NEEDS

The patient brings to the relationship a number of needs that eventually help to determine its character.

The patient's request for help usually centers on the presence of a *symptom* that manifests itself in the form of pain, disability, or some other type of discomfort. The patient needs assistance in finding a diagnosis, initiating and following a treatment process, and, in most cases, effecting a cure. The relationship essentially is over when the symptom disappears. Of course, the situation is not always this uncomplicated, but the description does provide an accurate general statement about what happens.

Part II, which discussed patients' problems, privileges, and value systems, revealed that there are implicit needs as well as the explicit one created by a symptom. The patient may need reassurance about a changing body image; understanding and guidance about an uncertain financial, vocational and personal future; and a means of adjusting a value system to make it viable. Reassurance has an integral function in "healing":

> Reassurance is essentially restorative . . . What is restored in the medical context is a former state of health. What is re-established is security, contentment, fortitude. Reassurance encourages hope and, through the confidence engendered, it enhances the . . . relationship so that partnership can work effectively. It makes patients better able to bear what must be borne, both of illness and of treatment, and helps them to concentrate upon recovery. There are few clinical situations in which reassurance is impossible, and successful reassurance promotes a patient's well being.[1]

To be sure, the desire to provide reassurance sometimes creates an ambiguous situation for the health professional. For example, consider the story of Mrs. Gleason and Sheryl Steinberg.

> Mrs. Gleason, a 70-year-old housewife, has had amyotrophic lateral sclerosis for just over a year. This is a progressive neurological disease in which all voluntary muscles of the body become weaker and weaker until the patient dies, usually of respiratory arrest. Mrs. Gleason has only a small amount of movement left in her legs but can get around in a wheelchair. She is in the hospital for treatment of pneumonia that is probably due to weakness of the swallowing muscles, allowing aspiration of mouth contents into the lungs. Her weakness has accelerated since hospitalization, even though her pneumonia is responding to antibiotics. She is very discouraged, knowing that the aspiration will continue, and that her present state will not allow her to go home. Her family is not willing or able to care for her at home, and yet none of them wants to see her end up in a nursing home. The physician has ordered extensive occupational therapy rehabilitation treatment, which improves Mrs. Gleason's spirits, although no one expects much improvement in strength. Sheryl Steinberg, the occupational therapist, readily assesses that occupational therapy will have very little therapeutic value as far as Mrs. Gleason's strength and endurance are concerned. However, Mrs. Gleason tells Sheryl that her daily visits are the only thing keeping her spirits up. She calls Sheryl, "the sunshine girl." The physician and family are delighted that Sheryl is such a source of reassurance.
>
> Sheryl is conflicted about visiting Mrs. Gleason because there is no real medical indication for occupational therapy treatments. She can't decide whether or not to charge Mrs. Gleason for these sessions, which serve the purpose of reassuring Mrs. Gleason.

What do you think Sheryl should do?

Why or why not?

Very often health professionals like Sheryl, who are sensitive to patients' needs, find themselves in a position of having to define the proper limits of their own involvement.

Whatever the needs resulting from the presenting symptoms may be, the patient is sure to have accompanying social and personal needs as well, each of which gives rise to a set of expectations. One study revealed that in the medical setting studied, latent needs included, among others, the need for catharsis, the need for help to cope with the future, and the need to attain status.[2] The patient, therefore, will be looking to the health professional with far greater expectations than those defined simply by the limits of the symptom itself.

PERCEPTIONS

In addition to the need for help, the patient brings his or her perceptions to the situation. The patient's eyes are as big as doorknobs when he or she enters the health facility or is visited by a health professional: They denote an alertness stimulated both by anticipation and by anxiety about what is going to happen. Every sense is attuned to the experience in much the same way as during an exciting vacation or in a time of danger.

The patient's perception of the illness often is much different than the health professional's. Patients are concerned primarily with what the illness signifies in terms of their daily lives, loves, and activities. Hardly ever is the technical aspect of what is wrong the governing factor. Baron suggests that health professionals are used to looking for the *abstractive* meaning of the condition: the chest sound, the laboratory findings, the x-ray, the sight of the skin or tone of the muscle. Contrary to this, the patient assigns *intuitive* meaning to the condition, related to and derived from his or her understanding of the disabling effects of the illness.[3] In John Updike's short story, "Journal of a Leper," the young man begins,

> Oct. 31. I have long been a potter, a bachelor, and a leper. Leprosy is not exactly what I have, but what in the Bible is called leprosy (see Leviticus 13, Exodus 4:6, Luke 5:12–13) was probably this thing, which has a twisty Greek name it pains me to write. The form of the disease is as follows: spots, plaques, and avalanches of excess skin, manufactured by the dermis through some trifling but persistent error in its metabolic instructions, expand and slowly migrate across the body like lichen on a tombstone. I am silvery, scaly. Puddles of flakes form wherever I rest my flesh. Each morning, I vacuum my bed. My torture is skin deep: there is no pain, not even itching; we lepers live a long time, and are ironically healthy in other respects. Lusty, though we are loathsome to love. Keen-sighted, though we hate to look upon ourselves. The name of the disease, spiritually speaking, is Humiliation.[4]*

Self-esteem, the extent to which one feels good about oneself at the moment, makes a difference in how one will perceive one's condition; for instance, self-esteem can determine whether a day is perceived as "partly sunny" or "mostly cloudy" when one small ray of sunshine peeks through the clouds. Everyone has days when he or she feels vulnerable and worthless, days in which everything is colored an ominous gray. Those perceptions usually reflect a self-esteem that for some reason is faltering on that day. Chapter 4 noted that loss of self-image, closely related to self-esteem, is a major problem for patients. Thus it is not surprising that their outlook is often more pessimistic and guarded than the health professional's.

Finally, the patient's role expectations can also make a difference in how observations will be interpreted. Patients have their own ideas of how the person offering them professional services should act, and they respond to the person accordingly. For instance, a "student" is supposed to be one who is just learning. Therefore, the patient may initially look anxious about being left with a student or express anger that he or she

---

*From "Journal of a Leper" by John Updike; © 1976 The New Yorker Magazine, Inc. Reprinted by permission.

has been assigned to a student. These reactions can be traced to the patient's expectation about what a student is. Occasionally a patient will have the opposite reaction because he or she believes that a student knows the latest information and will therefore be able to provide better care than the other people in the setting. Patients will also note and comment on the rapport (or lack of it) that exists among co-workers. Their role expectations cause them to have preconceived ideas about how professional colleagues are supposed to act among themselves. Patients are especially certain that they know how a professional person as "helper" acts; their role expectations derive from their previous personal experience and from television and books. The facts that not all physicians are Frankensteins or Schweitzers and that all health professionals have their good and bad days come as quite a shock to many. In short, all the roles assumed by a student during clinical education and throughout the professional career are interpreted sometimes quite differently by the patient than by the health professional.

Therefore, patients' perceptions are not interpretations made in isolation from a number of other factors. Similarly, the patient's conclusion about whether the health professional is working "for" or "against" the patient may depend on factors that have little to do with the health professional's actions.

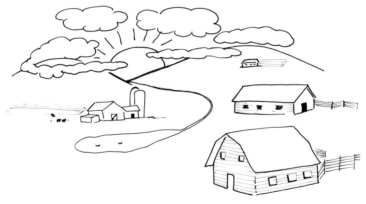

Half cloudy or half sunny day?

TRANSFERENCE

The discussion of authority-dependence relationships in Chapter 7 revealed that patients also come to the health professional–patient situation expecting certain kinds of behavior from an authority figure. I maintained in that chapter that the authority-dependence framework may not promote effective interaction in some situations. Elsewhere I have proposed alternative frameworks, such as the engineering, contract, and friendship frameworks, for some situations or for some periods of the interaction.[5] All four frameworks can be shown in schematic form on page 146.

Within any of the frameworks, the psychotherapeutic term "transference" can help one understand certain kinds of behavior shown by the patient toward the health professional. Transference is the process of shifting one's feeling about a person in the past to another person.[6] A young man, angry that his father "ruled with an iron hand," will think "Here it comes again!" as soon as the health professional does the slightest thing to remind him of his father. The health professional may have no clue as to what stimulated the patient's resistance to a suggestion or provoked his angry outburst.

Transference can be either negative or positive. The anger expressed by the young man is an example of negative transference. Positive transference, the good feelings the patient transfers to the health professional, can promote relatedness.[7] Chapter 4 maintained that a patient's past responses in authority-dependence relationships will be repeated in the health professional–patient interaction. "Transference" is one important mechanism by which this happens. The health professional should be aware that transference is taking place, though it may not be possible to identify with whom he or she is being associated in the patient's psyche!

The patient thus enters the relationship with a number of needs, perceptions, and past feelings about certain people. All of these factors influence the development of that relationship.

Enter, The Health Professional

The health professional, too, comes to the situation with a set of needs, perceptions and past feelings about certain people. Some of these factors have already been discussed, so the following paragraphs serve both as a reminder of some points and as an elaboration of others.

NEEDS

Chapter 3 was devoted to the role of the health professional as helper. The health professional's need to help is the greatest need he or she brings to the situation.

The health professional is eager to gain the confidence of the patient so that this helping can begin. No "relationship" is felt to have been established until the helping starts. In some instances, the health professional has but one meeting with the patient, which places tremendous pressure on him or her to develop this feeling quickly. In attempting to establish the relatedness, the health professional tries to show by both actions and words that he or she can be entrusted with that patient's health needs.

However, sometimes the patient incorrectly interprets the health professional's intent. The patient is overheard saying that he or she does not think the health professional is helping, that the person is casually indifferent, overly familiar, or disrespectful. Obviously, the health professional, despite good intentions, is exhibiting behavior that can be interpreted in more than one way. What, specifically, is this behavior?

Some of the most common actions that are subject to dual interpretations include the following: (1) The health professional shares some secrets or private jokes with the patient, and there is an exclusiveness about the relationship. (2) The health professional quickly encourages the patient to establish the relationship on a first-name basis. (3) The health professional tries to distinguish himself or herself from the other health workers by wearing a flower in his lapel or by bringing little presents to the patient. (4) The health professional spends extra time with the patient and appears to give him or her priority over the other patients.

Some patients tolerate these and similar kinds of behavior very well. Others, however, realize that they are being treated differently from other patients and are unable to understand it. Rather than being pleased by this extra attention, they may grow distrustful.

Trust, so central to relatedness, will be discussed in the last section of this chapter. The realization that attempts to quickly establish trust result partially from a need to help can be instrumental in understanding why these attempts sometimes don't work: One's own needs rather than the patients' are being attended to!

PERCEPTIONS

The health professional's perceptions of a situation are subject to as many influences as a patient's. Taken alone, the *concepts* learned by the student in the health professions influence how a person is perceived. For instance, there has been much criticism of the tendency to refer to patients as "the cardiac in Room 12" or "the hip fracture that comes at 1 o'clock"—at best a bizarre view according to the rest of the world's perception of the same people!

The value system of the health professions was discussed in Chapter 6. The author there raised the question of whether health care providers as a group hold values that conflict with those of society and of individual patients. If there is any such conflict, health professionals will perceive some aspects of any patient's situation differently than the patient would. Add to this the health professional's societally determined and individual values, and one begins to recognize that the health professional may filter the same perceptual inputs much differently than does the patient.

The health professional's own self-esteem enters the picture as well. On good days the health professional may believe the patient's response affirms that all is going well and that the patient is being helped. On bad days the same response from a patient is a sure sign that he or she thinks the health professional is a quack. In this case, the health professional is really responding to a faltering self-esteem because of some difficulty not related to the patient (e.g., a hoped-for promotion did not materialize). Certain that he or she is incompetent, disliked unjustly, or both, the

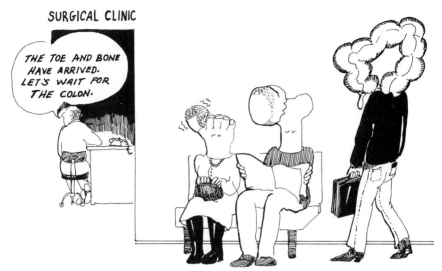

Professionals' view of patients. From Vård, Vårdare, Vårdad. Ruth Purtilo, W. B. Saunders Co. p. 139, © 1978.

health professional views the patient's response as an affirmation that this is so!

Finally, how health professionals interpret role expectations also influences their perceptions. Column four on the "Frameworks of Interaction" chart presented on page 146 helps to explain how role sets work. If a health professional adopts the "shaman" framework, as most do, and believes that it is proper to assume the role of authority figure, then he or she feels obligated to behave in a way that will meet the patient's "justifiable expectations." However, in order to fulfill the demands of those kinds of behavior, the health professional must screen out other information. For instance, in the friendship framework the health professional would believe the relationship was "working" (i.e., the patient was being helped) if the patient initiated activities other than those the health professional had planned. But within the authority-dependence framework, the patient's initiative is interpreted to mean that the health professional is not adequately doing the job nor is the patient fulfilling the health professional's justifiable expectations.

Therefore, the situation may look entirely different to patient and health professional, depending on what factors influence their perceptions of the situation. On the other hand, they may find that their perceptions are, after the filtering process, highly similar. In the latter case, the sense of relatedness is instantaneous and secure. Usually neither extreme occurs, and whatever similarity there is can serve as the foundation for further development of the relationship.

COUNTERTRANSFERENCE

Health professionals also engage in transference. In psychoanalytical theory the technical term is "countertransference," but in practical terms

SOME FRAMEWORKS OF INTERACTION IN HELPING RELATIONSHIPS*

Framework	Basis of Interaction	Characteristics		"Justifiable Expectations"
		Helper	Helpee	
Priestly (shaman)	Authority-dependence	Powerful, superior, has skill that helpee needs	Vulnerable, inferior	Health professional leads; defines, initiates, evaluates tasks; is not necessarily responsive. Patient follows; discloses much.
Engineering (engineer or architect)	Problem resolution and some authority-dependence	Designer, analytical	Flexible, has insight into own problems	Health professional defines and may initiate tasks; guides rather than leads; may be responsive, but discloses little. Patient may initiate tasks; is guided by helper; discloses little.
Contractual (business partners)	Shared benefits, fidelity, promise-keeping and some problem resolution	Decisions made by both as part of contract, openness to negotiation, cooperativeness		Health professional and patient: Expectations vary according to contract.
Friendship (friends, buddies)	Racial equality and some shared benefits, fidelity and promise-keeping	Few distinctions made with regard to roles, mutual interest maintained, trustworthiness		Health professional and patient: At times, each defines and initiates tasks; there is much mutual disclosure.

*All four frameworks operate, at some time or another, in the health professional–patient interaction. Value assumptions about how things "ought to be" influence interactions in any of these frameworks.

it is the same as the patient transference discussed previously. Counter-transference is an important psychological factor underlying the forma-tion of personal biases. A health professional not only attaches halos or horns according to stereotypes of "good" or "bad" *types* of persons; he or she also transfers feelings about an individual in the past to the present patient. Similar names, eye color, or age can increase the chance of transference. The health professional can determine whether counter-transference is taking place by tuning into feelings of affection, dislike, or anger that seem to go beyond what a situation would otherwise call for.[8]

Therefore, the health professional, like the patient, does not enter the relationship "empty-handed." Health professional and patient meet, each bringing a set of needs, perceptions, and past experiences. What relationship they will build in the moments, weeks, or months that follow will at least in part depend on these particular factors.

Trust and Relatedness

This chapter began with the assertion that a relationship does not just happen. The factors discussed so far constitute one important determinant of the type of relationship between health professional and patient. Both people also bring to their first meeting a number of other aspects of themselves, including personal interests, aversions, and skills (such as mechanical skills or the communication skills discussed in Chapters 8 and 9). There are so many variables that some maintain it is a mistake to talk about *the* health professional–patient relationship; rather, it is more accurate to discuss numerous health professional–patient relationships. I suggest this myself at the bottom of the "Frame-works of Interaction" chart. However, a basic underlying assumption in this book is that one can identify a kind of behavior that I have called "the therapeutic helping relationship."

One characteristic of that relationship is its authority-dependence framework. Trust in the relationship is built on the premise that the health professional will give the patient sufficient information to partic-ipate knowledgeably in the decisions made and that the patient's consent is required for the various procedures to be performed. The process of informed consent is the mechanism by which these criteria have been more fully met in recent years.

The idea of informed consent is currently receiving more attention than ever before in the history of medical thought. The recently com-pleted President's Commission on the Study of Bioethical Problems in Medicine devoted more space in its report to the issue of informed consent than to any other single topic, signaling the importance it assigns to the notion.[9] No major book or article dealing with the health profes-sional–patient relationship fails to include a discussion of it. Informed consent involves informing a patient of what is to be done to him or her and obtaining the patient's consent to the procedure.

BECOMING INFORMED

There is current debate over how much information must be provided to enable a person to make an intelligent decision regarding treatment. One school of thought in health care maintains that it is impossible to provide the information in all of its detail. Members of this group base their argument on the complexity of treatments, which, they argue, patients cannot understand. A second school maintains that it is inadvisable to provide information, that to do so can only harm the patient. This is a particularly delicate issue in the matter of treatments for mental illnesses in which the therapist believes a favorable outcome can be attained only by keeping certain information from the patient. Providing information is problematical, too, for health professionals who wish to use a placebo on a patient who is finding no relief from pain killers. The feeling is that as soon as a patient knows a sugar pill is being substituted for the prior medication, no hope of its working remains. Most often, the inadvisability of sharing information is discussed with regard to the allegedly negative effects of a patient's knowing that he or she is terminally ill. Proponents of a third view argue that information does not harm, but rather that knowledge sets a person free by allowing the patient to retain control over the events of his or her life. To rob the person of choice is to abrogate his or her *basic human right* of self-determination, or autonomy. A study authorized by the President's Commission showed that the patients interviewed believed that more information was desirable, and that the language with which the details were described should be personalized to maximize each person's comprehension. In other words, the standard used for determining the type and amount of disclosure should be one derived from the knowledge of each individual patient.

GIVING CONSENT

Giving consent ensures that the person is not being coerced into any course of action. Therefore, the basic human right of autonomy is retained, and the person's role as a voluntary agent is not compromised. Giving consent is also a means of enforcing the implicit rules of the relationship, which say that the health professional will neither harm the patient nor be unfaithful to the task of helping the patient. The implicit promise of help is made explicit by obtaining the necessary consent from the patient, who is the more vulnerable person in the relationship. Moreover, the idea of giving consent is a comment on the deep-seated belief that even though health professionals may have the best intentions about keeping their promises, they are nevertheless in the position of power and therefore need to be checked.

The idea that patients should have the right to refuse care is sometimes overlooked; still, patients do make that choice. The provision of good, even excellent, care is not enough if the patient does not consent

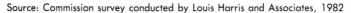

The Best Disclosure Standard:
Public and Physician Views*

Source: Commission survey conducted by Louis Harris and Associates, 1982

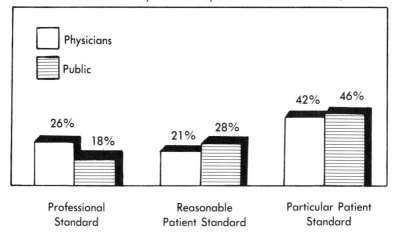

*1% of the public and 8% of physicians thought there should be no standard;
7% of the public and 4% of physicians were not sure what standard
they preferred.

to it.[10] Often what the patient considers best for himself or herself is not consistent with what the health professional considers best. When the patient refuses to grant consent, sometimes very perplexing situations ensue. Consider, for example, the story of Mrs. B.

> One morning while receiving the report from the third shift nurse, it was learned that a new admission to the hospital was scheduled for an angiogram. At that time, angiograms were not done at this hospital and patients were taken to a hospital in another town approximately 25 miles away from this service.
> Everything seemed normal until the nurse on duty saw the patient, Mrs. B., who was a large women weighing well over 200 pounds and who was very disturbed. The night nurse had tried to explain the procedure to her, but in her mental state she did not or could not comprehend. The nurses did not know if she was disturbed about having the angiogram or if she was disturbed for other reasons, but she was objecting very loudly to the procedure. . . .
> Mrs. B. would not listen to anyone. It was impossible to explain the need for the angiogram. When the physician was told that Mrs. B. was refusing the procedure, he went to see the patient, and then hastily said, "Aw, hell, we'll just snow her and take her on." One of the two nurses present told the doctor that this should not be done.[11]

If you were the nurse, what would you have done? Where did the breakdown in communication occur, and what could have been done to prevent this unhappy state of affairs?

Much more refinement of the concept and limits of informed consent still is needed in order for patients to be guaranteed a fully involved position in the decisions regarding their overall well-being and health. Nonetheless, all are agreed that great strides have been made in recent years toward recognizing and honoring patients' preferences as an integral aspect of health care decision-making.[12]

The process of gaining informed consent is designed to ensure that the health professional's promises to help and to not inflict harm are kept. However, daily interaction with the patient cannot depend on the health professional's acquiring written consent every step of the way. Underlying the consent process and whatever else goes on in the relationship is trust; it promotes the feeling of relatedness and allows the procedures to flow smoothly.

FROM CASUALNESS TO CARING

The existence of trust can be partially explained by the fact that individuals generally separate their lives into a private world of family and friends and a public world of institutional relationships.[13] Friendships are private-sector relationships, while the patient–health professional relationship belongs to the world of institutional interactions or public-sector relationships. The patient therefore enters the latter with different expectations than he or she does the former. The following explains a public-sector relationship: "Public-sector relationships, those between colleagues and with specialists or clients, are potentially temporary. The social distances established by public-sector usages function to permit rapid separation and recruitment, and to promote periodic cooperation. All public-sector relationships are characterized by abrupt changes from extreme remoteness to extreme nearness, potential temporariness, and the qualities imported into the relationship of both producer and consumer."[14]

When the health professional treats the patient as a casual friend, the patient does not know how to interpret it within the context of this public-sector relationship. Private jokes, a first-name basis, and other causal characteristics may occasionally be found in the health professional–patient relationship, but if they are misinterpreted, the patient will express it by withdrawing, becoming hostile, or showing other signs of distrust.

The confident professional person can, but knows it is often wiser not to, rely on causal mannerisms to express genuine concern for a patient. The patient readily discerns that these methods are being substituted for a deeper caring that only a more confident person dares express. When this happens the patient becomes caught in what Benjamin and Curtis have called "the compassion trap." The health professional in such a trap substitutes many diffuse but ultimately ineffectual behaviors for more thoughtful, patient-directed ones.[15] The result is that the patient becomes distrustful of the health professional.

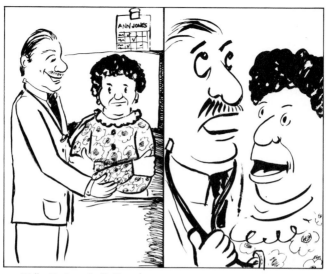

"Hello, Mrs. Jones, I'm Dr. Howard.
May I call you Nancy?"

"Sure, Howie!"

Genuine caring has been the subject of much consideration throughout the ages. One contemporary theorist has characterized care in direct opposition to apathy. The course of care, he feels, originates in one's own recollection of and sensitivity to pain, which then allows one to identify pain in others.[16] Caring is a kind of energy that one is willing to expend on another because one can remember, or vividly imagine, what it feels like *not* to be cared for. The quality of a person's life is largely determined by what he or she cares *about*. This is precisely what distinguishes care from sentimentality: Sentimentality stresses the awareness that a person has an emotion, while caring always involves concern about something or someone else.

Probably one of the most concise expressions of how to care for another human being, one that includes both feeling and the activity it generates, is found in Erich Fromm's *The Art of Loving*. He gives the following four basic elements on which to build a caring relationship:

1. Concern—encouraging the growth or progress of the other person.

2. Responsibility—responding to the other not simply out of duty but rather as a voluntary desire to meet the needs of the other person.

3. Respect—realizing the individuality of the other person. ("Respect" is from the Latin "respicere"—"to look at.")

4. Knowledge—trying to discover what is important to the other person.[17]

A striking distinction begins to emerge between casual "you-are-special" gestures and a deeper caring that results in benefit to the other person. Their complementary function is unmistakable, but to *substitute* the former for the latter is disastrous to the building of human trust. Trust, the basis for a feeling of relatedness, can grow only upon a foundation of genuine caring. The remaining chapters in Part IV are largely devoted to showing how genuine care can be expressed within the health professions.

REFERENCES

1. Kessel, N.: Reassurance. Lancet 1:1128–1133, 1979.
2. Shuval, J.: *Social Functions of Medical Practice: A Study of Doctor-Patient Relationships in Israel.* San Francisco, Jossey-Bass, 1970.
3. Baron, R. J.: Bridging clinical distance: an emphatic rediscovery of the known. *J. Med. Philos.* 6:5–23, 1981.
4. Updike, J.: From the Journal of a Leper. *The New Yorker*, July 19, 1976, pp. 28–32.
5. Purtilo, R. B.: *Frameworks of interaction in helping relationships.* A presentation at Workshop on Interactive Strategies in Supervision and Education. Medical College of Georgia, Augusta, March 11, 1977.
6. Freud, S.: *The Ego and the Mechanisms of Defense.* New York, International Universities Press, 1966.
7. Stewart, T.: Physical therapy and psychotherapy: common grounds. *Phys. Ther.* 57:279–282, 1977.
8. *Ibid.*
9. President's Commission for the Study of Ethical Problems in Medicine. Vol. 11. *Making Health Care Decisions.* Washington, D. C., U. S. Government Printing Office, 1982.
10. Affeldt, J. E.: Accreditation clinic: patients' rights. *Hosp. Med. Staff* 11:9–11, 1982.
11. Carroll, M. A., and Humphrey, R. A.: *Moral Problems in Nursing: Case Studies.* Washington, D. C., University Press of America, 1979, pp. 34–35.
12. Jonsen, A., Siegler, M., and Winslade, W.: *Clinical Ethics.* New York, Macmillan Publishing Company, 1982, pp. 51–60.
13. Taylor, C.: *In Horizontal Orbit: Hospitals and the Cult of Efficiency.* New York, Holt, Rinehart and Winston, 1970, p. 122.
14. *Ibid.,* p. 123.
15. Benjamin, M., and Curtis, J.: *Ethics in Nursing.* Oxford, Oxford University Press, 1981, p. 123.
16. May, R.: *Love and Will.* New York, W. W. Norton & Company, 1969, pp. 287–306.
17. Fromm, E.: *The Art of Loving.* New York, Harper & Row, 1956, pp. 22–24.

Chapter 12

IMPORTANCE OF MAINTAINING PROFESSIONAL DISTANCE

The ancient dictum of medicine, *primum non nocere*, meaning "first, inflict no harm," expresses the essence of what will be said in this chapter about caring. It correctly suggests that even people with highly developed technical skills can inflict physical or psychological harm. In keeping with this dictum, this general rule should be remembered: The emotional distance between the health professional and the patient must always be great enough to facilitate the patient's self-dependence. However, not all patients will want or be able to become self-dependent, and by encouraging the patient's self-dependence, the health professional will also more likely be able to maintain his or her own.

What Professional Distance is Not

As a preliminary to detailed discussion of professional distance, it is a good idea to define what it is *not*. This can best be accomplished by attacking a common misconception shared by many health professionals that being "professional" means being aloof, efficient, and coolly competent—and about as friendly as a fish and as warm as a frog in an icy pond. The idea that professionalism is synonymous with maintaining an impersonal distance from the needs of patients could not be further from the truth. However, to see how this misconception arises, it is necessary to examine the health professional's educational environment.

PROFESSIONAL AND PERSONAL QUALITIES IN TENSION

A student enters the professional curriculum with a desire to help others and a set of human qualities he or she believes will help accomplish this end. These human qualities enable the student to be close to other people and show them a caring attitude. Then "professional qualities" that sometimes create a vague feeling of "distance" are added. These qualities help the student show competence, objectivity, and efficiency. The student knows that both human and professional qualities are important but is confused because the two sets of qualities seem incompatible; human qualities promote the type of closeness he or she always sought in relationships, and professional qualities promote a sense of being denied any chance for intense intimacy. This confusion, which is usually subtle, is further compounded by the observation that health professionals do not seem cold and calculating.

A research paper entitled "Is Professionalism Interfering with Effective Health Care?", which was submitted by four health professions students, showed they were troubled by this apparent dichotomy between personal and professional characeristics and so decided to take the matter to the patients. In the opening paragraph was this query: "Should health professional students be wary of and question the impersonal character of professionalism?" The following four questions, posed to 65 adult patients at a private general hospital in a white middle-class section of a big city, formed the basis of their study:

1. Do you prefer to be called by your first or last name?

2. Do you think health professionals should be called by their first names?

3. Do you think topics of a personal nature should be discussed during the patient's treatment or test?

4. Do you think health professionals should wear uniforms or street clothes?

The patients' replies included the following:

1. Two thirds of all the patients said it did not matter to them whether they were called by their first or last names. Over 90 per cent of patients under 25 years of age preferred to be called by their first names.

2. Almost all the patients felt more comfortable addressing the health professional by his or her last name at their initial meeting.

3. All the patients thought that it was fine to discuss personal topics during a treatment or test as long as the patient did not feel forced to give information or to listen to things he or she should not be told.

4. About one half of the patients preferred that health professionals wear uniforms, and another 25 per cent preferred at least some easily visible identifying symbol. The other one fourth said they either had no preference or preferred street clothes.

To validate the students' findings, it would be necessary to have more information about the patients—their sex, age, diagnosis, length and type of contact with health professionals, and so forth. However, the important point here is not so much the specific findings of the students' study but rather their concept of professionalism that motivated it. Certainly, they should be wary of and question the character of professionalism, just as students should question every new concept presented to them. However, the students were puzzled about whether they should be suspicious of and question the *impersonal* character of professionalism. Somewhere they had become convinced that professionalism blocked the opportunity for expressing care as a human being. With that conviction, they devised a study that showed, at least to their satisfaction, that a more *casual* atmosphere was preferable to a more formal one, at least after the initial meeting.

While I agree that much could be done to create a more *humane* atmosphere, it is important not to equate the humane with the casual because, as the last chapter explained, casualness is not the primary means of expressing care or competence. If one views professionalism solely in a way that opposes it to a more casual or relaxed mode of interaction, the health professional is forced to assume two personalities—now being professional, now personable—as demonstrated in the following chart.

PROFESSIONALISM MISCONCEIVED

Professional Self	Personal Self
Uses last names	Uses first names
Is efficient	Cares; is unconcerned about efficiency
Always wears uniform	Wears street clothes
Is competent administrator	Is warm, enthusiastic human being
Avoids getting involved in conversations about patient's personal life	Asks patient questions concerning his or her personal life
Demands respect from patient	Encourages openness and honesty in patient
Places premium on sound application of technical skills	Places premium on social interaction with person
Protects self by maintaining distance	Risks self by encouraging closeness

If such a dichotomy really exists, the health professional must commit herself or himself not only to playing two roles but also to becoming two wholly different selves. There must be a better way to demonstrate both professional competence and care for the patient than by becoming a split personality!

PROFESSIONAL AND PERSONAL QUALITIES INTEGRATED

Where did the notion of a dichotomy between human and professional qualities originate? Perhaps it began in Greek legend, where life and death were in the hands of some distant, uninvolved god; or perhaps in the account of the God of the Israelites, who both smote and healed but whose face was never seen. Healing, now done by professionals, has a history of mysterious, *impersonal* power.

Few health professionals draw as complete a distinction between professional and personal qualities as set forth in the chart just presented, but many occasionally think of them as two separate or schizoid dimensions of themselves. This need not be the case, because professional and personal qualities can and should be integrated into one set of complementary qualities. It is important for personal well-being to have such an integrated set of qualities and to visualize oneself as a whole person. Moreover, it has been shown that this integrated personality is important for professional success. Health professionals who are more successful in establishing social relationships and adapting to changes in their everyday lives are also more effective in their therapeutic relationships.[1] The health professional's integration of professional and personal qualities, as shown in the following chart, allows him or her to proceed from a sound foundation of wholeness.

Personal-Professional Self

Decides whether to use the first or last name of each new patient; is cautious, knowing that casual use of the first name may be harmful; is relaxed in using the last names of patients.

Incorporates actions that communicate caring into the patient–health professional interaction; recognizes efficiency as a trait that can express caring when it does not impose rigid limits on the interaction.

Recognizes that, taken alone, wearing a uniform does not necessarily make a patient feel *less* cared for nor does the more casual appearance of street clothes make a patient feel *more* cared for.

Combines a pleasant approach with professional competence.

Shows interest in the patient as a person with values, needs, and beliefs but does not encourage a relationship that will lead to overdependence (detrimental dependence).

Is respected by the patient, who recognizes his or her integrity; acknowledges that complete, open, mutual sharing with each other is not necessarily conducive to the functioning of a public-sector relationship.

Maintains a balance between providing sound health care services and fostering friendly interaction.

Does not need to protect himself or herself; is not required to take unnecessary risks.

When the health professional can approach a patient in this integrated way, the patient will be able to feel cared for by the health professional. He or she also will be secure in the knowledge that the patient–health professional rapport is not merely a friendship but rather a therapeutic relationship in which a competent professional person is committed to meeting the health needs of the patient.

It should now be obvious that keeping a particular distance is in no direct way identical with being "professional," and neither is becoming close the same as being "personal." Rather, the health professional ideally approaches a patient with an integrated set of personal and professional qualities and then decides how much distance to maintain. In this connection, the health professional's main goal should be to leave the patient with the conviction that he or she was cared for within the distance established. This matter can now be examined in more depth.

Meaningful Distances

In human interaction, distance and closeness are highly relative. At one pole there is a complete lack of interaction, while at the other there is intimacy. At any point along this continuum certain professional and personal qualities are put into play, while others remain in the background. When the relationship becomes more intimate, other combinations of the qualities predominate. Behavior of health professional and patient will vary accordingly. For the purpose of further discussion, it is important to differentiate between some degrees of distance so that their effects can be compared.

The following five levels of communication or interaction in which people engage will prove helpful bases for later discussion.[2]

Level Five: Cliché Conversation. No genuine human sharing takes place at this, the most superficial, level. "How are you?", "It's good to see you," and "See you again" are said without thought, and standard answers are expected. The person who responds to "How are you?" with an hour of detailed description of how he or she really feels is frowned on or, more likely, left to talk to himself or herself. This level protects people from each other and increases the unlikelihood of any further involvement.

Level Four: Reporting Facts. Almost nothing personal is revealed at this level: Although some sharing does take place, only information about such subjects as baseball scores, fashions, or a book is shared.

Level Three: Personal Ideas and Judgments. People venture to give some information about themselves at this level. This may be done by expressing an idea, judgment, or decision, which is usually guarded and is monitored by the listener's response. If the listener looks disapproving, bored, or confused, the person probably will become anxious and will hesitate to share more at this level.

Level Two: Feelings and Emotions. Only people who share a deep trust reveal themselves at this level. Love between friends cannot grow unless there is a *mutual* sharing at this level, commonly known as gut-level communication. A person will not want to share at this level if he or she believes the other person is judging the emotions themselves as good or bad. The individual wants the other person to understand that the emotion being expressed is deep-seated.

Level One: Peak Communication. Mutual, complete openness and honesty are shared at this, the deepest, level. There is almost perfect mutual understanding. Obviously, not many human interactions take place at this level. It is an all-encompassing intimacy experienced rarely by most people and never by some.

These five levels, though arbitrary, are nonetheless valuable because they describe one set of behaviors from which comparisons can be made. Further reference to these levels will be made in this chapter and the next.

When Distance is Advisable

There are some specific situations in which interpersonal distance should be consciously created. In each situation, the professional person is trying sincerely to help the patient, whose problems the health professional is either unwilling or unable to resolve.

PATIENT LONELINESS

The first situation is often precipitated by patient loneliness, which almost every patient experiences. Quite often, a professional person who wishes to help the patient overcome loneliness becomes his or her companion. A problem arises only when the health professional and patient relate over a period of time. One-time encounters may enable the health professional to perceive the potential for responding to a patient's loneliness, but they do not create a problem like that illustrated in the following story:

> Jack Simms is a paraplegic. He has been a patient at University Hospital for six months. His affable, optimistic spirit has made him very popular with the staff. At 23 years of age, he was involved in a car accident in which his fiancée was killed. Some health professionals have long suspected that Jack's optimism is a veneer for the deep sorrow and frustration resulting from this sudden, dramatic change in his life. One day he tearfully tells Karen Morgan, a health professions student who has been treating him, that he is depressed and desperately lonely. Up to this point, their interaction has been full of banter and they have felt quite comfortable with each other. Karen does not divulge to the rest of the staff Jack's expression of depression and loneliness, but that night on the way home, she stops by his room to see him.
>
> In the following weeks, she begins to visit him more often. She finds him attractive, they share common interests, and he is obviously happy in her company. But during this time, Karen also leads her own private life, going on dates and interacting with a world of other people. But Jack lies in bed thinking about her and, in the afternoons, he counts the minutes until she arrives.
>
> During her Christmas vacation, Karen goes to visit friends in a distant city and has a marvelous time. When she returns, bursting with enthusiasm, she finds Jack sullen and angry at her for staying away from him for so long.

Jack's reaction indicates that he feels she has rejected him. He has now reached the point where leaving her to go to his own home will mean relinquishing an immediate, perhaps his only, enjoyment. Karen has thus unwittingly fostered detrimental rather than constructive dependence. In her attempt to be a bright spot in Jack's life, she has become for him life itself.

Her subsequent attempts to explain or her sudden withdrawal may have profound, lasting effects on Jack's entire recovery process. Instead of being an intimate friend as he had hoped she was, she becomes just another of a long line of rejections he has experienced. He has thus become far more dependent on her than she had intended or was able to manage. Karen's well-intentioned response to Jack's loneliness initiated the events leading to this tragic state of affairs. She responded with a combination of professional and personal qualities that led to behavior Jack did not understand.

Similar results can arise from circumstances in which the attraction is not the sexual attraction between a man and woman. A patient's loneliness can precipitate an intense need to cling to anyone who will lend a sympathetic ear. Unfortunately, this may be true even if he or she has been able to establish deep, meaningful relationships prior to the injury or illness.

PITY

The second situation in which distance may have to be considered involves a professional person who, in an attempt to respond well to a patient, gets so entangled in the apparent futility of the patient's plight that it becomes impossible to think about or act rationally toward the patient.

Most health professionals can name at least one type of illness or injury that involves them emotionally. Sometimes their feelings are so strong that they cannot bear to treat patients with that particular condition. In one study, 54 health professionals named blindness as the condition they felt would be the hardest for them to cope with.[3] This group may have had difficulty treating blind people because they felt so sorry for their patients. Other health professionals might have named cancer, severe burns, aphasia, or psychoses instead of blindness.

It is not at all unnatural for health professionals to become periodically so involved in the patients' dilemmas that they take these problems home with them. Almost any health professional can recall the time he or she had trouble falling asleep, or was moved to tears or laughter by a sudden tragic or joyful announcement touching a patient's life. There is, however, a significant difference between this depth of caring, which stimulates a purely human response, and fruitless or destructive entanglement. Again, the problem can be illustrated with a story:

> Michael Kader was admitted to the psychiatric ward of City Hospital after the police brought him there from his apartment. The police found him unconscious after a friend reported that he did not respond to her phone calls. Michael is a 26-year-old heroin addict, and a Vietnam veteran. His mother died when he was 12 years old, and he left home to live on the streets shortly after that. He recently learned that his father died of a heart attack shortly after he ran away from home.
>
> Craig Hopkins, a health professional student in clinical education, is 29 years old and is also a Vietnam veteran. His similarity to Michael Anderson, however, ends here. Craig Hopkins grew up in an upper middle-class home and served in Vietnam as an officer. He has never had close contact with an addict before, but he finds Michael very warm and human. They both chat when Craig has a few minutes, and over the weeks, Craig arrives at the conclusion that Michael has had more than his share of misfortune.

> One day when Craig goes into Michael's room, he finds the patient doubled up, writhing in agony. With a trembling voice, Michael tells him that the doctor has withdrawn his drug completely. To Craig's surprise, Michael grabs him by the wrist and pleads, "Please, Please, I can't stand this pain. If you will lend me five dollars, I can get just enough to make it over the hump. If I can't get a little relief, I will kill myself. The doctor is a sadist. . . ."
>
> Craig Hopkins tears himself away and leaves the room. That night, however, he cannot sleep. He is haunted by the picture of an asthenic man who has survived the death of his parents and the horror of war but has succumbed to the needle; he sees clearly the beads of sweat that cling to Michael's face as he speaks.
>
> The next day when Craig goes toward Michael's room, a nurse stops him, saying that Michael is asleep as he has been given a heavy sedative. "Last night he tried to hang himself in the bathroom by tying a sheet to the shower pole," the nurse says. "You've got to watch those fellows on the needle. They'll do anything to manipulate the staff to give them more of the drug. I think he was just trying to scare us."
>
> Craig remembers Michael's pleading eyes the day before and is overcome with a desire to make a sharp retort to the nurse's statements. He goes instead to Michael's room and deftly slips five dollars into the drawer of the bedside stand. He is not sure why he does this, but he quickly turns and leaves.

Clearly, Craig Hopkins has reached the point where he is responding instinctively rather than rationally because the situation is so painful to him. Such a feeling exceeds sympathy and is more closely related to pity. Because pity distorts the objective perspective necessary to resolve the real problem, he ceases to be of help. In fact, he may include himself among the patient's many problems.

Pity can be communicated to the patient in one meeting as well as over a period of time. Facial expression can instantly betray one's secret feelings. Quick nervous movements, coupled with a sudden departure, are sometimes correctly interpreted as expressions of pity. The desire not to talk about the patient's problem, and trite comments such as "It'll be fine, I'm sure," can also be interpreted to mean "Poor, poor you."

Again, the health professional cannot solve a problem arising from pity simply by acting aloof and "professionally" competent. The pity is in response to a real need of a patient. What is called for, therefore, is a combination of personal and professional qualities that allows the patient to know that his or her dilemma is acknowledged with sympathy. The problem occurs when the health professional, overcome by feelings about the dilemma, uses both professional and personal qualities to try to solve the problem in some irrational manner that results either in damage to the relationship or, as in the case just cited, in no help for the patient.

OVERIDENTIFICATION

The third situation in which distance must be maintained can also manifest itself at the first meeting between patient and health profes-

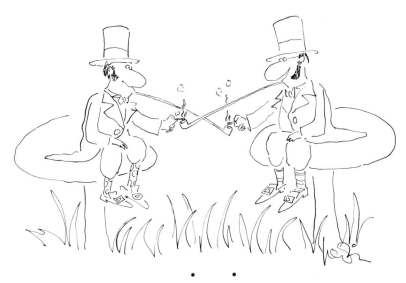

Drawing by Levin, © 1983 The New Yorker Magazine, Inc.

sional. The problem arises when the health professional has trouble seeing the patient as an individual, for a number of reasons: (1) The patient so perfectly embodies a stereotype that he or she becomes the stereotype. (2) The patient so reminds the health professional of someone else that the patient becomes that person (see the discussion of counter-transference, Chapter 11). (3) The health professional has had an experience so similar to the patient's that he or she believes the experiences to be identical. In all three instances such a reaction is called overidentification.

Having had similar experiences may actually *hinder* the effectiveness of health professional–patient interaction at times. Everyone has had the experience of beginning to relate a traumatic (or exciting) event only to have the other person interrupt with, "Oh! I know *exactly* what you mean!" and then go on to describe his or her own story. One feels cheated at such times, thinking, "No, that's *not* what I meant, but you are more interested in telling me about yourself than in listening to me!" The way such overidentification works within the health professions can be illustrated in a third story:

> Mrs. Garcia, an elementary school teacher, became interested in teaching language skills to deaf children after her third child, Lucia, who was born deaf, successfully learned to communicate by attending special classes for those with hearing impairment. Mrs. Garcia enrolled in a health professions course directed toward training teachers of deaf persons.
>
> During her clinical education, she was surprised and alarmed that some of the mothers requested that she not be assigned to their children. Finally, she approached one of the mothers whose child she had been working with and with whom she felt comfortable. "What's wrong?" she asked. "Do they think I'm incompetent because

I am an older student? Is it my personality? I want so much to help these children, and I can't understand what I'm doing wrong." The embarrassed mother replied, "Well, since you asked, I'll give you a direct answer. *I* don't feel this way, but some of the mothers think that you don't understand their children's difficulties because every time they start to tell you something about *their* children, you immediately interrupt with an experience that *your* child had."

In short, overidentification leads to an "I-know-how-you-feel" reaction that can be helpful or can convince the patient (or the family) of the complete opposite! The health professional who is astute enough to discern that he or she may be overidentifying will also be able to see that attempts to become close to the patient by pointing out superficial similarities between their experiences are being interpreted by the patient as the health professional's desire to talk about his or her own problem. The health professional should not be falsely led to believe that a closeness has been established. Rather, he or she should be willing to maintain greater distance until the uniqueness of the other person emerges.

How to Maintain Professional Distance

It is important to remember that the health professional can express genuine care for the patient by maintaining distance as well as by creating closeness between them.

In the first case report in the preceding section, the problem involved the health professional (Karen Morgan) who paid too much attention to the patient (Jack Simms). In such a case, it is always wise for the health professional to refrain from visiting the patient outside the treatment or testing situation until he or she is absolutely certain that the patient's feelings and life situation are such that a detrimental dependence will not result. This absolute certainty seldom can be established. Of course, if the health professional initiates the visits because he or she is lonely or infatuated with the patient, the latter will almost always be sensitive to this motive and may have extreme difficulty coping with it.[4]

One way for the health professional to avoid further development of an already too close relationship with the patient is to limit conversation to small talk and to matters pertaining to the patient's care (interaction at Levels Five, *Cliché Conversation*, and Four, *Reporting Facts*). However, it is more effective to mention personal topics (Level Three, *Personal*

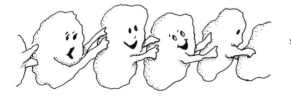

"You scratch my back and I'll scratch yours!"

Ideas and Judgments) that will remind the patient of the real situation between them. A young man, for instance, should know that the health professional he adores is engaged to someone else. By discreetly sharing with the patient personal incidents from everyday life, the health professional will be better able to maintain a distance in their relationship that will be helpful to both. In this case, the most important factor is not the level of the conversation, but rather the facts revealed at that level. It is the health professional's responsibility to give and receive pertinent personal information in such a way that workable limits are maintained in the relationship.

In the second case report, Craig Hopkins responded to Michael Kader because he pitied him. But patients abhor pity, even if it serves some small immediate purpose. This is well known to any health professional who even once has experienced a patient's bitter response to pity. Pity is destructive and belittling to the patient, who recoils from it.

When pity is the chief motivation in a relationship, there usually has been extensive interaction involving conversation at Levels Three (*Personal Ideas and Judgments*) and Two (*Feelings and Emotions*). The patient who is in pain will not know how or when to limit personal revelations when he or she finds a professional person with a sympathetic ear. The health professional can monitor the extent to which the patient reveals confidences by simply asking if he or she really wants to tell so much, since the health professional is in no position to solve most of the personal problems. In addition, the health professional can and should refer the patient to someone—such as a person in the clergy, a psychologist, or a social worker—who *can* probably do something about them. The health professional makes a mistake by responding with a display of overwhelming emotion—pity, in this case—while failing to put the person in contact with other means of support.[5]

When troubling personal feelings or biases seem to be surfacing in the patient–health professional relationship, it is generally wise for the health professional to avoid interaction at any more intimate level than Level Four (*Reporting Facts*). The patient needs interaction at a deeper level, but it should be with someone other than the health professional. The incident between Craig Hopkins and the nurse is a case in point. She told him that Michael Kader was simply manipulating the hospital staff, to which accusation Craig responded antagonistically. The nurse made a generalized statement that is often correct of such patients but was questionable in this particular circumstance. However, if Craig had listened to what she said, he might have gained a clearer insight into this patient or into others like him. Rather, he became defensive and was unable to listen objectively; in addition, he did nothing that might have helped the nurse attain a better understanding of Michael's situation.

Co-workers can be valuable in a situation in which the health professional's close relationship with the patient prevents him or her from seeing the patient objectively. Another professional person working with the patient may view the situation from a different perspective and thus provide some insight into the health professional's troubling responses. When the health professional refers a patient to someone else or shares disturbing feelings with co-workers, he or she is maintaining a distance from the patient by bringing other people into the relationship. However, unless some confidence is breached in the process, the act also shows that he or she genuinely cares about that patient.

In the third case report, Mrs. Garcia's effectiveness as a teacher of deaf children was hindered by her own previous experiences, which led to overidentification. Overidentification, once a part of the health professional's thinking, cannot be easily erased. However, an important step toward adequate interaction is *initially* to refrain from sharing stories of similar experiences with the patient and his or her family. Effective interaction is achieved when the health professional first stresses the uniqueness of the patient's experience and only then allows comparisons with the health professional's own experience.

The health professional, then, should at first usually restrict communication to the more impersonal level, Four (*Reporting Facts*), while the patient communicates at more personal levels, Three (*Personal Ideas and Judgments*) and Two (*Feelings and Emotions*). This gives the patient an opportunity to describe fully his or her unique experience and express the feelings attached to it before the health professional superimposes any similarities on it. Then as the health professional shares his or her own ideas and judgments, the patient will begin to realize that the health professional's own account reveals concern about and insight into the patient's problem.

In all three case reports, maintaining professional distance does not mean a cold or impersonal approach should be used. Indeed, such an approach would only increase the person's loneliness and self-pity and strengthen the conviction that he or she was not understood by the health professional. The health professional is faced with the challenge of carefully structuring the individual situation so that the dignity of both health professional and patient is preserved. While in these cases dignity depends on the health professional's wisdom in maintaining an appropriate distance, the next chapter emphasizes situations in which the challenge is one of creating appropriate closeness.

REFERENCES

1. Dopson, L.: The key is adaptability. Nurs. Times 79:35–36, 1983.
2. Powell, J. S. J.: Why am I Afraid to Tell You Who I Am? Chicago, Argus Communications, 1969, pp. 54–62.
3. Janicki, M. P.: Attitudes of health professionals toward twelve disabilities. Percept. Motor Skills 3077–3078, 1970.
4. Derlega, V. J., and Margulis, S. T.: Why loneliness occurs: the interrelationship of social-psychological and privacy concepts. In Peplau, L. A., and Perlman, D. (eds.): Loneliness. New York, John Wiley & Sons, 1982, pp. 152–156.
5. Young, R.: The family-illness intermesh: theoretical aspects and their application. Soc. Sci. Med. 17:395–398, 1983.

Chapter 13

CHALLENGE OF CREATING PROFESSIONAL CLOSENESS

In patient–health professional interaction, professional closeness is yeast in bread, wind in a sail, oxygen in a flame. At the right time, in the proper place, and with the necessary skills, the health professional can create this closeness, indicating that he or she has achieved the optimal mode of interaction between patient and health professional.

What Professional Closeness is Not

First, professional closeness is *not* merely a casual or informal approach, as shown in Chapter 11. A patient will not necessarily be more trusting of a health professional who uses first names indiscriminately or tries to make the test or treatment situation more interesting by abolishing structured schedules, by being inappropriately cheerful, by constantly joking, or by humming the latest rock tune. Patients are usually seeking, besides health care, a feeling of security in their dependent state, and these actions do not necessarily contribute to this end. In one study in which 15 female subjects were each allowed to choose a helper, they chose not the most interesting people they knew, but people who they perceived to be authoritative, trustworthy, and steady.[1]

Second, professional closeness is *not* intimate entanglement in the patient's interests and problems, as illustrated in Chapter 12. Intimacy in any relationship implies that both parties contribute equally to that relationship, even if it results in detrimental dependence. It is possible, of course, that the health professional and the patient, as individuals, have the potential to become intimate, but their present relationship is one in which the patient voluntarily seeks the specific services of the health professional, which he or she needs and will pay for. Thus, such a potential is not lacking, but "to everything there is a season, and a time to every purpose under the heaven" (Eccles. 3:1). The purpose of the patient–health professional relationship is to improve the state of the patient's health by the use of professional skills, and other goals should not be substituted.

Third, professional closeness is *not only* the health professional's reassurance, although this is a vital component of it. Alone, verbal reassurance or a pat on the shoulder can frighten as much as console. In

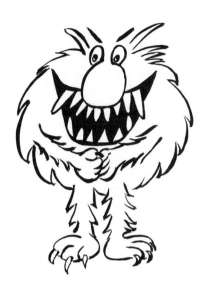

Inappropriate cheerfulness will not be reassuring to the patient.

I Never Promised You a Rose Garden, Deborah hears the ward administrator tell her, "It [the cold pack] doesn't hurt—don't worry," and she thinks, "Watch out for those words . . . they are the same words. What comes after those words is deceit."[2]

Finally, professional closeness is *not* automatically found in the relationship that develops from prolonged contact between patient and health professional. This distinction is especially important because professional closeness can be created between the health professional and the patient who meet only once. The possibility of creating professional closeness in this single meeting or during a short period of time may be easier today than ever before.

The rapid social change that modern society is undergoing is attracting the attention of anthropologists, theologians, sociologists, and psychologists, who ponder the question: How will this rapid transition in human relationships affect people? Some thinkers are very pessimistic, prophesying a generation of automatons and depersonalized "humanoids." However, others suggest that the present barriers to human relationships will be broken down, thus increasing the possibility of relating immediately, intensely, and without traditional social props. Such a trend can be observed in the move toward candidness and honesty, qualities that are increasingly valuable today. The health professional can develop professional closeness with a patient in a short period of time if he or she wisely uses these qualities.

Professional closeness in the patient–health professional relationship is based on mutual respect and dignity. When a person's lifestyle is changed suddenly by disease, accident, or injury, he or she begins to ask, "Am I still worthy to be included among human beings as one of them?" Psychologists call this phenomenon "cognitive dissonance"—that is, a person's past self-image is not in harmony with the present one.

Chapter 4 discussed this feeling as a serious problem faced by patients. They sense that the illness may require some radical changes in their lives, and understandably they become very anxious. Such anxiety is repeatedly observed in patients—a man is afraid he may not be able to return to his job as a bricklayer; a woman is afraid she may lose her opportunity for tenure at the university where she teaches; a child is afraid the other children will laugh at her because she has scars on her face and neck.

The cause of so much anxiety in the man, woman, and child is that their *dignity* is threatened. Like everyone else, they need to preserve their dignity, which will enable them to accept the other adjustments made necessary by their illness or injury

The health professional can play an important part in helping a patient preserve his or her dignity, but because of society's current standards, the health professional can also unwittingly destroy it. Because society is geared largely to manipulating objects to its own advantage, the health professional must also manipulate objects in his or her personal everyday life; the danger is that patients will be manipulated in the same impersonal manner and be robbed of their human dignity. The many ways in which patients feels themselves "depersonalized" and therefore robbed of dignity are illustrated in May Sarton's account of the woman Laura being admitted to the hospital during a bad episode of a long illness.

> . . . they were silent as the ambulance turned off the drive, proceeded through dirty city streets, and drew up at the Massachusetts Memorial Hospital. Laura closed her eyes. The very look of it was appalling, cold, a jail for the sick. "Ann, stay with me," she said.
>
> "Of course. That's why we're here. We're not going to abandon you, dear Laura."
>
> With the knife thrust of fear Laura realized that she wanted their help. She had to admit that. In this dreadful impersonal place. She hated the thought that the young man would leave her now. Already she was being lifted from the ambulance stretcher to a hospital one

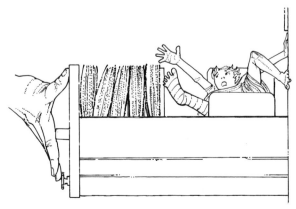

The health professional who manipulates objects in everyday life is in danger of manipulating the patient in the same impersonal manner.

on wheels. "Good-by," she called, and the young man turned and waved. "Good luck," he said with a smile. As he went through the door Brooks came in.

"Take it easy, Mother. You know what hospitals are like. It may be a while before we know where you're going." Ann was standing by the stretcher holding Laura's hand.

"It's good of you to do this," Laura said. Then she closed her eyes. A voice came over the public address system, "Dr. Warner. Dr. Warner." Feet shuffled past, subdued voices, the sound of a typewriter. Laura felt she was in the middle of a huge, empty world, a center of loneliness among strange, busy sounds. And she was terribly tired.

"Ann, is my suitcase there?"

"Right here, Laura."

"Mother, we'll need your Blue Cross number." Brooks had returned from somewhere, very businesslike and calm.

"Look in my purse, Ann. I think it must be there, somewhere among the credit cards."

Laura had broken out into a sweat—papers, things one had to have! She had not put her mind on all this. She had let herself be bundled away to a hospital without even thinking of these necessary preparations.

"Here, I've got it," Ann said in triumph.

"Thanks. I'll be right back."

"And indeed in a very short time Brooks was there with an orderly to wheel the stretcher to room 103 on the fifth floor. She was wheeled into a huge elevator, Brooks and Ann on either side of her. Brooks had the suitcase now.

There were two nurses and an intern in the elevator. They talked in loud voices and laughed about the food in the cafeteria. It was as though Laura on her stretcher simply did not exist. The voices hurt her ears. "After all," she thought, "I might be dying."

"Can't you be quiet," Brooks whispered furiously. "My mother is very ill."

"Oh, sorry," said the intern. Laura opened her eyes and caught his lifted eyebrow and a muffled giggle from one of the nurses, and she hated them.

The elevator crept from floor to floor, an interminable progress, now made in complete silence, a self-conscious silence, exposing Laura, she felt, to incurious resentment. What do they care? She thought. I'm just another body to be carted around and done things to. Why did I ever allow Jim to persuade me? To be trapped like this. Very far away down an interminable tunnel she evoked the apple tree in flower in her garden, Mary waving at the door. Would she ever see them again?

"There, at last!" Ann breathed, as Laura was wheeled out on the floor and into her room. "And it's a single room, thank God."

"And you can look out on some pretty dreary roofs," Brooks added. "But at least there's some sky."

Ann meanwhile was unpacking the suitcase. She took the transistor out, set it at the station with classical music, and laid it beside Laura under her pillow.

"Now I have some hiding place down here I'll be all right," Laura said. "It was just that awful feeling when we were dumped in the hall!"[3]*

---

*Reprinted from *A Reckoning*, by May Sarton, by permission of W.W. Norton & Company, Inc. Copyright © 1978 by May Sarton.

If health professionals avoid manipulating the patient as a means to their own ends (such as to make money for the department, organization, or themselves, or to learn more about an interesting disease), they will allow the patient to retain his or her dignity. With dignity intact, the patient will have reason to trust the health professional and will likely want to be trusted in return. This mutual trust was described in Chapter 11 as that which forms the basis for the feeling of relatedness between health professional and patient when they first meet. It becomes even more important as the relationship progresses. Not all patients treated with dignity will reciprocate in their attitude toward the health professional. Human relationships are not always so ideal and simple. Nonetheless, the health professional's approach should always promote trust.

Let us now consider some of the many positive ways a health professional can act to preserve a patient's dignity and promote trust.

The Health Professional Defines Limits

Defining the limits of a relationship gives it direction, providing the parties involved with knowledge about the relationship, one of Fromm's four characteristics of caring listed in Chapter 11.

Since caring is central to developing professional closeness between people, it follows that defining limits can actually help to create professional closeness in a patient–health professional relationship. Two kinds of limits are immediately evident in the relationship: one imposed by setting, the other by time.

SETTING

The physical setting in which the patient–health professional relationship develops is likely confined to an area in which at least one other type of health professional is employed, except in the case of home care. Most often, the setting is further confined to (1) the patient's bedside or (2) a testing or treatment area. In either case, the surroundings are easily distinguishable from a cocktail lounge or hotel lobby, where purely social interactions take place.

The health professional helps to create this setting. He or she works in the health facility and spends leisure time elsewhere. There is usually at least one other professional person in the area who is performing a similar or complementary function. They both may wear the same kind of uniform or other identifiable symbols. At first the patient may see the health professional only as someone capable of rendering a specific service, since the health professional was not chosen on a personal basis.

The patient also helps to create the setting. The health professional's services are needed to help him or her recover from a specific malfunction. If an inpatient, he or she interacts primarily with the patients and hospital staff. Unlike the health professional, who only works here, the patient lives here for the duration of the illness. Whether inpatient or outpatient, he or she comes to regard the health professional as an important part of the daily routine. Furthermore, the illness or injury has created many other problems with which he or she must try to cope. Limitations imposed by the setting are thus related to why, where, when, how, and between whom the interaction takes place. The patient who is visited in his or her own home does not have the benefit of some of these limits that guide other patients, and the health professional may have to make a greater effort to help define the limits.

TIME

Time also limits the relationship. The health professional should devote to the patient time to which he or she is entitled, but not at other patients' expense. It is not always easy for the health professional to do this, because patients may begin to feel that they are forced into rigid little time slots; furthermore, every health professional knows that on some days a particular patient needs some extra time to work through a problem or just to talk. However, there is the patient who, because of loneliness or simple enjoyment of the surroundings, tends to linger every day and make small talk with the health professionals. It is this person who is more likely to divert time and energy that should be directed to other patients; he or she may also show excessive dependence on the health professional or setting and may need to be gently weaned from it.

The tactful but firm defining of time limits can thus help to prevent the development of a relationship that could be destructive to both patient and professional person. This establishment of time limits is the health professional's way of saying, "The time I spend with you helps to determine the amount of involvement that we should have with each other."

Although it is good to set time limits for the patient, ironically it more often seems that the health professional has *barely adequate* time for a patient. The hectic pace in most health facilities makes it difficult to focus attention on just one patient during the time rightfully belonging to her or him! The health professional's goal in this case would be to set limits on distractions that detract from the time spent with a patient. The health professional who fails to do this does as much to deter the development of professional closeness as the one who rigorously enforces reasonable limits on the time a patient is allowed to spend with the health professional.

The following guidelines help the health professional make the most use of the time spent with a patient, regardless of whether the meeting is the first or the fiftieth. You, the health professional, should:

1. Remove the patient from hospital traffic or other area where distractions are likely to occur.

2. Sit down when talking to the person to give the impression that he or she is the only patient in the world who needs care.

3. Refrain from calling attention to how busy you are, or you will seem to be paying even less attention to the patient than you are. If there

was an unavoidable delay in getting to the patient, explain why; or if you cannot hide your distraction, explain that too.

4. Approach the patient slowly and graciously, even though you may have to run to the patient's room to be on time.

5. Look the patient in the eye when conversing, instead of glancing all around the room. A lack of eye contact communicates lack of interest and further increases the patient's feeling that his or her time with the health professional is being dissipated.

6. Protect the time that you have with the person by telling other people in the area that you are busy and will be happy to talk with them later. The patient who is scheduled to spend 15 minutes alone with the health professional, but shares them with ten intruders or telephone calls, will feel more cheated than one who spends five uninterrupted minutes with him or her.

Neither setting nor time limits should be viewed as inflexible boundaries. If they are, the health professional will begin to see patients as objects to be manipulated within a given area in a prescribed time. Rather, the health professional is encouraged to be aware of natural boundaries that help to give both the patient and him or her a sense of direction. In this way, the dignity that belongs to them both is enhanced, and the patient will be spared the hurt or embarrassment of misinterpreted intentions.

The Health Professional Attends to Detail

An important way to enhance a person's self-worth or dignity is to acknowledge little details. These too often go unnoticed. This particular method of developing closeness was described by a former student of the author's in the following conversation:

"Jane," the author said. "You've been working [at the health facility] for six months now. What is the most important thing that you have learned in these six months?"

"Well," she replied. "There are many things. I have learned the importance of lighting a cigarette, listening to the ninth inning of a baseball game between parts of a treatment, getting water, wiping a nose. Perhaps these things sound silly to you, but I know that I could not be getting the good results I am seeing if I had not mastered these skills along with my technical ones!" After a pause, she added with a smile, "I guess I have learned to *nurture* my patients a little!" Jane had learned that attention to detail—nurturing, as she put it—was an effective way of showing a patient that he or she mattered as a person.

Nurturing is divided into the following broad categories:

Personal-Hygiene Detail. When the patient has a hygienic need, attention to it will make him or her very grateful. This is not to suggest that the health professional should wait on the patient with toothbrush, mouthwash, and nail clippers in hand, nor that hygienic activity should in any way compromise time that should be spent utilizing professional skills. However, sometimes a simple act, such as providing a Kleenex when the patient needs one, makes the difference between an embarrassed and an attentive patient.

Personal-Comfort Detail. The patient sometimes experiences a certain amount of discomfort in a treatment, diagnostic, or testing situation. There are, however, many ways a patient can be made more comfortable; they may involve crossing the room to straighten or clean the patient's glasses, supporting the arm while drawing blood, or running for an extra towel.

Personal-Interest Detail. This includes asking the patient about the noon menu; listening, as Jane did, to the ninth inning of the ball game; admiring a vase of flowers, a bathrobe, or a pipe; reminding a teenager that her favorite rock artist has a special show on TV that night; and spelling Mr. Schydlowski's name correctly on his appointment slip. Birthdays and holidays are also important dates to remember. On Mr. Arnold's birthday, write "Happy Birthday, Dick Arnold" in bold letters on the schedule board or on a poster in his booth; he will work as though he were ten years younger rather than one year older.

Expanding-Awareness Detail. The health professional who has been confined to a hospital or bed knows how quickly one loses track of time and becomes out of touch with the rest of the world. By sharing an incident observed on the way to work, by reviewing a play seen the evening before, or by taking the patient to a window to see a child and dog playing together, the health professional can extend the patient's environment beyond the immediate area, bringing him or her in contact with the outside world. I once brought apple blossoms into a four-bed

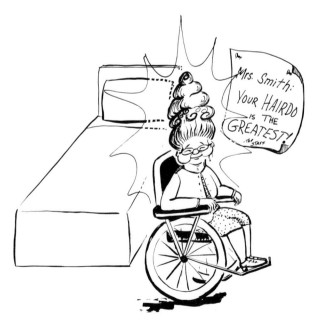

ward in an extended care facility only to have two of the patients burst into tears. When I asked with surprise what I had done wrong, they both admitted to missing the smell of apple blossoms more than anything else during their springtime confinement.

The danger of paying attention to any or all kinds of detail is that they may be substituted for actual professional services. The professional person who would rather fluff pillows than proceed with a treatment, or would rather chat than work, cheats the patient. He or she may be a casual friend to the patient, but the substitution of detail for professional skills denies the patient the one thing he or she needs most.

Self-Revelation by Health Professional and Patient

THE HEALTH PROFESSIONAL

Once a basic trust, which promotes a feeling of relatedness, has developed between health professional and patient, the groundwork for creating professional closeness has been laid. Now the challenge for the health professional is to reveal to the patient who and what he or she is in such a way that the patient–health professional relationship will be constructive and will grow.

Previously, the reader has been reminded of danger signals such as infatuation, pity, and overidentification. It was suggested that, in these cases, the health professional should not restrict interaction unnecessarily, but should guide communications so that further misunderstanding or overdependence can be prevented. If danger signals are not readily apparent, the health professional need not be so concerned about maintaining distance and can discreetly proceed to create professional closeness with the patient.

In the absence of danger signals, how much personal information about oneself should be revealed to a patient? In order to establish some basic guidelines, it is expedient to refer again to the five levels of communication outlined in Chapter 12.

Interaction at Levels Five (*Cliché Conversation*) and Four (*Reporting Facts*) can be comfortably maintained in one-time meetings, such as with acquaintances on a bus trip or with people at a coffee house. Restricting the conversation to these levels can assure adequate distance when pity or overidentification arises as a potential problem.

These two levels are useful for creating professional closeness only when patient and health professional are initially trying to get to know each other. They can be used afterwards but do little to create further trust between the two people. At Level Three (*Personal Ideas and Judgments*), the health professional begins to reveal a more personal self to the patient. Used wisely, this level is almost always acceptable from the very beginning and should be avoided only when the danger signals are present. An example of this level of communication, which is used widely by health professionals who see patients over a period of time, is found in the comments made about the patient's progress: "That's better" and "You will have to work harder than that."

At Level Two (*Emotions and Feelings*), the health professional reveals himself or herself at a level commonly called "gut level." It is important to note that the author of these five levels, in stating that mutual revelation is desirable at this level, was referring to mature friendship between peers. The health professional will certainly want to express some degree of feeling in relating to the patient. The potential difficulty lies in stressing the emotional aspect to the point where the patient is unable to retain his or her own independence and dignity or to recognize them in the helper.

The health professional should therefore excercise great care as to when and how his or her emotions are revealed to the patient. A sudden outburst of anger or tears can completely unnerve a patient. It is unfair to make the patient responsible for reacting with understanding and insight when the health professional explodes with emotion.

Finally, Level One (*Peak Experiences*) does not pertain to the patient–health professional relationship. With rare exceptions, the occurrence of peak-level interactions indicates that the relationship has moved beyond what is defined as the health professional–patient relationship. When patients see the person behind the professional role, they will be convinced that they, too, are worthwhile human beings in a dynamic human relationship. The health professional need not bare his or her soul or engage in highly charged emotional encounters for this to happen.

At any of the communication levels described, the health professional can also reveal himself or herself simply by responding consistently and honestly to the patient's actions. The health professional should let the patient know that certain topics and kinds of behavior are unacceptable in their professional relationship. Interaction at Level Four may include jokes that are crude or have ethnic or sexual overtones. In Level Three interaction, the patient may divulge personal details that the health professional judges better left unshared, while at Level Two, he or she may pout, become fresh, or exhibit childish outbursts of anger.

These types of behavior very often surface within minutes after a health professional introduces himself or herself. They do not necessarily wait for the relationship to be firmly established. The health professional should make the patient aware that he or she objects to such behavior. The patient's behavior is monitored for two reasons: to prepare him or her to return to society; and to ensure that the health professional is treated with the same respect he or she shows the patient. After all, mutual respect is vital to constructive dependence.

Confronting the patient with the unacceptable behavior may embarrass and upset the person initially, but will obviate unspoken tension between them that may hinder the effectiveness of the test or treatment.

It is equally important that the health professional express delight and approval when he or she is happy about something the patient does. If the patient compliments the health professional, the latter should accept the compliment graciously. A small, appropriate gift also is acceptable, though the health professional must be exceedingly careful not to allow the patient to use it as a means of trying to ingratiate himself or herself. The patient will then be encouraged to display this positive behavior to others, and the present relationship will be improved.[4]

Showing disapproval, delight, gratitude, or any other response for the purpose of establishing a *consistent* and *honest* interaction with the patient is one way of telling him or her how other people may also react.

The patient's trust grows in proportion to self-awareness as a social being. If, however, the health professional expresses disapproval, delight, or gratitude for the purpose of coercing the patient into doing something not ultimately to the patient's benefit, the health professional is manipulating the patient, thereby potentially harming him or her.

A health professional thus reveals himself or herself to the patient in the following ways: (1) by clarifying how he or she perceives the relationship instead of exchanging irrelevant personal information with the patient or displaying uncontrolled emotion; (2) by revealing his or her own personality; and (3) by making the patient aware of behavior judged to be acceptable, which is accomplished by maintaining a consistent response to the patient's many tentative actions.

THE PATIENT

Meaningful human interaction cannot take place if one party reveals himself or herself but the other does not. Thus it is important that the patient also be able to engage in self-revelation. However, many health professionals hesitate to let patients talk about themselves because they are uneasy about discussing topics they feel could be better handled by a psychologist.

Such health professionals should be reminded that every day they are involved in situations that require them to use the principles learned in basic psychology courses. While the helpful and unique role of the psychologist in the health care setting should not be underestimated, the health professional who refuses to engage at all at a personal level with a patient readily will convince the patient that the health professional does not care. In other words, the health professional *must* learn to allow the patient to reveal himself or herself. The question then arises: How much revelation should be encouraged? In discussing this question, the five levels of communication and interaction again prove helpful.

Levels Five (*Cliché Conversation*), Four (*Reporting Facts*), and Three (*Personal Ideas and Judgments*) are used by most patients within a short period of time. Level Three is important because it allows the patient to talk about his or her health condition and about health care in general. Some patients talk about themselves in order to manipulate the health professional. For instance, in the previous chapter, the nurse was suspicious of the motives of the heroin abuser, Michael. She had obviously known patients to do and say things of a very personal nature in order to gain the hospital staff's sympathy.

But in spite of an occasional problem, it is a good general rule to encourage a patient to engage in self-revelation at Level Three. One way people reveal much is through story-telling. Four categories of questions can be asked to encourage the patient to talk about himself or herself, although these need not be followed verbatim as listed here:

1. What *wounds* or hurts do you resent having suffered?
2. What *gifts* were you given for which you were grateful?
3. Who are your important *heroes* and models?
4. What were the crucial *decisions* for which you were responsible?

Keen, who makes these suggestions, contends that "these categories focus attention not only on the remembered facts which constitute the raw material of autobiography, but on the way in which memory functions to justify present attitudes, such as resentment or gratitude.[5] At any age, it is one way by which a patient reveals important personal ideas and judgments.

Patients also often express themselves emotionally to the health professional. Here the inequality of the relationship becomes more readily apparent. The health professional consciously monitors the type and amount of Level Two communication (*Feelings and Emotions*) that he or she displays in the presence of the patient. But the patient is usually unable and should not necessarily be encouraged to hide emotions from the health professional, even during a one-time meeting.

One of the hardest emotions to express is the gut fear, the blood-sweat-and-tears terror the patient experiences from time to time when thinking about his or her uncertain future. That this is a problem for many patients has been mentioned several times now. Many health professionals discourage such emotional expression because it is uncomfortable for them to watch an adult break down and sob. Without saying a word, the health professional can prevent the patient from expressing his or her fears; a "don't-tell-me" smile, an "I'm-too-busy" shrug, a "you're-above-that-kind-of-thing" wink, and a pleading "I-won't-know-what-to-do-if-you-cry" look will deter the most desperate patient.

However, if professional closeness means deep caring of one human being for another, then the patient should have the option of sharing his or her fears with the health professional. Furthermore, the health professional should be prepared to be understanding but should try not to become completely entangled in the situation.

Patients especially afraid to reveal themselves are those with qualities that are unacceptable to a large segment of society. The feeling of rejection accompanying the illness is added to the stigma they bear because of an unacceptable social role. One such person is the prostitute. Another is the member of a small but zealous religious sect, such as a Jehovah's Witness or Hari Krishna, who has ideas not consistent with those held by the health care provider. The health professional, however, need not agree with a person's lifestyle or behavior in order to feel responsible for maintaining that person's dignity as a human being and helping to destigmatize them within the health care context.[6]

People are understandably distressed by their unhappy situations, socially unacceptable characteristics, or undesirable images. This is illustrated in the great Hermann Hesse novel, *Steppenwolf*.[7] One is moved by the wicked wolf's sad eyes, and later discovers they are sad because the wolf is really the dark side of the hero, Harry Haller. The patient will likely feel remorse or regret after revealing this dark side, but the health professional can help the person to overcome those feelings in the following manner:

First, it is crucial to recognize that the patient has an emotional or feeling-level problem. This is not always easy to do because the patient, afraid and embarrassed, may have clever means of disguising true emotions. What does the patient really feel? Is it anger, hurt, or fear?

Second, the health professional should verbalize to the patient what emotion the latter appears to be expressing, by saying the following: "Mr. Lee, you seem sad today," or "Mrs. Cerosi, I think you must be angry about something. Am I right?" The patient may readily admit to the emotion. If the health professional's guess is wrong, the patient may blurt out what he or she is really feeling. But in some cases the person will, at least initially, deny that anything is the matter.

Third, the patient should be allowed to express his or her true emotion. This, of course, does not mean the patient should be allowed to take advantage of the health professional, to begin throwing objects across the room, or to engage in a "free-for-all!" As in any such relationship, an underlying foundation of mutual respect must be maintained and honored by all involved.

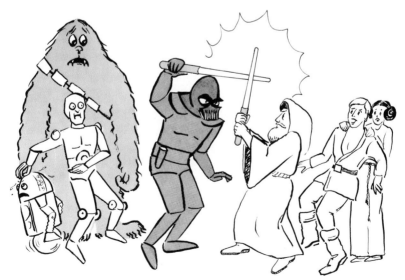

Allowing the patient to express emotions does not mean encouraging a "free-for-all."

The health professional should try to identify common purposes. For instance, the emotion (anger, fear) may be directed toward the health professional or toward some part of the professional services he or she administers. It may be necessary to decide whether the patient's anger will be allowed to interfere with his or her goals. If the emotion has nothing directly to do with the health professional, he or she can direct the patient to someone who can help solve the problem and allay the fear or hostility. In some cases, the pent-up emotion will simply dissipate itself because the health professional is willing to listen to the patient.

The patient is thus in a situation in which he or she may need to reveal some deep-seated feelings without fear of rejection or ridicule. He or she may also need to know that the health professional will try to offer help.

In some instances, then, a patient will reveal himself or herself simply by telling the health professional about personal matters. In other instances, more emotionally charged matters will eventualy erupt. The health professional's response helps to assure the patient that he or she is worthwhile. In that assurance lies the key to professional closeness at its best.

REFERENCES

1. Duryee, J. S.: The therapeutic qualities of professional and non-professional helpers. *Diss. Abstr. Int.* 31:2227, 1970.
2. Greene, H.: *I Never Promised You a Rose Garden.* New York, Holt, Rinehart & Winston, 1964, p. 56.
3. Sarton, M.: *A Reckoning.* New York, W. W. Norton Company, 1978, pp. 200–202.
4. Drew, J., Stoeckle, J. O., and Billings, J. A.: Tips, status and sacrifice: gift giving in the doctor-patient relationship. *Soc. Sci. Med.* 17:399–404, 1983.
5. Keen, S.: *To a Dancing God.* New York, Harper & Row, 1970, p. 73.
6. Conrad, P., and Schneider, J. W. P.: *Deviance and Medicalization. From Badness to Sickness.* St. Louis, C. V. Mosby Company, 1980.
7. Hesse, H.: *Steppenwolf.* Rev. ed. New York, Holt, Rinehart & Winston, 1970.

Part IV Summary

Both health professional and patient enter their potential relationship with a number of needs, expectations, and perceptions. They each also engage to some extent in transference. All these factors are important determinants of the character a given relationship will assume.

The idea of consent is central to the health professional–patient relationship because it is a means of ensuring the patient's liberty in the situation. Also important is the trust between health professional and patient, which produces a feeling of relatedness. In trying to establish trust, the health professional sometimes confuses casualness with closeness. If the health professional and patient act casually toward each other, either no sense of relatedness or a dependent relationship that will be detrimental to one or both of them develops. In some instances, health professionals think that qualities traditionally equated with professionalism create distance in patient–health professional interaction, and that their results will be better if they try to maintain some personal qualities as well. Professional and personal qualities need not be considered incompatible, because they are both complementary components of an integrated whole.

The following are some instances in which professional distance should be maintained: (1) When a patient's loneliness causes him or her to depend on the health professional for more than the latter can or wants to give; (2) when professional persons recognize that they are becoming so involved with a patient that they begin to feel pity for the patient; and (3) when the health professional overidentifies with the patient because of similar problems.

Professional closeness results when there is mutual trust between the patient and the health professional. The latter can promote trust by demonstrating that the patient is a worthwhile person who deserves to be cared for. The health professional can communicate this to the patient by: (1) defining the natural limits of the relationship; (2) paying attention to details that are important to the patient; (3) engaging in self-revelation in such a way that the patient knows what to expect in the relationship; and (4) encouraging the patient to engage in self-revelation, then responding to these revelations in such a way that the patient's worth as a human being is affirmed.

Part IV Questions for Thought and Discussion

1. Mr. Zachary has been treated for several weeks by the attractive young intern Ms. Montgomery. On her birthday, he slips her an envelope as he goes out the door. When she opens it, she finds a birthday card and a check for 25 dollars.
   (a) How should Ms. Montgomery interpret the gratuity?
   (b) What problems may arise between patient and health professional if she returns the money?
   (c) What problems may arise if she keeps the money?
   (d) What details, if any, may you want to know about Mr. Zachary or Ms. Montgomery in order to better interpret Mr. Zachary's action?
2. Mrs. Walters comes to your department for a test. Within the first five minutes that you are with her, she tells you that she is a friend of your co-worker and thinks you should know that your co-worker is sexually promiscuous. According to Mrs. Walters, your co-worker has had three illegal abortions and is currently having an affair with one of the prominent politicians in the city. Your co-worker is pleasant and well liked by both her patients and her colleagues and, as far as

you can discern, she is professionally competent. She does make sure she takes all her sick time whether or not she is sick, but so do a lot of the others.

(a) What should you say to Mrs. Walters when she confronts you with this information?

(b) Should you tell your co-worker what Mrs. Walters has told you? If you do, are you wrongfully betraying what Mrs. Walters has told you in confidence?

(c) What, if any, difference will this information make in your attitude toward your co-worker?

Part V

EFFECTIVE INTERACTION: WORKING WITH PATIENTS IN THE MIDDLE AND LATER YEARS OF LIFE

Part V

In this poem, McKuen proposes a contrast: the raging energy of younger years and the adventure of middle age with a bleak, disintegrating picture of old age. In the next three chapters we will more closely examine the patient who has begun the journey into middle age and the one who has crossed that meadow, into old age. The student will become more aware that neither middle nor old age is all adventure or all bleakness—each has its hills and valleys, and each presents itself as a weighty challenge to the individual.

Part V begins with Chapter 14, which describes the "middle years". It is only in recent times that this life period has been given more than a cursory glance by researchers, and there is still a dearth of information about what happens to people physically, psychologically, and emotionally during these years. It is a complex and important period that the health professional should understand. This chapter also serves as a basis for comparison with the following chapters, in which some issues related to the older population are examined: Chapter 15 discusses some major biological, intellectual, and psychosocial processes that ordinarily take place; and Chapter 16 provides practical applications based on material presented in the previous chapters.

The problems of middle-aged and elderly people are singled out for attention not because they are in any way more important than those of children or young people but because (1) they are less often discussed directly in textbooks of this sort and (2) they often require the attention of a wide range of health professionals.

The information and techniques of effective interaction presented in previous chapters are general enough to be applied to any number of patients. Part V demonstrates how they can be applied specifically to the middle-years and elderly patients. By studying, the reader should more

---

*From Listen to the Warm. New York, Random House, 1967, p. 92. Used by permission of Random House, Inc.

readily be able to understand which factors must be considered in applying the techniques to other types of patients.

In Part V much of the emphasis is on the factors that influence how each type of patient responds to the world. Such factors undoubtedly have a strong influence on the patient during interaction with the health professional.

Chapter 14

THE MIDDLE YEARS

Rod McKuen's poem at the beginning of this Part portrays the middle years* as achievement-oriented, relationship-directed, and adventure-some. His images of "roaring rivers to be crossed" and "wild oats to sow" do correspond closely to the way these years have often been stereotyped, and in many ways the stereotype reflects the actual experiences of this period.

If it is true that of all the life periods the unique facets of this one have been least understood, it follows that health professionals will probably be least adept at interacting effectively with persons in this age group. The relative ease with which health professionals initially approach such people does not ensure that the needs of a person of middle years will then automatically be better met. While ease of initial interaction is an important ingredient in effectiveness, it is not in itself sufficient. For that reason it is important to examine some vital issues concerning life as a middle-years adult in this society.

Most of the critical experiences during the middle years revolve around the concepts of *responsibility* and *achievement,* both of which can be defined in a number of ways. Some "midlife crises" (see page 197) seem to stem from a person's having adequately assumed responsibility and realized his or her achievement potential, while others arise when the individual has failed to do so. Thus, the first section of this chapter examines the ways in which this happens. The second section explores the little understood but important phenomenon of *boredom* as it occurs in the middle years. The third section examines the idea of a midlife crisis or crises. These three sections, taken together, should serve as a useful basis for comparison with the discussion of old age in the next chapters. The final section focuses on some key components of effective interaction between a middle-years patient and the health professional.

Responsibility and Stress

RESPONSIBILITY

A profile of a person in the middle years of life will necessarily involve a consideration of his or her sense of "responsibility." When we

---

*The term "middle years" still really suggests nothing more than a stretch of time existing between the two more significant periods of adolescence and old age. I have adopted this term, however, because of its current usage in the literature.

ask if someone is willing to "assume responsibility," we are concerned with acts that the person *can* and has *voluntarily agreed to do*. Given these conditions of ability and agreement, we want to know whether the person can be trusted to carry out the acts, regardless of whether the agreement was *explicit* (i.e., a promise to abide by the terms of a contract) or *implicit* (i.e., a promise to provide for one's young children once one has brought them into the world).

Underlying the idea of acting responsibly is an assumption that the individual is a free agent who is willing and able to act autonomously. That is, a person coerced into performing an act is not considered to have accepted responsibility for it.

During the middle years, there is another aspect to acting responsibly: It involves having a high regard for the welfare of others. The acts may flow from a free will, but the will must operate in accordance with the reasonable claims and justifiable expectations of other people. The claims of society on a person peak during the middle years, so "acting responsibly" must be interpreted in terms of how completely the person fulfills the conditions of those claims. This seems true not only of our own culture but also of others. For instance, in Hindu culture one stage of acting out a *karma* involves active engagement in the affairs of family and business. Only when one has successfully completed these tasks does one move on to higher, more contemplative levels of existence.

One way to view the matter in our culture is to recall the discussion of values in Chapter 6. The basic value of self-respect was discussed at some length and shown to be among the most essential ingredients of "the good life." During the middle years, most people perceive self-respect as vulnerable to the judgments of others: One's self-respect at least partially depends on the extent to which one commands the respect of one's employer, family, and friends, an idea related to our concept of "reputation"; and one commands respect by giving due consideration to society's claims. Hiltner notes, correcty I believe, that to a large extent even the *personal* values of the middle years must include a regard for others. For most it is a highly social period when interdependencies are complex and pervasive.[1]

Several roles characterize the middle years, giving rise to certain claims upon the person of middle years. However, before examining them in more detail, there is one observation to be made about the present-day person of middle years that distinguishes him or her from like persons in other periods of history: Today some of the psychological components of adolescence are extended to a much later age than during other historical periods. Thus, the 25-year-old individual who feels some of the weight of the societal claims placed on people of middle years may still be financially dependent on his or her parents (or spouse), may still be in school, may be living in the family home, and may still be actively exploring sexual preferences and lifestyles. It is common for a person who attended college and graduate school to be assuming his or her first bona fide work position at age 35. An extended psychological adolescence is more likely to be associated with people in educational programs, though not exclusively so. The delayed acquisition of independence, combined with the earlier physical maturation characteristic of modern cultures and the pressures on young people to "grow up fast," creates much stress both for children who have now reached their middle years and for their older parents.[2] At best, one can conclude that the line between adolescent and middle-year life periods is by no means distinct!

We are ready to turn now to the roles that most fully characterize life during the middle years.

Primary Relationships. It is almost always during the middle years that one decides with whom lasting relationships will be developed. Fortunately, an increasing number of old people are also developing new relationships, but they are usually the ones who were able to sustain deep and lasting relationships in the middle years as well.[3]

The primary relationship takes priority over all others, with the most common type being the relationship with a spouse. Choosing a spouse or other permanent companion and becoming better acquainted—that is, exploring the heights and depths of knowing the person and discovering the potentials and limits, the similarities and differences, and the compatibilities and incompatibilities of the relationship—are processes interwoven with the more basic activities of eating, sleeping, acquiring possessions, working, worshiping, relaxing, and playing together.

Those who do not enter into a marriage relationship sometimes develop deep and lasting involvement with a friend or sibling. One of the health professional's first tasks, especially in an ongoing relationship with the patient of middle years, is to find out if there is a key person and, if so, who he or she is. Too little credence is given to the obvious fact that almost no one exists as an island; particularly in times of crisis that key person is looked to for comfort, sustenance, and guidance. However, sometimes the person whom the health professional assumes would be the most supportive is not the key person. Consider the story of Mary Ogden and Pam Carlisle:

> Mary Ogden, age 51, is a retired single school teacher who is hospitalized for treatment related to severe diabetes. She is adored by the entire small community where she has resided and taught school for 35 years. Through the years she has received numerous awards for community service. She is a cooperative, cheerful person, who, in spite of her illness, continues to be an inspiration to everyone. She is especially fond of Pam Carlisle, the head nurse on the unit where Mary has been treated.
>
> On the afternoon prior to the patient's planned hospital discharge, an unscheduled visitor comes to the nursing desk insisting that she needs to speak to Pam about a highly personal matter. The visitor is Agnes Ogden, an elderly lady who informs Pam that she is the sister (and only living relative) of Mary. The visitor seems sincere and asks that Pam provide details of her sister's condition in order that she might be better prepared to aid her with both her physical illness and her personal affairs. Pam complies with her request, actually feeling

relieved that there is someone to share this burden with her. The following morning Pam visits Mary's room and finds her profoundly irate for the first time. She informs Pam that she has not been on speaking terms with her sister for many years, that she considers her sister to be untrustworthy, and that she thoroughly resents her sister having the knowledge of her personal affairs and illness.

After that, Mary's distrust of Pam never diminished. She became depressed, agitated, and uncooperative.

How could Pam Carlisle have acted differently to foster the trust between her and the patient rather than to destroy it?

What different types of action could Pam Carlisle have taken when Agnes came to her requesting information?

What would you have done?

Parenting. A second role involves caring for children. The current sex role stereotypes assigned to mothering and fathering are breaking down in many families, and the whole range of parenting skills is shared by both parents. The concept of parenting is being expanded, too, by the "single parent," who, because of divorce, death, or having adopted a child as an unmarried person, is providing the full care usually shared by another. Finally, a small but growing number of people are attempting to live within extended family situations in which parenting is shared by several persons. Whatever the difficulties of the various arrangements, all of these people share the awareness that theirs is a society that believes the child's welfare depends on the quality of parenting. The age-old recognition that a child's physical well-being depends on adult care is now buttressed by more recent assertions that the child's potential for fulfillment and satisfaction in later years is also determined by the parent. This position is set forth in the following remarks by an investigator in the area of child development:

> It is my deepest conviction that we must meet the needs of children in our society as they develop. . . . Parents have the capacity to create loving human beings who are productive in society; they also have the capacity to create destructive human beings who commit destructive acts against society. We can usually trace an individual's attempt to gain self-esteem through destructive acts to early parent-child relations.[4]

It is such beliefs that create the overwhelming feelings of guilt in some parents when their children do not follow the path these parents believed was the most beneficial. The complex interplay between parent and adolescent is poignantly portrayed in the diary of a young woman who repeatedly runs away from home and finally dies of a drug overdose. In the book that records her diary, *Go Ask Alice*, the young woman reflects:

> I finally talked to an old priest who really understands young people. We had an endlessly long talk about why young people leave

home, then he called my Mom and Dad. . . . Mom answered the phone in the family room, and Dad ran upstairs to get the extension, and the three of us almost drowned out the connection. I can't understand how they can possibly still own me and still want me, but they do! They do! They do! They were glad to hear from me and to know I am alright. And there were no recriminations or scoldings or lectures or anything. . . .

I don't know how I can treat my family like I have. But I'm going to make it all up to them, I'm through with all the shit. I'm not even going to talk about it or write about it or even think about it anymore. I am going to spend the rest of my entire life trying to please them.[5]*

The least that can be said of parenting relationships is that they are among the most enduring and complex of human interactions. The health professional who fails to consider them in an ongoing relationship with a patient neglects an integral part of the patient's identity.

Work. A third critical role involves the work situation. The achievement aspects of that role will be discussed in the next section. We are here concerned with the responsibilities created by the work role.

The form this responsibility actually takes will depend, of course, on the person's specific environment, job title, and position within a hierarchy. For some, work is primarily in the home; for a great many others, it entails a significant amount of time away from home. Adults in the middle years are judged to spend about a half of their waking hours engaged in work. The kind of work they do largely determines their income, lifestyle, social status, and place of residence.[6] Because of the amount of time and energy expended, the type of factual information one acquires over a lifetime is often largely determined by the working situation. Studies of professional socialization suggest that at least for the white-collar and professional worker the kind of work done also defines the world view.

Work-related responsibilities sometimes differ for men and women. By "work-related" is meant the responsibilities incurred and privileges gained by being a member of the labor force, and not only of the "housewife" force. The reader undoubtedly has observed what most women experience in their work roles: the "reasonable expectations" include not only doing a job equally as well as men but also maintaining the quality and amount of work previously done in the home. This leads many to burnout.[7]

Two types of responsibility are associated with the work role: (1) to do one's job well and (2) to fulfill the reasonable expectations of employer and peers. The professional relationship has the added dimension of helping: One is expected to *help* those who need professional services. These relationships are different from simple friendships in a number of ways, though work relationships can be as lasting, deep, and complex.

---

*From *Go Ask Alice.* © 1971 by Prentice-Hall, Inc. Published by Prentice-Hall, Inc., Englewood Cliffs, New Jersey.

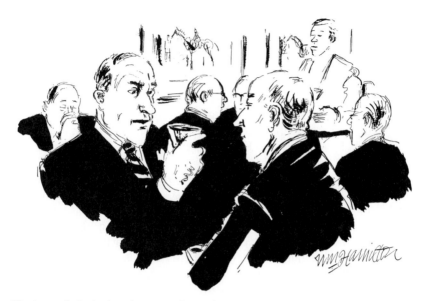

"I've learned a lot in sixty-three years. But, unfortunately, almost all of it is about aluminum."

From *The New Yorker,* November 11, 1977, page 27. Drawing by Wm. Hamilton; © 1977 The New Yorker Magazine, Inc. Used with permission.

(The car pool phenomenon is an intriguing combination of the two; here people who are grouped together for the purpose of getting to and from work also engage in camaraderie over a considerable period of time and more regularly than with their own family members. I have known some car pool members who interact as friends or acquaintances during the commute, then assume their "proper" role with each other within a hierarchial working environment. A study of this phenomenon could lend valuable insights into the work and social relationships characteristic of the middle-years group.)

The health professional's task is to assess how the patient views his or her work situation, particularly the relationships in it. Whether a patient's work involves providing quality child care, laboring on the section crew to replace railroad ties, or presiding over a meeting in the Oval Office, the work entails responsibility toward a job to be done and toward other human beings. Treatment goals must be tailored to help the patient either carry out these responsibilities or accept the fact that it is no longer possible to do so.

Political and Social Activities. Involvement in political and social organizations has traditionally been at a peak during this period. Responsibilities stemming from membership in such organizations are often second only to work in terms of energy consumption and personal commitment. A middle-years person's sense of identity may depend heavily on belonging to a particular political party, religious group, service organization, or honorary society. A telling comment on the significance attached to such associations is the proportion of space given to the listing of them in obituary columns! That old people are making greater efforts to no longer be excluded from such organizations is further testimony to the importance of such affiliations in this society.

There are, of course, other sources of claims on a person in the middle years, but those just listed constitute some highly significant ones.

One additional dimension of the responsibility concept should be discussed briefly. So far I have emphasized responsibility in terms of relationships in the middle years, and have suggested that self-respect during this period is largely determined by meeting the justifiable expectations of others. However, self-respect unquestionably also depends somewhat on believing in and being true to oneself. Thus the person of middle years who meets all the society's expectations can still be unfulfilled.[8] That, in fact, is precisely the plight of many people today who have not pursued personal interests and goals at all, or very minimally. This situation can be viewed as an inability or unwillingness to assume responsibility toward onself, and it leads to a form of the "midlife crisis," which is discussed in a later section. Accepting the consequences of one's behavior is vital; all of us share, to some extent, the problem expressed by the motto on President Truman's desk, "The buck stops here." The sense of "being somebody," such an integral part of adolescence, must in the middle years become more fully defined. In this period one is expected to be able to show more clearly who one is and what one is able to contribute to the welfare of one's loved ones and to society.

STRESS

The more responsibilities one assumes, the more vulnerable one becomes to stress.

Major problems associated with stress of the middle years are finally gaining the attention of investigators, businesses, religious groups, and counseling services. Stress is recognized as a threat to the well-being of the present generation and one that will grow if not stopped.

Chapter 1 discussed some aspects of student stress. Middle-years stress, in its most general form, is somewhat the same. The specific sources differ, but the means by which the child and young person have learned to deal with stress will be carried into adulthood. One significant difference is that in the middle years there is often no clearly defined end to the source of stress—no "gracious exit" out of an impossible situation. The stress attending next week's exam can be more easily managed than that arising from the realization that one has a stressful lifestyle in general.

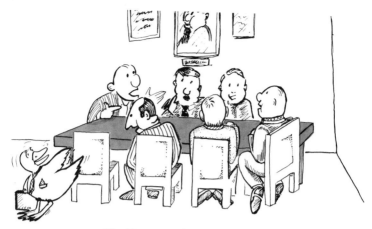

"Ducking out early again, Fenwick?"

Some stresses result from personal life choices. The responsibilities assumed in marriage (and other primary relationships), child-rearing, and work all create stress, as do unemployment and some factors in the social structure itself. Each will be discussed separately.

Primary Relationships. Marriage relationships during the middle years have been studied more extensively than other types of primary relationships, but it is reasonable to believe that they all produce stress situations. Common sources of stress in the marriage relationship include nonfulfillment of role obligations by a spouse, lack of reciprocity between marital partners, and a feeling of not being accepted by one's spouse. Illfeld maintains that sources of stress that are damaging to the marital relationship are composed of an ongoing state of affairs instead of a discrete event. He further proposes that these common mundane stressors in every day life take more of a toll in suffering than does the impact of a dramatic life crisis.[9] Couples with children often experience stress around the departure of "the kids":

> The departure of their children provides a critical challenge to their adaptive faculties, giving an opportunity for new or reclaimed intimacy or increasing distance and chronic loneliness. At the same time the current urban living pattern whereby adults interact but little with the departed children . . . places an even greater demand for intimacy and dependence upon the marital partner. Paradoxically, this requirement occurs at a time when cultural patterns allow greater autonomy and independence to both men and woman. This shift in middle life to an isolated married pair, both members being subjected to forces which they do not share in common, represents a major challenge to the stability of the marriage bond in contemporary life . . .[10]

A more violent expression of stress, the primary source of which may not arise from the relationship itself but is acted out within it, is the "battered spouse" syndrome. Such people are finally receiving attention from self-help groups and other organizations and may well be present among one's patients. For generations they have remained hidden and silent, victimized by the fear of stigmatization and of having no place to go. "Refuges," as they are called, are now springing up around the country, and an increasing number of health professionals are volunteering their services for the treatment and rehabilitation of these women and men.

Parenting. The heavy weight of responsibility associated with parenting also leads to stress situations in the middle years. Child abuse, which is on the increase (or, perhaps, more systematically being reported), is another tragic example of what happens when stress gets out of control. Most stress related to child-rearing leads to less deplorable results, but nonetheless does take its toll on both parent and child.

Work. Finally, stress related to work is, for many individuals in the middle years, primary, manifesting itself in a wide range of disorders. The source of stress may be job dissatisfaction in general, coupled with the notion that there is nowhere else to go. It may be that the job is basically satisfactory but that some component is an ongoing source of stress, such as a co-worker who is a continual "thorn in the flesh." Some jobs are in themselves highly stressful: One of the most studied is employment in an intensive care unit, and another is work in the control tower of an airport.

We will examine, briefly, two of the most serious manifestations of stress in the United States, myocardial infarction (heart attack) and chemical (especially alcohol) abuse. It is difficult to determine all the factors contributing to these disorders, but for many people of middle years, work-related stress is certainly a key one.

Myocardial Infarction. Cardiovascular disease is the number one killer in the United States, responsible for one half of all deaths. Myocardial infarction itself accounts for one third of all deaths[11] and many more persons suffer myocardial infarctions than die from them. Men are especially prone to heart attacks.

The probability of a myocardial infarction occurring is associated with the presence of several risk factors besides being male. Serious risk factors include (1) elevated levels of blood lipids (cholesterol, triglycerides), (2) obesity, (3) hypertension, and (4) cigarette smoking; other significant factors are (5) family history of myocardial infarction, (6) gout, (7) diabetes, (8) physical inactivity, (9) Cardiac Type A Personality, and (10) living in an area where the drinking water is soft. If any two or more of these factors are present, the risk increases dramatically.[12] Purtilo observes:

> The vulnerability of males is maximal between the ages of 35–55 years, the so-called myocardial infarction–prone years, During this time in life the male:female ratio is 5:1. Beyond 55 years the ratio becomes equal.[13]

The "Cardiac Type A Personality" mentioned as a risk factor has been studied extensively. Friedman et al. formulated their and others' findings into one syndrome they called "coronary-prone behavior syndrome." A person exhibiting the symptoms of the syndrome is called a "Type A Person." The traits of this Type A Person include achievement orientation, perfectionism, inability to relax easily, commitment to a job or profession, high energy, aggressiveness, and a sense of time urgency. Not all aspects have to be present for a person to be considered Type A.[14]

A number of studies have been conducted to assess the psychological effects of myocardial infarction. One discouraging finding is that the heart attack itself is a source of additional stress.[15] Stress is also increased by loss of job and other securities, and especially by the threat of the heart attack to self-esteem:

> Typical was a 40-year-old accountant who cheerily greeted the consultant with the information that his admission was "a big hoax." He was healthy all his life, he said, so much so that his friends referred to him as "the bull," but as he talked he became sober and his face fell. "When I get back home, I'll be walking down the street and someone will point me out and whisper, 'there goes another guy with a heart attack at the age of 40, check him off the list!' "[16]

Clearly, the physical and psychological dynamics of myocardial infarction need still to be much explored. It is certain, nonetheless, that the health professional who works in an adult health care facility or treats adult patients in their homes will meet those who have suffered myocardial infarctions and should therefore bear in mind their special needs.

Alcoholism. A second major stress-related disorder is abuse of alcohol. It, too, is a highly complex disorder with physical, mental, and social dimensions.[17] Although by no means exclusively a problem for the person of middle years, the majority of the at least 4 million alcoholics in the United States are in this age group.

A pervasive theme in American society is the illusion that alcohol is an "enabler" and a means of decreasing stress, a point not missed by cartoonists and other social commentators. Nonetheless, more persons in their fifties die from alcoholic cirrhosis than at any other age, the mortality rate during this period being 50 per 100,000 in the United States.[18] It is supposedly higher for black people than for white below the age of 45. It is also generally maintained that alcoholism is higher in men than in women, though those statistics are being questioned by some who suspect that it is reported more often in males. Alcoholics Anonymous, suspecting this to be true, has recently waged a campaign urging women to "come out of the closet" about their drinking problem. This group and others are aware of the special fear, shame, and social stigma that women alcoholics experience and that discourage them from

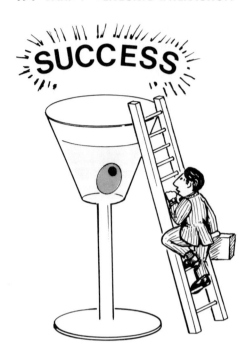

seeking help. In fact, the stigma attached to being an alcoholic is undoubtedly one reason why the disorder is allowed to progress so far before help is sought by both men and women.

Why some people are especially prone to alcoholism is largely still an open question despite the wealth of research being conducted in this area. Better understood are the wide-ranging physical symptoms, the most common of which include cirrhosis of the liver, pancreatic dysfunction, peripheral neuropathies, and encephalopathy.[19]

Alcoholism manifests itself in such social symptoms as accidents, crime and family disruption. The person who presents with alcoholism at the health facility will be bringing not only physical symptoms but also social symptoms.

Thus, myocardial infarction and alcoholism account for an immense amount of suffering in the middle years. Both are known to be responses, in large part, to stress.[20] The reader thus should become acquainted with the latest information on the theory, diagnosis, treatment, and care of both disorders beyond what has been included in this book.

Unemployment. A particular form of stress related to the work role is caused by the *inability* to work. Unemployment, a major problem of the present decade, is taking its toll in human resources. The increase in admissions to mental hospitals in the last five years has been greatest among men in their middle years who have lost their jobs and cannot find work. Moreover, in a society that rewards its members for gainful employment, the stress of working seems no less threatening to health and well-being than the stress of being unemployed.

Social Structure. In addition to *personal* stress in the middle years, yet another source of stress arises from the changing social structure. For instance, a medical journal recently had on the cover: **Watch out, guys! The women are c~~oming~~ here!**[21]

Affirmative action, equal opportunity employment policies, and an overall increasing consciousness of the importance of including all types of persons in the labor force are pushing at long-held prejudices and conceptions of the "place" of women, blacks, old people, and others.

Societally induced stress is produced by the awareness that institutional arrangements are changing: Young people are living together without getting married; the Roman Catholic liturgy is sung in English instead of Latin; schools don't teach what they used to, and much of what they do teach is done on a computer. Basic organizational foundations that have always been taken for granted in the person's life are, like Humpty Dumpty, breaking apart. The fear is that they, again like Humpty Dumpty, cannot be put together again.

Thus it becomes evident that the middle years, in which a person is in many ways at his or her prime, are also years of responsibility and stress. Although these years are sometimes characterized as a plateau, they are much more varied than that: They are packed, instead, with alpine meadows, treacherous cliffs, cool blue pools, and swift undercurrents.

Boredom

The assumption of responsibility toward others and oneself best characterizes the primary task of the middle years. We have noted that taking on responsibility sometimes creates stress, at great cost to one's body and spirit. But the end result of accepting responsibility is achievement and the hope of reaching one's goals is enough to spur most people on.

There is, however, an apparently "unmotivated" type of person who may have been well on the way to meeting his or her goals and may have even achieved them. But this person has genuinely lost sight of what all the excitement was about! Such people are suffering from a pervasive but little understood phenomenon of the middle years, *boredom*. It must be emphasized that these are not people who have had no goals; rather, these are individuals whose energy to continue their pursuit of goals suddenly and inexplicably dissipates. A feeling for all that was important suddenly goes numb.

It is characteristic of a Pollyanna society such as ours to believe that satisfaction and happiness flow down to refresh one on the endless treadmill of pursuit. Entirely missing from such conceptions is the possibility that, even in success, a shadow that chills rather than refreshes creeps over the spirits of many people. The French call it *ennui*. The ancient Romans referred to it as *taedium*. One contemporary theologian suggests that in modern society it is "the common cold of the psyche."[22]

Basically, boredom is a type of stress, though it is seldom thought of as such. Like all types of stress, it is perceived to exert a power over our lives: We so often say, "I was bored to death" or "This boredom is driving me to tears." Anyone who has seen Beckett's play *Waiting for Godot* knows how much tension can build between two men sitting on a park bench with nothing to do but wait!

Almost everyone has looked back at some experience and wondered why it seemed so important at the moment, in light of what one feels about it now! Boredom is that state in which a person's reflection on the whole of his or her life is met with the same astonishment. A man may ask, "Is that what all that striving has been for? Is this *it* for me?" He scatters his resources around his feet, like toys from a toy box, and now gapes into the empty void for that one surprise that would have captured his attention but isn't there.

Not much is understood about boredom or the toll that it takes on an individual's life. There are now efforts to assess the causes and effects of boredom related to certain jobs such as assembly line work or tollbooth collection, but it remains to be understood why many people in apparently interesting positions also experience it.

Some investigators believe that future generations of middle-years adults will be yet more susceptible to boredom than the present ones. Their prediction is based on the observation that ours is increasingly a society designed to alleviate the first hollow surge of boredom with a distraction of some sort: As children, we go to computer camp, or sports camp, or music lessons, or football practice or ballet, or to the computerized games room at the shopping mall. As adults, we switch on the

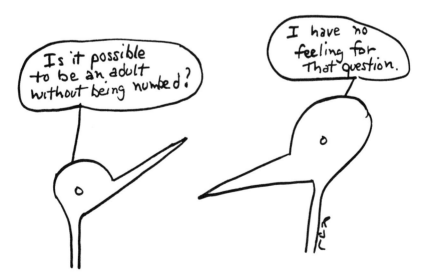

Cartoon by Robert Jay Lifton from *Living and Dying* by Robert Jay Lifton and Eric Olson. © 1974 Robert Jay Lifton and Eric Olson. Permission to reprint granted by Praeger Publishers, Inc., a Division of Holt, Rinehart and Winston.

TV, run to the shopping center, call someone on the CB radio, or get stoned. But investigators are concerned because these stopgap measures do little but assuage a superficial symptom while the underlying problem, whatever it may be, deepens.

Of course, all age groups experience periods of boredom. But it appears that the boredom of the middle years is more tenacious and profound. Fortunately, not everyone experiences it, but those upon whom it settles like a cloud are among the most unhappy people in this age group. They find it especially hard to gain sympathy because they are often people who *apparently* "have everything one could want," or are in a survival situation where there is little time for such "luxuries" as feeling sorry for someone who has the "blahs."

Like depression, this form of stress is difficult to overcome because one's energy is too low to remember what to do to get out of the situation! One of the most important things the health professional can do is to persist in trying to help the patient get interested in some task, if even for a brief period. This effort may facilitate any possible move out of the void and into new or revitalized activity.

Doubt at the Crossroads

The task of assuming responsibility and its attendant stresses, the great desire to achieve, and the boredom that overtakes one may all combine at some critical moment to create a genuine crisis situation. The feeling accompanying the experience is most clearly expressed as *doubt*. It differs from the vacuous zero-point of boredom and lacks the volcanic fervor of other types of stress. Doubt allows no rest; indeed, it is a relentless churning that nakedly reveals almost all the dimensions of one's life. The masks that have allowed the masquerade to go on, the clatter that has accompanied the parade, the walls that have kept fearful monsters from view all suddenly evaporate and leave a pregnant silence. The self stands alone.

This midlife crisis has received more attention than many other components of existence during the middle years. Numerous theories have been set forth to explain what happens, most of them reflecting, as I have just done, that it is a period of expanding more fully into one's life-space. It is a head-on look in the mirror.

It is widely agreed that almost all people of middle years experience the crisis in one form or another. Judith Viorst, a poet, describes various facets of the experience, all of which are summed up in the title of her collection: *How Did I Get to Be Forty and Other Atrocities.*[23]

The experience itself, characterized by doubt, has a paradox built into it. The paradox is expressed more aptly by the German phrase *Torschlusspanik* than by any comparable English phrase I can find. *Torschlusspanik* means "the panic (or rush toward) the gates." Ostensibly, the state-owned apartments in parts of Germany are locked at 11 o'clock, and any hapless resident who fails to return home by then must find a park bench for the night. Thus, as 11 o'clock nears, those residents still on the outside muster tremendous energy in an effort to get everything done and still make it to the gates before it is too late. On the one hand, the challenge is terrific; on the other, the dread is overwhelming. The experience is one in which both the potential for completing or achieving one's goals and the clearly defined limits of those goals are brought simultaneously into focus.

Sheehy, who more than any other person has brought the crisis of the middle years to public attention, concludes from her research that the *Torschlusspanik* happens between the ages of 35 and 45 for most. She calls it the "deadline decade," brought on by the moment of confronting the certainty of one's own death for the first time.[24]

More central to Sheehy's work, and worthy of consideration here, is her basic assumption that the middle years are *not* marked by one great "middle-age crisis" as previously believed, but rather by a whole series of such "passages." Adults, like children and adolescents, progress through a series of developmental stages, each with its particular form of what I have been calling "doubt." Time and again, she contends, we call into question where we are, molt parts of our old skins, peer gingerly at new possibilities, and deal with new limitations.[25] Judging from the number of people in their middle years who have responded to her book by commenting, "It's nice to be understood by a book," she has probably contributed significantly to the understanding of life processes in the middle years. It may be the catalyst that has been needed to further the work of Erikson, Freskel, Brunswick, Mead, and a few others who, all along, have been suggesting some of the things she has made more explicit.

Although some people never resolve the ambivalent factors brought into focus during the crises of the middle years, fortunately most do. Some emerge from the process with a new job, a new mate, and a new life view. Others gain a revitalized perspective of life as it existed before that struggle.

It was mentioned earlier that some people, particularly married women in this society, never really establish an identify for themselves. For them, therefore, the struggle is not one of reclaiming the vision of their lives, but rather of claiming their vision for the first time. In essence, they combine some parts of the adolescent and middle-years passages into one short furious burst. Regardless of whether a vision is being claimed or reclaimed, however, it seems that surviving the throes of the experience prepares the person of middle years in a dramatic way for the adjustments and opportunities still to come.

Working With the Patient of Middle Years

The reader has by now ascertained that this chapter deals almost exclusively with the psychosocial processes of the middle years rather than with biological and intellectual processes. The fact is that, to a large extent, the problems associated with the middle years are primarily psychosocial ones.

This is not to suggest that intellectual or biological processes in the middle years are of no concern to the health professional. To the contrary, they can become preoccupations of a patient, especially if they are perceived to be weakening. Take, for example, some physical factors. It is during this period that the pure joy of physical activity experienced in younger years acquires a sober edge. My husband, who for years has enjoyed running just for the sport of it, told his friend the other night, "Yeah, my running will probably guarantee that I live five years longer, but I will have spent that five years running!" Certainly, the person who experiences a myocardial infarction similarly thinks about exercise and physique in a new light. Finally, smoking brings on a number of physical problems that cause concern. The adverse effects of smoking on health increase significantly in the 45 to 55 year range, with the death rate for smokers increasing more than twice as much as that for nonsmokers.[26]

However, in spite of all these concerns related to physical processes, the psychosocial ones are still primary to the person of middle years. Of what consequence is this to the health professional?

First, consider the physical processes. The person of middle years who arrives at the health facility is, in almost all cases, experiencing a *physical* symptom. Because existence during the middle years is not "supposed to be" characterized by physical symptoms, at least to the extent that aches and pains are expected to be part of old age, such a person may feel especially angered or confused by this physical intrusion into the work of being a responsible person and pursuing goals! A woman of middle years who was being interviewed recently in a seminar reported that she had "bow-and-arrow" disease. The doctor had told her that she had multiple myeloma, a bone marrow disease, but the way she heard her diagnosis more accurately expresses how many people experience their illness or injury. The images of "being struck down" in one's prime and of the "untimely accident or death" are pervasive for this age group. The denial, hostility, depression (and usually all three) that patients feel about being so attacked are factors to which the health professional will have to give much attention, whether the meeting occurs only once or extends over a long period of time. Recall, for instance, the "bull" in the earlier section of this chapter who initially insisted to the hospital personnel that his admission was a big hoax! Simply treating such a person as though he were crazy does nothing to help him move toward recovery or adjustment.

Second, because the psychological and social processes are preeminently important for the person of middle years, treatment must be attuned to them. Of all the losses described in Chapter 4, the loss of independence most epitomizes the overall loss experienced by the patient in middle life. Of course, the former self-image is greatly threatened too, but this is almost a direct outgrowth of the loss of independence: The patient who no longer can go about meeting the responsibilities expected of him or her and pursuing the numerous life goals now established will usually feel trapped, vulnerable, and frustrated. The primacy of these concerns in adult middle life helps the health professional to understand why a patient is seemingly overconcerned about having to get a baby sitter for an hour or having to be home at a given time, or why he or she is willing to forgo treatment rather than take time from work for a trip to the health facility.

Furthermore, the patient experiencing acute stress, including the type expressed as boredom, poses special problems and challenges. Each patient must be treated according to the particular manifestations of the stress, and a suggestion for helping the bored patient was provided. In general, however, the most important thing to keep in mind is that many patients of middle years will be experiencing the types of stress discussed. Part of the health professional's role is to assess how much of the physical symptom arises from the stressful situation itself. This, of course, must often be done with a psychiatrist, but not always. Indeed, listening to what is on a patient's mind may not only help to decrease his or her anxiety at the moment but also enable the health professional to make minor adjustments in schedule, routine, or approach that will further diminish it.

Many of the suggestions made throughout this book apply to all age groups. However, the alert health professional who is keyed to some of the central concerns and roles of middle life may well find that effectiveness with the patient of middle years is heightened.

In the next chapter we will examine some changes that are faced by the person who has successfully lived through the middle years. As the reader will see, these changes involve some of life's biggest challenges, both positive and negative.

REFERENCES

1. Hiltner, S.: Personal values in the middle years. In Ellis, E. O. (ed.): The Middle Years. Acton, Mass., Publishing Sciences Group, 1974, pp. 27–34.
2. Pearlin, L. I.:The social contexts of stress. In Goldberger, L., and Breznitz, S. (eds.): Handbook of Stress: Theoretical and Clinical Aspects. New York, The Free Press, 1982, pp. 324–375.
3. Huyck, M. H.: Sex gender and aging. Humanitas 13:83–89, 1977.
4. Salk, L.: Parenting—the hope of the future. In Ellis, E. O. (ed.): The Middle Years. Acton, Mass., Publishing Sciences Group, 1974, pp. 47–60.
5. Go Ask Alice. Englewood Cliffs, N. J., Prentice-Hall, 1971, p. 105.
6. Tasto, D., and Colligan, M.: Health consequences of shiftwork. DHEW (NIOSH) Publication No. 78-154. Washington, D.C., U.S. Government Printing Office, 1978.
7. McGow, J.: Women and the history of American technology. Signs: A Journal of Women in Culture and Society. 7(4):798–828, 1982.
8. Moos, R. H., and Billings, A.: Conceptualizing and measuring coping resources and processes. In Goldberger, L., and Breznitz, S. (eds.): Handbook of Stress: Theoretical and Clinical Aspects. New York, The Free Press, 1982, pp. 212–230.
9. Illfeld, F. W.: Marital stressors, coping styles and symptoms of depression. In Goldberger, L., and Breznitz, S. (eds.): Handbook of Stress: Theoretical and Clinical Aspects. New York, The Free Press, 1982, pp. 482–495.

10. Smith, D., and Bierman, E. (eds.): *The Biologic Ages of Man: From Conception Through Old Age.* Philadelphia, W. B. Saunders Company, 1973, p. 156.
11. Purtilo, D. T.: *A Survey of Human Diseases.* Menlo Park, Calif.: Addison-Wesley, 1978, p. 261.
12. *Ibid.*, p. 264.
13. *Ibid.*, p. 264.
14. Eliot, R. S.: *Stress and the Major Cardiovascular Disorders.* Mount Kisco, N. Y., Futura Publishing Company, 1979.
15. Roskies, E.: Stress management of type A individuals. In Meichenbaum, D., and Jaremko, M. E. (eds.): *Stress Reduction and Prevention.* New York, Plenum Press, 1983, pp. 261–288.
16. Cassem, N. H., and Hackett, T. P.: Psychological rehabilitation of myocardial infarction patients in the acute phase. *Heart Lung* 2:382–388, 1973.
17. Pohorecky, L. A., and Brick, J. (eds.): *Stress and Alcohol Use.* New York, Elsevier Biomedical, 1983.
18. Smith, D., and Bierman, E. (eds.): *Op. cit.,* p. 160.
19. Pohorecky, L. A., and Brick, J. (eds.): *Op. cit.*
20. Institute of Medicine: *Report of a Study: Research on Stress and Human Health.* Washington, D.C., National Academy Press, 1981, pp. 217–221 and 244–246.
21. Howard, R. B.: Watch out, guys: the women are coming here. *Postgrad. Med.* 73(4):13–19, 1983.
22. Keen, S.: Chasing the blahs away: boredom and how to beat it. *Psychology Today,* May 1977, pp. 78–84.
23. Viorst, J.: *How Did I Get to be Forty and Other Atrocities.* New York, Simon & Schuster, 1976.
24. Sheehy, G.: *Passages: Predictable Crises of Adult Life.* New York, E. P. Dutton & Company, 1976.
25. *Ibid.*
26. Office of Smoking and Health: *The Health Consequences of Smoking: Cancer.* A Report of the Surgeon General. Publ. #82-50179. Washington, D.C., U.S. Government Printing Office, 1982.

Chapter 15

THE LATER YEARS

There are three generations of people over 65 years of age in the United States; about 26 million of these are 65 years or older, 10 million are older than 75 years, and 2.25 million are older than 85 years.[1] In many instances, the younger generation of the two cares for the older. One of the grave problems confronting this author and anyone who attempts to speak of old people is the inability to define whether or not a person is old. According to many statements on social policy, eligibility for financial and other supportive benefits begins at age 65, but the usefulness of this age as a distinguishing line ends there. In fact, people's feelings that they are "old" may be as much determined by the presence of sickness, disability, or other factors as by their chronological age.[2] In the following chapters, the ages for study groups will be given when possible, but in most cases 65 was used as the age dividing young and middle years from old.

Almost every generality advanced about the old person is quickly countered by an individual's personal experience with a chronologically old man or woman. To the generalities necessary in a book of this sort, the astute reader will find exceptions from his or her own experience. However, some *processes* taking place in a person as he or she advances in years basically differ little from one individual to another. Whenever possible, these basic processes will be emphasized so that aging can be viewed as a process that begins at birth and ends with death. In that perspective, the *aged* will be those people in whom the process has taken place over a period of many years. Aging involves biological, intellectual, and psychosocial processes. This chapter is devoted to a brief explanation of each, with an emphasis on the psychosocial processes, especially as they are relevant to effective interaction.

Biological Processes of Aging

Some theories that attempt to explain why biological aging takes place are as follows: (1) Genetic theories state that changes are due to genetically controlled activating and deactivating mechanisms. (2) Counterpart theories propose that changes are due to pressures imposed upon a species. Aging processes are counterparts to earlier developmental processes that were put into motion before the individual was born. (3) Accident theories assume that changes are due to the wear and tear or to all the random accidents inflicted on the body, mind, and environment. Many researchers combine parts of these theories to form other new theories. All of them, however, consider the aging process to be universal, decremental, and progressive.

One's first impression that a person is old is often based on physical appearance; one may say: "He looks old for his age," "To look at her you'd never guess she was that old," "He certainly has aged in the last couple of years."

The search for possible means of slowing down biological aging is a lucrative business today. Currently, several pharmaceutical companies are known to be conducting tests with a series of compounds in attempts to identify an agent that will affect the basic processes of aging. Serious ethical questions can be raised about a drug whose side effects may include (1) an increase in the size of the labor force, (2) a change in the lifestyle of the population, (3) the creation of new intergenerational family relationships, and (4) the bankruptcy of the Social Security Administration![3] At any rate, a key question posed by researchers, clinicians, and gerontologists is: What actually causes the biological changes associated with the aging process?

One biological-aging theory presently receiving considerable attention was advanced by Nobel laureate F. M. Burnett. He suggests that aging is due to an autoimmune process in which there is an exhaustion of the cell quota for the body's immune system; the body thus becomes more vulnerable to attack from both outside and within.[4]

The health professional should be aware of research being conducted in geriatrics. As more is understood about biological aging, the health professional can do more to diminish its detrimental effects. Indeed, biological aging traditionally has been thought of as essentially irreversible and intrinsic to all members of a species, such that with the passage of time, they become increasingly unable to cope with the stress of the environment. This idea of the relentless march "downhill" is being questioned by many today. As one writer puts it,

> As we scan the time slope of our existences, it seems wise to inquire, at least occasionally, whether the decay curve contains within it any elements that may be subject to active intervention. It is clearly important to differentiate the intrinsic, as yet inscrutable, time-dependent forces that underlie aging from those extrinsic factors that have an impact on the aging organism. As recently as a few years ago, arteriosclerosis was held to be an inevitable consequence of the aging process that was, in effect, an expression of "God's will." We now identify arteriosclerosis as a disease, as surely as tuberculosis, and thus subject to precise definition and prevention.[5]*

During professional preparation, the student will undoubtedly study the specific biological changes in the process of human development and aging in detail.

---

*From J.A.M.A., 248:1203, 1982. Reproduced by permission of the American Medical Association.

Intellectual Processes of Aging

There is a myth that intellectual deterioration is an inevitable consequence of being old, resulting in senility or second childhood. This destructive stereotype of the aging process is false. Under some circumstances, intellectual functions decline. However, recent research indicates that old persons who remain physically well are less likely to have a marked decline in intellectual functioning and that the intellectual changes vary in rate from one individual to another. One recent estimate is that approximately 10 per cent of persons 65 years and older have clinically important intellectual impairment.[6] The health professional is well advised to approach each patient with an open mind about this matter.

LEARNING ABILITY

People learn at different rates, but this difference in rate is not always due to differences in age, rather being attributable to the whole gamut of human differences. Rigidity is one deterrent to effective learning at any age. With increasing age, the majority of individuals do become more rigid or "set in their ways" as one way of coping with stress.[7]

There is some difference of opinion about the basis for an older person's rigidity. Carl Eisdorfer suggests that an older person's reluctance to engage in risk-taking behavior may be due to a fear of failure:

> . . . The possibility that "fear of failure" replaces the "need to achieve" as a motivating force in older individuals cannot be ignored. It has fairly dramatic implications for the general behavior patterns of older individuals. If an achievement-oriented motivation characterizes much of middle and upper-middle class Western behavior, then it might be expected that in older individuals, when positive reinforcement begins to be replaced by negative feedback (through loss of abilities, social change, displacement of the job by younger, better-trained persons, or whatever) a shift from a more aggressive posture to a more defensive posture might be to defensively limit the response in order to avoid failure rather than to respond in the hope of being successful.[8]

The health professional must set up treatment or diagnostic situations that pose no major threat to the patient's faltering self-esteem. This can be achieved by assessing the older person's abilities and by pacing the amount and content of information so that success is almost guaranteed, particularly in early attempts.

A second insight to be gained from these studies on learning and anxiety is that an older person should not be *expected* to be anxious in a new situation. The health professional must not project anxiety onto the older person. There are many ways in which older people are products of self-fulfilling prophecy, and the health professional's expectation that the older person will be anxious may be enough to convince him that he *should* be.

ACQUISITION OF SKILLS

Many aspects of health care are concerned with helping people to acquire skills to function adequately in society. These skills range from functional or diversional psychomotor skills to those in communications and interpersonal relationships.

An important distinction must be made between learning ability and acquisition of skills. Learning is a *process*, while skill is a *performance*. Therefore, a person may have ability to process information necessary for acquiring a skill, but may not actually be able to perform the skill. Conversely, some people need to have information given more slowly or repeated many times, but once they get the idea, they are perfectly able to perform the skill. Thus a direct relationship does not always exist between *ability to learn* and actual *performance* of a skill. In working with older people, it is important not to confuse their learning ability with their performance ability. One or both functions may be impaired, but the two must not automatically be interchanged.

Some older persons appear to have decreased learning ability because they are physically slow. This is not at all a decrease in ability but a slowing of motor function or performance. Speed of perception, of initiating a response, and of movement are all affected by the neural changes due to aging.[9]

The inexperienced or impatient health professional may give up on a person long before maximal performance has been reached, or may interpret the patient's test results incorrectly because physical slowness has been interpreted as inability to perform a given skill. This is damaging to the patient's self-esteem and may be detrimental to his or her potential for better functioning.

In conclusion, some facets of intellectual functioning generally decrease with age, but these are not the same for, and do not progress at a given rate in, every individual. The danger lies in stereotyping the patient's responses rather than discerning whether there is some difficulty with the *ability* to learn or some motor problem hindering *performance* of the skill.

Psychosocial Processes of Aging

The days of over-the-river-and-through-the-woods-to-grandmother's-house have disappeared in large segments of today's society. Indeed, grandmother often discourages the visit because it will interfere with her scuba-diving lesson or her scheduled speech at a meeting concerning newly proposed city ordinances.

Where did grandmother go? Did the big bad wolf eat her? Did she at last find the Fountain of Youth? Neither grandmother nor grandfather has gone anywhere. They are both where the old person has always been—at the other side of time. It is society that has gone somewhere; the rapid societal changes taking place around older people give them greater opportunity for divergent roles than ever before. If they are unable to take advantage of these opportunities, as many are, then they are burdened with greater insecurity and more complex problems than were any of their predecessors. However, if they can make the best of these opportunities, their potential for an active and meaningful old age is excellent. One such fortunate person is Margaret Ray. An article in the *New York Post* reports:

> Mrs. Ray, 80, made her nightclub singing debut last night after "75 years of preparation." She has a rather unique perspective on time. . . . Accompanied on piano by John Wallowitch, Mrs. Ray came equipped for the three-night engagement with such hits as "The Baggage Car Ahead," and "She's More to be Pitied Than Censured." Both tunes go back to the 1880's. "I always wanted to sing," she said. "I just never had time before. It takes time to raise three children."[10]

Some basic psychological and social processes are evident in the widely divergent lifestyles of today's older people. Erik Erikson proposes that the success with which an older person can make psychological and social adjustments will depend on his or her ability to meet the major crisis of old age—that of integrity. Integrity is characterized by total acceptance of one's past and present ways of life, with no substitutions. The older person's integral strength "takes the form of that detached yet active concern with life bounded by death, which we call wisdom in its many connotations from ripened 'wits' to accumulated knowledge, mature judgment and inclusive understanding. . . ."[11]

Health professionals are delighted, sometimes awed, by an older person who expresses the breadth and depth of acceptance described by Erikson. These older people readily accept the psychological and social adjustments that confront them. However, older persons often seem to despair of being old; the psychological and social adjustments of old age overwhelm them, and they find little from their past to support them in their present situation. These people have not succeeded in meeting the crisis of integrity. Key psychological and social processes assist in or deter from achieving a sense of wholeness and integratedness in old age. Some of these are discussed on the following pages.

FRIENDSHIP AND FAMILY TIES

Older people vary greatly in the amount of contact they maintain with their families and friends. Many persons lose a valuable source of natural physical contact and companionship with the diminution of friendship and family ties, while others remain actively involved. The health professional should learn to assess how much of the patient's need for physical contact, among other needs, is still being met by friends and family.

Friendships. Until the present ultramobile way of life, the acquisition of a single set of friends continued throughout early life and tapered off when one settled down in a community. One's job seldom changed during the entire period of employment, and, as a result, the community (and the friends therein) remained the same up to old age. In one sense, this is a secure mode of existence, but reliance on lifelong friendship carries with it the risk that if these friends all die, the person will be left alone. Many people dependent on lifelong friendships find it impossible to make new acquaintances at 70 or 80 years of age.

One theory of aging, the disengagement theory, suggests that even before their friends die, some people contribute to their own isolation. Henry and Cummings, who first proposed the theory, define "disengagement" as "an inevitable process in which many of the relationships between a person and other members of society are severed, and those remaining are altered in quality."[12] They view disengagement as a normal process that occurs earlier for some than for others, depending on the person's physiology, temperament, personality, and life situation. Retirement, they proposed, is society's permission for men to disengage, while widowhood serves the same purpose for women; the disengaged person eventually develops a high morale.[13]

Subsequent studies have challenged the conclusion that "disengagement" is desirable. Perhaps the old people in the Henry and Cummings study were well adjusted in that state, the doubters assert, but they were all white, middle-class, healthy, and economically independent. Levine concluded from her own study that disengagement by the elderly in low-income neighborhoods was involuntary, caused by the individual's inability to make new contacts (because he or she could not afford transportation, was not asked to join in activities, and so forth) and resulted in a low morale.[14]

These disengagement studies have been conducted on an elderly population who grew up in an era when mobility was not the way of life it now is. It will be interesting, in 20 or 30 years, to note the engagement patterns of older people who have known nothing but mobility. Already a new pattern can be seen in the movement toward retirement or senior citizen communities. Middle- and upper-middle-class old people are moving to those parts of the country whose climates are conducive to their health. In the process, whole cities are being created. The possible result of this new pattern is that these old people will not disengage from others their own age, but rather only from younger generations. However, it can be speculated that persons economically or physically unable to become a part of such communities will continue to live alone, with families or in low-income housing, unless they join the thousands of old people already living in nursing homes. Thus, unfortunately all but those in upper-middle-class retirement communities will continue to live in an environment generally not favorable to the development of new and lasting friendships. If this is the case, the increased mobility of society will benefit only those who are well-to-do.

The old person's ability to make new friends depends partly on the extent to which friendship has been considered an important individual value throughout life and therefore on the extent to which friendship skills have been cultivated. Another important determinant is the type of friendships the person established in younger years. The quality of relationships seems key:

> It seems that it is not "how often" or with "how many" one interacts, but rather under what circumstances, for what purposes, with what degree of intimacy and caring the interaction takes place that will have its impact on morale. As in other areas of life, we have been working from the assumption that "more is better." In the case of social involvement, we find that abundance is not necessarily associated with the more positive life adjustment of older people.[15]

There are basically four types of friendship, which vary in number and importance over the years: (1) *Fusion* friendships, fused to other roles such as those involving family or occupation, increase or decrease in importance according to the person's present situation. (2) *Substitution* friendships are those into which the person channels energies that formerly were directed toward someone or something else. (3) *Complementary* friendships develop from situations in which another role (such as that related to occupation) and the friendship are mutually supportive. (4) *Competition* friendships are those that compete with another role.[16]

Therefore, an older person whose *fusion* or *complementary* friendship, made at an early age, centered on his or her occupation may find that after retirement the friend is very much alive but their friendship is dead. Conversely, a *substitution* or *competition* friendship may thrive after retirement, because energy directed elsewhere can now be devoted to the friend. In this sense, the basis of a friendship is an important determinant of its longevity.

Family. For most people in Western society, the immediate family includes a spouse and children, and participation in that unit is one of the most lasting and significant roles a person assumes.

In the early years of marriage, a husband and wife spend much time alone together. When their children are born, the attention is transferred to them, and for the next 20 years or more, much of the husband-wife communication takes place in the presence of at least one child. Only after the children have left home are the man and woman alone again. Their attempts to re-establish direct communications are often futile, causing them to withdraw, literally or symbolically, from the family structure. Either of them may leave the spouse or commit suicide, may become absorbed in a hobby or social organization, or may escape into reminiscence about the good old days. (The great importance of reminiscence in helping a person to accept old age is discussed later in this chapter.)

Many parents find it difficult to remain deeply involved with their grown children. Some are afraid that a situation involving close contact with their children denotes dependence or loss of self-dependence. Others find that family relationships are too demanding; the older person who cannot communicate effectively with his or her spouse after the children leave home may find that communication with adult children is also strained.

In the present older population, married women are generally less equipped to cope with financial and other business affairs because, in their day, it was considered improper for them to be thus involved. But men tend to die younger than women (there are four women to every three men over 65 years of age in the United States),[17] so the unfortunate result is that many widows are totally unprepared to manage alone in their later years.

A discussion of aging and family relationships must include a look at who is most likely to provide support for older people in times of illness. A recent study of 167 post-hospitalized patients aged 65 years and older showed that a "principle of substitution" dominated the support system; that is, family members were available in serial order rather than acting all together as a shared-functioning unit.[18]

It is usually assumed that older people with children can look to the children for support. Therefore, consider the position of the adult children of today's elderly people. Although the stereotype of the children who ruthlessly abandon their old parents to nursing homes is sometimes justified, more often children do try to take care of needy parents and are caught in the middle financially: Both their elderly parents and their own children are economically dependent on them. The health professional is often consulted by a distressed person attempting to figure out how to provide for a chronically ill parent while trying to send his or her own children to college. In all cases, the health professional can listen sympathetically and can often direct the person to a social worker, charitable organization or other resource.[19]

Although much emphasis is placed on the offspring's capacity to provide support, the spouse is the major deterrent to institutionalization and is expected to be the primary caregiver even if he or she also is somewhat incapacitated.[20] Among the widowed, the child is the one who gives support, more often than do siblings or friends.[21] Only among the unmarried childless are other relatives (and friends) observed to provide at least perfunctory care.[22]

Health professionals sometimes don't realize that a relative other than a spouse or child can be central to the elderly person's life. Failure to acknowledge this can damage the relationship between health professional and old person; in addition, the health professional may be overlooking an important resource in the patient's treatment.

LOSSES

In the following section, the losses described in Chapter 4 will be discussed as they apply specifically to the old person today.

Loss of Former Self-Image. Many older people, deprived of meaningful family, friendship, or occupational ties, and experiencing the stigma of old age, feel they are relics from another era, whose only use is to be displayed for the entertainment of the present generation. In John Updike's novel, such a feeling is expressed by the elderly inhabitants of the poorhouse, as they watch the townspeople coming through the gates for the annual poorhouse fair:

> Heart had gone out of these people [the fairgoers]; health was the principal thing about the face of the Americans that came crowding through the broken wall to the poorhouse fair. They were just people, members of the race of white animals that had cast its herds over the land of six continents. Highly neural, brachycephalic, uniquely able to oppose their thumbs to the other four digits, they bred within elegant settlements, and both burned and interred their dead. History had passed on beyond them. They remembered its moment and came to the fair to be freshened in the recollection of an older America, the America of Dan Patch and of Senator Beveridge exhorting the Anglo-Saxons to march across the Pacific and save the beautiful, weak-minded islands there, an America of stained-glass lampshades, hardshell evangelists, Flag Days, ice men, plug tobacco, China trade, oval windows marking on the exterior of a house a stair landing within, pungent nostrums for catarrhal complaints, opportunism, church going and well-worded orations in the glare of a cemetery on summer days. . . .[23]*

The older person's assumption that he or she is different and is therefore no longer worthwhile as a human being sometimes manifests itself in a variety of ways. We all develop elaborate "coping mechanisms" for dealing with stress, and three common ones seen among old people are (1) extreme defensiveness, (2) false jocundity, and (3) withdrawal. Yet a fourth group becomes frankly dependent, giving up all efforts at coping.[24] The old person adopting the first mechanism views the environment as full of threats, challenges, and dangers that must be overcome. Use of the second mechanism reduces the old person to the role of court jester in the Kingdom of the Young. If employing the third mechanism, the individual simply withdraws from any big challenges, choosing to remain in his or her own small world at all times. Whether defensive, jocular, or withdrawn, the older person's interaction is based on ambivalence and thus does not enhance his or her self-esteem. T. S. Eliot expresses this well:

> And indeed there will be time
> To wonder, "Do I dare?" and, "Do I dare?"
> Time to turn back and descend the stair,
> With a bald spot in the middle of my hair—
> [They will say: "How his hair is growing thin!"]
> My morning coat, my collar mounting firmly to the chin,
> My necktie rich and modest, but asserted by a simple pin—
> [They will say: "But how his arms and legs are thin!"]
> Do I dare
> Disturb the universe?

---

*From John Updike: The Poorhouse Fair. New York, Alfred A. Knopf, 1958, pp. 158–159. Used by permission of Alfred A. Knopf, Inc.

. . . . . .

But though I have wept and fasted, wept and prayed,
Though I have seen my head [grown slightly bald]
    brought in upon a platter,
I am no prophet—and here's no great matter;
I have seen the moment of my greatness flicker,
And I have seen the eternal Footman hold my coat,
    and snicker,
And in short, I was afraid. . . .[25] (Poet's brackets.)*

Retirement poses a threat to the former self-image (and, subsequently, to the self-esteem) of many older men and women. For most, retirement not only involves a substantial reduction in income but also signals the end of a whole identity. Therefore, even people who may have found that their jobs take a toll on their physical or emotional well-being may be reticent to retire. To be sure, the amount of satisfaction a person has found in his or her work, along with a variety of other personal factors, will determine the significance of retirement. However, for many people,

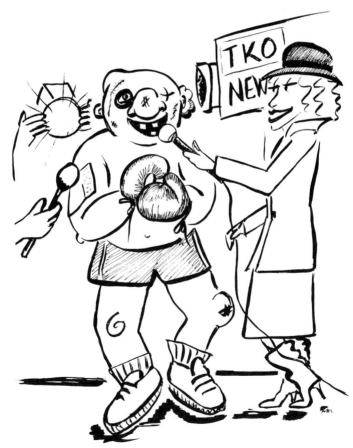

"I ain't retirin', boxin's been good to me!"

*From "The Love Song of J. Alfred Prufrock" in *Collected Poems 1909–1962* by T. S. Eliot, copyright 1936 by Harcourt Brace Jovanovich, Inc.; Copyright © 1963, 1964 by T. S. Eliot. Reprinted by permission of the publisher.

their dignity is associated with their vocation, and retirement is the time when a person can say, "I have seen the moment of my greatness flicker."

In order to maintain their former image of themselves as useful members of society, old people need to be engaged in some kind of ongoing activity. This may be a job, a hobby, a volunteer service, or a club. Regardless of what it may be, they do need to have something to look forward to, and to feel that they are needed in a certain place at a certain time. All too often, such activity is not provided for the older person. However, there are some other good reasons why many older people do not take advantage of the activities available to them: (1) They are shy about meeting new people, particularly if they have maintained one set of friends and acquaintances for many years. (2) They are physically too ill to go to these functions. (3) They have no way to get to them. (4) They cannot afford to go. (5) They are afraid to go out at night or alone. One or more of these reasons may also prevent them from seeking ongoing health care.

Fortunately, older people are becoming increasingly involved in continuous activities. Politics is one area in which the elderly population is gaining a voice. In this sense, their occupation during retirement is crusading for the rights of their age group, and their occupational associations are maintained through political conventions and attendance at hearings or caucuses. Political involvement by the elderly should facilitate progress in legislation regarding them, as well as provide a broader perspective for legislation regarding society as a whole.

Losses Associated with Institutionalization. Chapter 4 explained how the losses of home and privacy can have a detrimental effect on any patient. The health professional should bear in mind that these losses may have already occurred for the old person simply because he or she is old rather than because of illness or injury. Thus, any further losses in these areas may have a greater significance for old people than for those of any other age group. For example, an old woman who has been forced to move out of her long-established place of residence into a nursing home may be completely "undone" by being asked to make another move to a hospital room, where yet more separation from familiar surroundings and objects is experienced. The thoughtful health professional will take these factors into consideration and will be patient in helping the old person adapt accordingly. Sometimes the most the health professional can do when visiting an individual who has had to make such a move is first to recognize that the old person mourns the loss of home and privacy and then to extend sympathy and comfort to him or her.

Loss of Independence. The sick person's loss of independence is closely related to a feeling of decreased self-worth. This is also true for the older person in danger of losing his or her independence. The fear is not unfounded.

A parallel between the dependent state of young children and that of old people is often vividly drawn in literature, as in Dylan Thomas' "Under Milk Wood":

FIRST VOICE: All over the town, babies and old men are cleaned and put into their broken prams and wheeled on to the sunlit cockled cobbles or out in backyards under the dancing underclothes, and left. A baby cries.

OLD MAN: I want my pipe and he wants his bottle.[26]

Edward Albee, another playwright, takes the dependent role of the old person to its natural extension, so that Grandma becomes the child of her own daughter and son-in-law:

(The MUSICIAN enters, seats himself in the chair, stage left, places music on the music stand, is ready to play. MOMMY nods approvingly.)

MOMMY: Very nice; very nice. Are you ready, Daddy? Let's go get Grandma.

DADDY: Whatever you say, Mommy.

MOMMY (leading the way out, stage left): Of course, whatever I say. (To the MUSICIAN) You can begin now. . . .

(After a moment, MOMMY and DADDY reenter, carrying GRANDMA. She is borne in by their hands under her armpits; she is quite rigid; her legs are drawn up; her feet do not touch the ground; the expression on her ancient face is that of puzzlement and fear.)

DADDY: Where do we put her?

MOMMY (the same little laugh): Wherever I say, of course. Let me see . . . well . . . all right, over there . . . in the sandbox. (Pause) Well, what are you waiting for, Daddy? . . . the sandbox!

(Together they carry GRANDMA over to the sandbox and more or less dump her in.)

GRANDMA (righting herself to a sitting position; her voice a cross between a baby's laugh and cry): Ahhhhhh! Graaaaaa!

(Banging the toy shovel against the pail) Haaaaa! Ah-haaaaa!

MOMMY (out over the audience): Be quiet, Grandma . . . just be quiet, and wait, (GRANDMA throws a shovelful of sand at MOMMY).

MOMMY (still out over the audience): She's throwing sand at me! You stop that Grandma; you stop throwing sand at Mommy! (To DADDY) She's throwing sand at me. (DADDY looks around at GRANDMA, who screams at him.)

GRANDMA: GRAAAAA!

MOMMY: Don't look at her. . . . Just sit here . . . be very still . . . and wait. (To the MUSICIAN) You . . . uh . . . you go ahead and do whatever it is you do.

(The MUSICIAN plays. MOMMY and DADDY are fixed, staring out beyond the audience. GRANDMA looks at them, looks at the MUSICIAN, looks at the sandbox, throws down the shovel.)

Grandma does not know that she has been left in the sandbox to die, nor does she express a fear of dying. What she does fear about her predicament, and what we all fear about being in a dependent state, is fully expressed at the end of the quote:

GRANDMA: Ah-haaaaaa! Graaaaaa! (Looks for reaction; gets none. Now . . . directly to the audience) Honestly! What a way to treat an old woman! Drag her out of the house, . . . stick her in a car . . . bring her out here from the city . . . dump her in a pile of sand . . . and leave her here to set. I'm eighty-six years old! I was married when I was seventeen. To a farmer. He died when I was thirty. (*To the* MUSICIAN) Will you stop that please? (*The* MUSICIAN *stops playing.*) I'm a feeble old woman . . . how do you expect anybody to hear me over that peep! peep! peep! (*To herself*) There's no respect around here. (*To the* YOUNG MAN) There's no respect around here![27]*

We believe that once our ability to command respect is gone, so is our bargaining power as a member of the human community. Being regarded as somehow less human than those in positions of power can compromise our rights, dearest hopes, and most basic needs.

The loss of independence is thus of consequence to the old person; self-respect and the power to command the respect of others depend on it. Though we may react with apprehension to this portrayal of Grandma, Albee unfortunately has done little more than capitalize on the attitudes many adults have toward old, dependent people in society. Sandboxes come in the form of nursing homes, back rooms, walk-up apartments, and low-cost housing. Attitudes, too, can create the *feeling* of a dependent, sandbox existence even for the old person who is provided with the most luxurious of physical surroundings.

Old Age and Agism

The particular form of stigma associated with being old is related to the prejudices of an "agist" society. "Agism" has been coined to designate the discriminatory treatment of old people (like "sexism," which describes the systematic devaluation of one sex on both an individual and a societal basis). Of course, the stigma of old age can combine with other types of stigma: Old women, for example, feel the effects of both agism and sexism, while old black women experience the "triple whammy" of stigma in a society that discriminates against people on the basis of race, sex and age.[28]

Old people are constantly confronted with the handicaps of agism. In order to be acknowledged by society at all, they must in some way excel, and in doing so, they run the risk of still being "different" from other people by virtue of their excellence. That is, the double bind of being either looked down upon or placed on a pedestal creates a situation in which simply "belonging" is nearly impossible.

ECONOMIC DISCRIMINATION

The most blatant form of discrimination against old people is economic. While the situation is complex and the overall standard of

---

*Reprinted by permission of G. P. Putnam's Sons from *The Sandbox* by Edward Albee. Copyright © 1960 by Edward Albee.

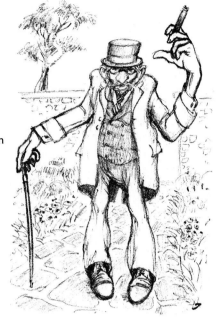

(".... as long as they don't think I'm poor....")

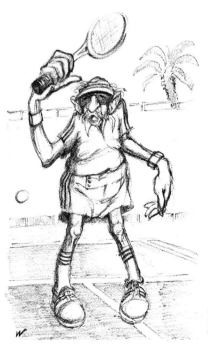

(".... as long as they don't think I'm old...")

Illustrations from In Our Time by Tom Wolfe. Copyright © 1979, 1980 by Tom Wolfe. Reprinted by permission of Farrar, Strauss & Giroux, Inc. These drawings first appeared in *Harper's*.

living of old people in the United States is higher than most places in the world, the report of the 1981 White House Conference on Aging noted that 3.6 million (or about 15.1 per cent) of the elderly population live at or below the official poverty level.[29]

A person is ready to disengage when he or she (1) becomes aware of the shortness of life, (2) sees increasing constriction in the roles and activities available to him or her, and (3) recognizes a decreased energy for involvement with others.[13] More than half of persons holding jobs today still are not going to be provided for in old age by private pension plans. Even those who, upon retirement, will be among the pensioned elite are not protected from the threat of inflation, which will potentially erode their benefits. Clearly, we may be taking giant strides toward better provisions for old people, but we are by no means out of the tall grass yet.

BELITTLING STEREOTYPES

The stigmatization of old people manifests itself in ways other than economic discrimination:

> It has become almost a cliché to deplore the plight of our aging population and to point out clusters of ailments, disabilities, and socioeconomic limitations that being old signifies. To feel one's age means to feel bad. People are told to "act their age," not that they are growing up to their age. Always the emphasis is upon holding back time, as if time had one and the same linear meaning for everyone under every circumstance. We are always asking "When?" or "Do you remember?" not "What is it like?" Old age means obsolescence, decline, deterioration, frailty, uselessness, as if there were no place to go, nothing else to do, and certainly nothing to become, regardless of one's solvency, economic, physical or mental.[30]

One of the most damaging effects of being an older person, and one that is associated with stigma, is the deprivation of human physical contact. These people are already isolated by the death of loved ones or are separated from those who formerly fulfilled this basic human need. With few exceptions, the present population of older people had more inhibitions about touching and more limitations imposed on them by society than younger people have today. Often the only acceptable touching took place between husband and wife, among family members, or in organized team activities. The death of a spouse, separation from grown children, or inability to participate in group activities sometimes isolates the older person from all human contact. Furthermore, a stigmatized person is often thought "untouchable" or "unclean" (recall the leper throughout history). Thus many people find the old person undesirable to touch, usually because of scaly skin, noxious odors, or other physical characteristics reminiscent of death and decay.

Often the old person will look to the health professional to satisfy

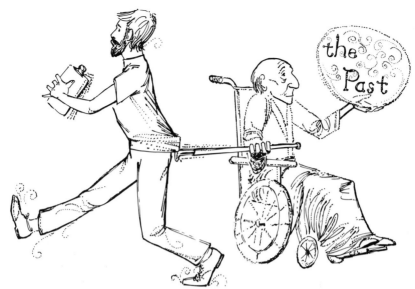

The need for physical contact between the elderly patient and the health professional.

this need for physical contact. The desire not only for actual *physical* contact but also for the *social feeling of acceptance* that attends it may come into play. In an attempt to realize the social gains discussed in Chapter 5, such people may even resort to malingering.

Sexual functioning is assumed to decrease in old age, if one is to believe the stereotypical image of the old "spiritual" person. Contrary to this, the majority of old people desire continued sexual activity and are physically capable of it. A damaging stereotype is that old people who continue to desire sexual involvement are "crazy" or "oversexed," or in some other way deviant, to continue sexually active lives into the 70s or 80s. The "de-sexed" role of old people is reinforced in fiction, cartoons, and jokes. All of this convinces the old person that he or she is, in yet another way, "different" from other people. Of course, a number of old people find themselves and their potential sexual partners repulsive because they have been so instilled with the idea that only the young are beautiful. These persons, probably agists when younger, have now grown into that which they deplored and reject themselves as well as those like themselves. Fortunately, some activist groups of old people such as the Gray Panthers are waging campaigns to help break down this and other destructive stereotypes of old age. By discovering that people can acquire new insights and levels of feeling during a lifetime of lovemaking, they propose the view that there is a developmental potential to sexuality that continues to grow into old age.

Continued sexual functioning can thus be a means for ensuring that old age will be a rich and fulfilling period. In addition, physical contact through socialization can help prevent the isolation and loneliness often experienced by old people in today's agist society. The fact is that old people frequently experience a decrease in physical contact of *all* kinds—a sad comment on the extent to which agism has taken its toll.

Depression and Reminiscence

Almost every major textbook dealing with the psychological processes of old age lists depression as a major problem. It is the most common of functional psychological disorders in older people. Recent estimates are that elderly persons in the community have a prevalence rate of depression of approximately 10 per cent.[31] A brief examination of depression in old age may help the reader to better understand some responses from old people that otherwise seem inappropriate.

Depression is believed to be a response to loss. Charatan, writing on this topic, concludes, "The psychopathology of depression can be summarized in the single word, loss—whether actual, threatened or fantasized.[32] Among the losses he lists as examples are those of sensory input, physical prowess, loved ones, peer group association, status, and location.

The most profound loss in old age is that of a spouse. Grief reactions to this loss are especially prolonged, often leading to self-neglect, malnutrition, and alcoholism. In addition, the suicide rate for elderly white men is four to six times as high as the average suicide rate in the United States; Charatan believes that there is a correlation between this high rate and loss of spouse.[33]

To overcome losses, the old person must have a great many inner resources; the same society that tends to rob the old person of a sense of self-worth unfortunately does not provide support for a process of self-renewal. Most old people direct their energy entirely toward maintaining a meager physical subsistence and an emotional equilibrium, leaving little time for creative renewal.

What are the signs of depression? Depression has both biological and psychological manifestations. Biological signs may include insomnia, weight loss, constipation or diarrhea, and hypochondriasis, while the psychological signs commonly are profound sadness and withdrawal.[34] There is a reduced participation in activity, a slowing of speech and thought processes, a loss of sexual desire, and a decreased involvement in interpersonal relationships.[35] Usually patients will exhibit most of these general signs.

It should be noted that the type of depression in older *disabled* people is believed to be somewhat different from that of younger disabled people, mainly in terms of the object or situation to which the patient attaches his or her depression. The older person will more likely connect the feeling of sadness with external losses.[36] Thus, an older disabled person can generally be expected to be openly hostile about a physically limiting symptom and may direct the hostility to the health professional involved in diagnosing or treating the disability. Steger reminds the reader that depression and its attendant hostility are understandable in such situations:

Aging already has stripped them of family, companions, vocation, recreation, finances, belongings, prestige and social roles, as well as physical health. Disability often is the final blow to tenuously maintained independent living, so that acceptance of a dependent, institutionalized status becomes unavoidable.[37]

Steger's comments should not be interpreted to mean that depression is either acceptable or inevitable. Older people all too often are not referred to a psychiatrist or to other supportive and counseling services because depression is considered somehow "normal." It must be emphasized that the older person suffers from depression as much as anyone else, and a failure to help alleviate it is a failure of one's commitment to the relief of suffering. The health professional who observes the old patient becoming increasingly withdrawn and sluggish, or complaining and aloof, can ward off a deeper depression by immediately helping the person find the necessary professional help.

One important resource the older person has for overcoming the threat and suffering of depression is to engage in reminiscence.

Two relatively new theories about reminiscence have developed: (1) It is the older person's way of daydreaming; and (2) it serves the purpose of a life review in preparation for death. Daydreams are important foundations of hope for what we would like to become. In the future-oriented Western society, it is only natural that people's greatest hopes lie in what is ahead of them. But older persons cease to be future-oriented, reminiscing about the past becoming their hopes, their daydreams.[38] Rather than thinking, "One day I will be . . . ," the older person thinks hopefully, "One day I was . . ." Sometimes the reminiscence is evoked by a person or place in the present. A 91-year-old man wrote in his diary: "Yesterday I saw a woman who evoked memories of fifty or more years ago. I was upset and have not got over it yet."[39] Everyone has these "flashbacks" or "associations" that have the power to produce the most painful or joyous emotions unexpectedly. The older person, who has many years of life behind him or her, experiences these more often, and their significance increases as orientation to the future diminishes.

Reminiscing serves a second function for the aged person; it gives him or her one last opportunity to reorganize attitudes. The person can probably face death more easily if there is a clear idea of the image he or she is leaving behind. Robert Butler terms this verbal autobiography "the life review."[40] This review sometimes leaves no stone unturned. The old man is back in the schoolroom where he sat as a child; he recalls with horror the traumas of his young life, and may burst into tears at the sudden recollection of a pet or playmate who has long since disappeared from his life. He is in love again. Old religious beliefs, long abandoned, haunt him; songs from his youth delight him once more; and the taste of homemade bread again pleases his palate.

Some of his reminiscing relates to his present life situation. In this sense, it is not merely a review but, as Butler stresses, also a reconciliation. The old person recalls an unfair deed he committed and fears he will now receive similar treatment. If, in the past, he tried to be generous to those around him, he may feel grateful that he is currently the recipient of generosity or, conversely, that he is being cheated.

Once the old person's inhibitions are lowered, the long-suppressed memories return at such a torrential rate that it may be difficult to integrate them except in a haphazard fashion. This may lead an observer to conclude that the patient is confused or disoriented. A 94-year-old woman describes her feelings about being called confused when she is engaged in her life review:

> My mind slips rapidly and I know this, but I cannot prevent it. What I remember best are things that happened in the past, only they seem to be really happening now. To me, there is no past, present, or future; the 1960's or 1900's are equally current with me, I look for my mother. Or my babies are small and need care. "Confused, disoriented" the nurses say, not knowing the inner workings of my mind.
>
> Actually I am well aware of most situations but with things flashing through my mind the way they do, I'm likely to speak of my school days in the same breath as I talk about traffic outside my window. I know it's confusing to others but I can't help it. I cry out in desperation, "What's happening to me?" I wish the nurses wouldn't write me off as "not in touch." . . .[41]

It is enlightening to listen to this 94-year-old woman analyze her own confusion. The fact that such people are almost always considered "senile" will be discussed in the next chapter. There are lapses of recent memory to which even she admits, but she is also aware that the past is significant in her analysis of who she is now.

If an older person's reminiscence is viewed in terms of daydreaming or life review, the health professional should pick up important clues from the person's stories. An alert health professional will listen intently and learn to meet the patient's need to continue the story in the time they spend together. One of the most important components of constructive dependence may be the health professional's sensitivity to how important the story actually is to the patient.

In conclusion, the psychosocial processes of older people do vary from one individual to the next. However, some elements present in many aging people are due to their family and social functions, and reflect an era when hard work and lifelong friendships were the norm.

REFERENCES

1. Brotman, H.: Supplement to the Chartbook on Aging in America. Washington, D. C., U. S. Government Printing Office, July 1982.
2. Lawton, M. P.: Environment and other determinants of well-being in older people. Gerontologist 23:349–357, 1983.
3. Case study discussed at the General Meeting of The Hastings Center, Institute of Society, Ethics and Life Sciences, Dobbs Ferry, N.Y., June 17–18, 1977.
4. Burnett, F. M.: An immunological approach to aging. Lancet 2:358, 1970.
5. Bortz, W. M.: Disease and aging. J.A.M.A. 248:1203–1208, 1982.
6. National Institutes on Aging Task Force: Senility reconsidered. Treatment possibilities for mental impairment in the elderly. J.A.M.A. 244:259–263, 1980.

7. Ratzan, R. M.: 'Being old makes you different': The elderly as research subjects. *Hastings Cent. Rep.* 10:32–40, 1980.
8. Eisdorfer, C.: Intellectual and cognitive changes in the aged. In Busse, E., and Pfeiffer, E. (eds.): *Behavior and Adaptation in Late Life.* Boston, Little, Brown & Co., 1969, p. 246.
9. Hardin, W. B.: Neurologic aspects. In Steinberg, F. U. (ed.): *Care of the Geriatric Patient.* 6th ed. St. Louis, C. V. Mosby Company, 1983.
10. *New York Post,* June 7, 1977.
11. Erikson, E.: *Identity, Youth and Crisis.* New York, W. W. Norton & Company, 1968, pp. 139–140.
12. Cumming, E., and Henry, W. E.: *Growing Old: The Process of Disengagement.* New York, Basic Books, 1961, p. 211.
13. *Ibid.,* p. 216.
14. Levine, R. L.: Disengagement in the elderly: its causes and effects. *Nurs. Outlook* 17:28–30, 1969.
15. Conner, K., Powers, E., and Bultena, G.: Social interaction and life satisfaction: an empirical assessment of late-life patterns. *J. Gerontol.* 34:116–121, 1979.
16. Riley, M. W. (ed.): Friendship. In *Aging and Society.* Vol. 3, A Sociology of Age Stratification. New York, Russell Sage Foundation, 1972, pp. 362–370.
17. Brotman, H.: *Op. cit.*
18. Johnson, C. L.: Dyadic family relations and social support. *Gerontologist* 23:377–383, 1983.
19. Brody, E.: Women in the middle and family help to older people. *Gerontologist* 21:471–480, 1981.
20. Shanas, E.: The family as a social support system in old age. *Gerontologist* 19:169–174, 1979.
21. Lopata, H.: Contributions of extended families and the support system of metropolitan widows: Limitations of the modified kin network. *J. Marriage Family* 40:355–364, 1978.
22. Johnson, C., and Catalano, D.: Childless elderly and their family supports. *Gerontologist* 21:610–618, 1981.
23. Updike, J.: *The Poorhouse Fair.* New York, Alfred A. Knopf, 1958, pp. 158–159.
24. Stotsky, B.: Coping with advancing years. In Brown, L. E., and Ellis, E. O. (eds.): *The Later Years.* Acton, Mass., Publishing Sciences Group, 1974, pp. 116–128.
25. Eliot, T. S.: The Love Song of J. Alfred Prufrock. In *T. S. Eliot: The Complete Poems and Plays 1909–1950.* New York, Harcourt, Brace, 1952, pp. 4–6.
26. Thomas, D.: *Under Milk Wood: A Play for Voices.* New York, New Directions Publishing Corporation, 1954, p. 41.
27. Albee, Edward: The Sand Box. In *Two Plays by Edward Albee.* New York, Signet Books, 1959, pp. 10–14.
28. Sontag, S.: The double standard of aging. *Sat. Rev.* 55:28–33, 1972.
29. U. S. Department of Health and Human Services: Introduction, Final Report. *The 1981 White House Conference on Aging.* Vol. 1. Washington, D. C., U. S. Government Printing Office, 1982.
30. Weisman, A.: Does old age make sense? Decisions and destiny in growing older. *J. Geriatr. Psychiatry* 7:84–93, 1974.
31. Freichs, R. R., Aneshensel, C. S., and Clark, V. A.: Prevalence of depression in L. A. County. *Am. J. Epidemiol.* 113:691–699, 1981.
32. Charatan, F. B.: Depression in old age. *N. Y. State J. Med.* 75(4):2505–2509, 1975.
33. *Ibid.,* p. 2506.
34. Blazer, D. G.: *Depression in Late Life.* St. Louis, C. V. Mosby Company, 1982.
35. *Ibid.,* pp. 19–31.
36. Gordon, S. K.: The phenomenon of depression in old age. *Gerontologist* 13:100, 1973.
37. Steger, H. G.: Understanding the psychological factors in rehabilitation. *Geriatrics* 5:68–73, 1976.
38. Rich, T., and Gilmore, A.: *Basic Concepts of Aging: A Programmed Manual.* Washington, D. C., U. S. Dept. of Health, Education and Welfare, SRS Administration on Aging, Publication No. 274, 1969, p. 117.
39. Butler, R. N.: The life review: an interpretation of reminiscence in the aged. *Psychiatry* 26:42–47, 1963.
40. Butler, R. N. Psychiatry. In Rossman, I. (ed.): *Clinical Geriatrics.* Philadelphia, J. B. Lippincott Company, 1979, pp. 532–553.
41. Hahn, A.: It's tough to be old. *Am. J. Nurs.* 70:1698, 1970.

Chapter 16

WORKING WITH THE OLDER PATIENT

In the opening paragraphs of Chapter 15, it was proposed that aging be considered a developmental *process*. It should be reiterated at this point that the aged person is one in whom the process is well advanced; the old person, then, is not to be considered only in terms of his or her chronological age.

Working with an older person is, in many ways, no different from working with a person of any other age. The principles for creating professional closeness, outlined in Chapter 13, apply to this situation as well as to any other. However, a few minor differences can enhance the health professional's success in working with older people. Some have already been mentioned: (1) recognizing the heightened role of storytelling, (2) recognizing that the greatest conscious fear of many older people is that of losing their independence, and (3) recognizing differences in sensory or motor acuity that may affect their responses.

Some health professionals who are many years younger than their old patients fear they have nothing in common with these people. If this were true, effective interaction would understandably be hindered. However, some investigators maintain that there are striking parallels between people of college age and their grandparents. Richard Kalish, for instance, says that both groups are adjacent to but not part of the group in control, and neither one has much influence in making decisions. This, he feels, accounts for the tremendous need for independence experienced by both age groups.[1]

A second study, using three groups of male subjects, was based on Seeman's five components of alienation (powerlessness, meaninglessness, normlessness, social isolation, and self-estrangement).[2] It showed that the middle generation had the lowest alienation score; the sons, the highest score; and the grandfathers, the intermediate score.

A third study compared the values of three generations of women and found that, in many of their attitudes, the old and middle generations differed more than did the old and young.[3] These studies all suggest that persons in their forties and fifties are more apt to retain stereotypes of older persons than are younger and older persons. The potential for truly understanding older people may be found in the young.

Assembling the Parts

A high percentage of older people have defective sight, hearing, taste, smell, touch, or position awareness. As the previous chapter explained, loss of the sense faculties is among the most traumatic losses, producing depression in many persons. Sometimes the older person "adjusts" to the losses with graciousness. An example is the exchange the author had with her 92-year-old neighbor, Tom Coughlin. As she walked into his living room, where the television announcer was blaring the Red Sox' latest play, she was surprised to see Tom planted in front of a blank screen. "Tom!" she shouted above the clamor, "There's no picture!"

"Picture tube went about a month ago!" he shouted back. "I can't see the screen anyway; it's cheaper to watch the game when you're 92!" (Tom, in spite of his eternal optimism, would probably concede that the savings on the picture tube was not worth the price of failing eyesight.) For people with sensory impairment, the entrance into each day must seem like, as Shakespeare put it, the "Last scene of all,/That ends this strange eventful history . . ./Sans teeth, sans eyes, sans taste, sans everything" (*As You Like It,* Act II, Scene 7).

Perhaps the closest a person can come to imagining this sensory-deprived experience is to begin a day with eyes blindfolded, ears plugged, mouth gagged, and legs tied together. For such a person, "getting up" includes not only getting out of bed but also putting on glasses, inserting a hearing aid, putting in dentures, and locating his or her cane.

An older person sometimes goes all the way to the health facility without one or more of these extensions in place! The alert health professional will make a quick mental check to see whether the patient has come equipped with glasses, hearing aid, and cane. Both literally

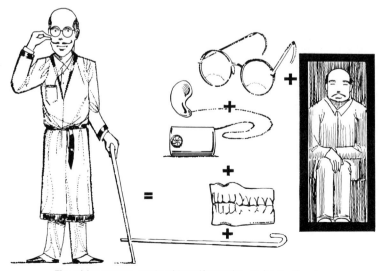

The older person getting himself together to begin the day.

and figuratively, the health professional must come in loud and clear to the sensory-defective older person in order to ensure effective interaction.

A related issue is the cosmetic threat that the loss of teeth or necessary addition of a hearing aid or glasses causes to many. To highlight the power of these visual signs of a "failing" body, consider the following excerpt from the novel *Diary of a Mad Old Man* by Japanese Nobel Prize–winning author, Junichiro Tanizaki. The old man's daughter-in-law implores him to remove his false teeth before going to bed, to which he replies:

> "It's more comfortable to have them out at night, but it makes me look horribly ugly. I don't mind being seen by my wife or Miss Sasaki, though."
> "Do you think I've never seen you like that?"
> "Maybe you have."
> "Last year you were in a coma for half a day, remember?"
> "Did you see me then?"
> "It doesn't matter whether you wear false teeth or not. But it's ridiculous to try hiding it!"
> I'm not eager to hide it, I just don't want to be unpleasant to others."
> "But you think you can hide it if you don't take them out!"
> "All right, I *will*! You'll see what I look like."
> I got out of bed and went over to stand before her. Then I took out both my upper and lower plates, put them in the denture box on the night table, and clenched my gums hard, shriveling up my face as much as I could. My nose flattened down over my lips. Even a chimpanzee would have been better-looking. Time after time I smacked my gums open and shut, and licked my yellow tongue around in my mouth. Satsuko kept her eyes fixed steadily on that grotesque spectacle.
> "Your face doesn't bother me in the least!" She said, taking a mirror out of the night-table drawer. "But have you ever had a good look at yourself? Let me show you. . . . See!" She held the mirror up to my face. "Well? What do you think?"
> "It's incredibly ugly."
> After looking at myself in the mirror, I looked at Satsuko. I could not believe that we were creatures of the same species. The uglier the face in the mirror, the more extraordinarily beautiful Satsuko seemed. If that ugly face were only uglier, I thought regretfully, Satsuko would look even more beautiful.
> "Come on, let's go to sleep, Father. Back to bed, please."[4]*

Understandably, attention to detail in helping the older person "assemble" for the day and then reassurance that the person is worthwhile are critical components of effective interaction with the elderly person. But there are additional means of fostering effective interaction, some of them addressed on the following pages.

*From *Diary Of A Mad Old Man* by J. Tanizaki. Translated by Howard Hibbett. Excerpted by permission of Alfred A. Knopf, Inc.

Establishing a Time and Routine

All patients benefit from the security of a set schedule, and this may be especially true for the old person. First, the security arises from the knowledge that at least in this one small area he or she is in control of the environment. Even if this control extends no further than telling the taxicab driver to hurry because he is scheduled to be in speech therapy in 13 minutes, an old man's self-respect will have been bolstered by exercising that control.

More important, it is a way of helping an old person maintain a proper orientation to the environment. Some retired or hospitalized elderly patients become confused about the time of day and the date because they have few clues to orient them, compared with the person who works five days a week and has more ongoing routine activity. It is possible that the older person is also greatly confused by reminiscing or by forgetting recent events. Besides asking him to be there at the same time each day, the health professional can increase the older patient's time awareness by bidding him good-bye with "Mr. Cubie, I'll see you again tomorrow at 2 o'clock."

One group of investigators hypothesized that if geriatric persons could improve their time awareness, they would be less disoriented about other factors in their environment. In a study designed to test this hypothesis, a small group of hospitalized geriatric patients were presented each morning with a magnetic board that had colored letters displaying date, day, month, and year. As a result, the patients' orientation was improved, thus supporting the hypothesis.[5]

Besides setting a time, the health professional can state the time limit of a certain treatment or test. For instance, if an old man will be in the testing situation for a half hour, he should be told this at the onset and at the end of the test, and a clock should be provided so he can check the time in the interim.

Any method the health professional can devise to call older people's attention to the time, without insulting their intelligence, will help them maintain a correct orientation.

An elderly person's sense of security, control, and orientation can be further enhanced if, in addition to being treated at the same time each day, the routine of the treatment or test is kept reasonably stable from one day to the next. If the treatment or testing situation varies significantly every day, the patient may feel that nothing about it is familiar; it may be a new and anxiety-producing experience every time the person reports to the health professional. Anxiety can greatly decrease the person's performance and have a detrimental effect on both the relationship and the patient's progress.

Establishing a routine does not imply that the treatment should be exactly the same each day. Monotony or boredom can be just as detrimental to the patient as anxiety. Rather, the ideal situation is a balance between the patient's need for stability and his or her continuing interest in life and need for stimulation.

Interacting With the "Senile" Patient

There is much disagreement about what the term "senile" means. As Robert Butler points out: "Senility is a wastebasket term . . . we have no measurable indicators for it. So-called senile symptomatology raises the following possibilities: the beginning of a depression, showing itself as confusion; the development of a reversible brain disorder with the five main signs [disturbance of intellection or comprehension, memory, orientation, and judgment, and the instability or shallowness of affect]; or a chronic brain disorder that may remain stable or that may progress at various rates of speed. . . ."[6]

Hawker disagrees with this interpretation, suggesting that the terms "senile" and "senility" are erroneously used: "Their frequent use in the context of the older patient conveys an impression of irreversible physical and mental degeneration. Yet the dictionary defines senility as old age and its adjective senile as characteristic of old age. Thus, by no stretch of imagination can senility be termed a pathological process and consequently its use as a clinical diagnosis is entirely inappropriate."[7]

These two citations represent the extreme positions in the debate over how the term should be applied: Butler simply lists the several clinical diagnoses encompassed by this one term, while Hawker denies its use as a diagnostic term at all. With much research being conducted in the area of organic brain syndrome in the aged, it is reasonable to expect that the previously applied term "senility" will become obsolete altogether. At the very least, all other possibilities should be ruled out before a patient is considered senile, even if the health professional is told by others that this is so.

What are these "other possibilities"? We have already seen that an old person's confused speech patterns may result from anxiety about strange surroundings, or from some types of expressive aphasia. Moreover, the example in Chapter 15 of the old woman who did not want the nurses to "write her off" revealed that reminiscence can sometimes lead the older person to speak confusedly during a free flow of consciousness. In addition to these possibilities, Butler suggested that confused utterances often signal the beginning of depression and the actual breakdown of coherent thought processes. Stotsky includes confused speech among the techniques of coping that are considered pathological and maladaptive, suggesting that immediate psychiatric intervention may be needed to prevent it from worsening. Such speech may take the form of confabulation, tangential thinking, echolalia, and perseveration.[8] Finally, loneliness causes confused responses. Glasser maintains that much of what we call senility is simply the reaction of old people to physical or emotional isolation.[9]

If the term "senile" is to be used at all, it should be limited to those organic brain syndromes that directly affect the thought and speech processes. In these cases, confusion is usually continual and increasingly profound, though this does not rule out, by any means, the possibility that the health professional can help diminish the confusion at any given moment. In fact, the distinction that was just made between actual senility and other types of confusion is of no great importance. Of far more significance is the common denominator shared by these people: their confusion and probable fear. Therefore, at the start the health professional should respond similarly to each such patient, with the goal of sorting out any confused-sounding parts of the message. That is, it is important that the health professional not support the older person's constantly confused ideas, unless correcting them causes him or her to become violent or deeply agitated. (In such instances a psychiatrist may be needed. But in many cases the confusion is not that profound.) If an old man thinks he is in a hotel, the health professional should correct him. If he confuses the health professional with someone else, his mistake should be corrected by showing him the health professional's name tag. Chances are he will be less frightened if the people around him are willing to help him clear up his mind, if only for a few minutes. It is a good general practice to correct the person each time he or she makes a confused statement. However, the health professional should remember to listen with interest and politeness to the patient. Listening will help the health professional to determine when apparently confused people are making sense in some context not immediately clear. For example, consider the story of Alex Myers and Anthony Carnavello:

Alex Myers, a physical therapist, has just begun work in a large municipal nursing home. The facility has a reputation of not maintaining high standards of care. Therefore, when Alex was interviewed for the position, he made a thorough tour of the home and talked to several employees. Everything seemed "in order," and he took the job.

One day, near the end of his second week of work, Alex goes to the nursing home office to read the personal chart of a patient he will be treating for the first time after lunch. He learns that Mr. Anthony Carnavello is 76 years old and is a diabetic. He has recently had an amputation of his leg following complications from an accident in which his left femur was fractured. According to the chart he fell in the corridor of his home after tripping over a chair. Reportedly he is "confused" most of the time, and is kept quite heavily sedated to prevent him from becoming "violent." He is almost blind.

Alex decides to introduce himself to Mr. Carnavello before going to lunch. When he finds Mr. Carnavello's room he is surprised to see a shriveled up little old man staring at the ceiling. Alex introduces himself, and tells Mr. Carnavello that he will be treating him in the afternoon.

Mr. Carnavello squints in an effort to see Alex. Abruptly he raises up on one elbow and says, "I'm so scared! They keep giving me shots and pills that make me crazy! Can you help me get out of here?"

Just then a nurse comes into the room with a syringe on a tray. "Anthony!" she says, in a firm, loud voice. "Turn over on your side, please! It's time for your shot!"

Mr. Carnavello protests that the pills and shots are making him "crazy as a hoot owl." But the nurse has exposed one loose-skinned buttock and is deftly injecting the solution before Mr. Carnavello succeeds in resisting. He tries to take a swipe at her, but she backs off quickly. She pats his bony hip, says, "There now," and leaves immediately. Mr. Carnevello lies back on the pillow and sighs. He grabs the bed rail, pulls himself up towards Alex, and says, "See what I mean!" Alex thinks that Mr. Carnavello looks genuinely anguished. He reaches out to pat Mr. Carnavello's hand but Mr. Carnavello pulls it away and falls back against the sheet.[10]

What is your assessment of Mr. Carnavello's behavior? What, if anything, should Alex do to relieve Mr. Carnavello's obvious suffering in this situation?

The seemingly confused person should be treated kindly. Such treatment should never be condescending, but should show the gentle authority that gives the patient a sense of security. Goals for these confused people must be adapted according to what they can comprehend. Some patients may be unable to remember the simplest tasks from one testing or treatment period to the next and may never grasp the most elementary verbal instructions, while others will be able to follow astonishingly complex procedures. It is the responsibility of the health professional in such situations to approach each person as an individual and not to take for granted that all confused utterances are signs of senility. If the confusion is extensive and continuous, the patient may need the services of a psychiatrist, and in some cases the confusion will increase no matter what is done. However, none of these complications should deter the thoughtful health professional from first attempting, in a kind way, to correct the inaccuracies. In a great number of cases, this humane act is all that is needed.

Assessing the Patient's Value System

The specific suggestions for helping the elderly patient made thus far in this chapter are, in themselves, empty gestures. The mechanics of adjusting a hearing aid, setting a schedule, or correcting a confused-sounding statement must all be done in a way that supports the old person's value system. Otherwise, the person is reduced to nothing more than an object to be efficiently manipulated.

Chapter 6 listed some of the primary societal and personal values cherished by people in this society. Old people as a group can be expected to hold the same range and variety of values; no particular value can automatically be ruled out on the basis of age. However, the topics treated so far in Part V can help the health professional understand

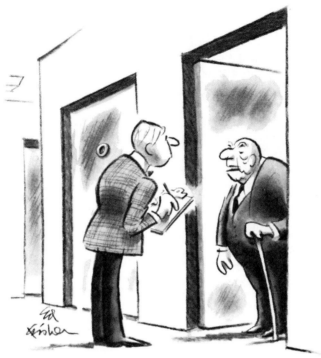

"That was back then. I now espouse gerontocracy."
Drawing by Ed Fisher. © 1983, The New Yorker Magazine, Inc.

why a large number of old people adhere to some values more than others.

For instance, the primary good of self-respect will often be a more consciously prized value for old people because they perceive, correctly, that they are subject to loss of self-respect in an "agist" society. Security, both financial and physical, may also be highly prized by older people because, again, the hold on it is more tenuous. Further, continued independent functioning is valued dearly when commitment to a nursing home threatens or when activities that can be performed alone become increasingly limited. Listening for which values the old patient expresses as the most precious and then trying to set treatment goals accordingly will greatly enhance one's success.

In working with the elderly, the most important challenge confronting the health professional is that of fighting the tendency to stereotype the older person. Society's expectations of older people, many of which are inaccurate and outdated, are propagated through literature, television, and other popular media. It is *not* true, as the previous chapter showed, that old people inevitably value only the spiritual aspects of existence and lose all interest in physical, sensual, and aesthetic matters.

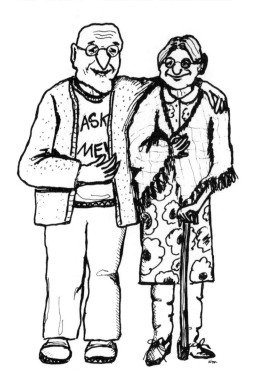

Time-proven data banks.

The health professional can learn to appreciate individual differences among aged persons by increasing his or her contact with people who are 65 years old or more. Programs sponsored by churches, private organizations, and the government offer volunteer services ranging from transportation to recreational activity to hot meals for the home-bound person. Some cities have foster-grandparent or foster-grandchild programs. Hospitals, extended care facilities, and other institutions for the aged welcome young people who are interested in volunteering their services or in visiting the older patients.

Whether through volunteer services, organizations, or contact as health professional, the reader is challenged to develop an acutely discriminating eye for individual differences. The secret to successful interaction with older people is to keep their age-related problems in mind but to concentrate on their individuality.

REFERENCES

1. Kalish, R.: The old and the new as generation gap allies. *Gerontologist* 9:83–89, 1969.
2. Bengston, V. L., and Martin, W. C.: *Aliention and Age: An Intergenerational Study*. Paper presented at the 23rd Annual Meeting of the Gerontological Society, Toronto, October 22, 1970.
3. Kalish, R., and Johnson, A. I.: Value similarities and differences in three generations of women. *J. Marriage Family* 34:49–55, 1972.

4. Tanizaki, J.: *Diary of a Mad Old Man*. New York, G. P. Putnam's Sons, 1965, pp. 100–101.
5. Sanders, R.: Improvement in time orientation in hospitalized geriatric patients. *J. Am. Geriatr. Soc.* 13:1013, 1965.
6. Butler, R. N.: Clinical psychiatry in late life. In Rossman, I. (ed.): *Clinical Geriatrics*. Philadelphia, J. B. Lippincott Company, 1971, p. 445.
7. Hawker, M.: *Geriatrics for Physiotherapists*. London, Faber & Faber, 1974, p. 73.
8. Stotsky, B. Coping with advancing years. In Brown, L. E., and Ellis, E. O. (eds.): *The Later Years*. Acton, Mass., Publishing Sciences Group, 1974, p. 124.
9. Glasser, W.: *Reality Therapy*. New York, Harper & Row, 1965, p. 8.
10. Purtilo, R. B., and Cassel, C. K.: *Ethical Dimensions in the Health Professions*. Philadelphia, W. B. Saunders Company, 1981, pp. 25–26.

Part V Summary

Aging can be viewed as a developmental process that begins at birth and ends with death. The middle years, usually considered to be the "prime of life," constitute a period of achievement and stresses, often culminating in a series of "crises." From the middle of life onward, most biological processes of aging are detrimental to the functioning of the individual.

Intellectual changes due to aging vary widely from one person to the next. There is evidence to support the theory that older people become more rigid with age. Some of them may experience a decrease in learning ability, in motor speed, or in both. Any of these can cause an apparent inability to acquire a skill. Most older people also experience some memory changes.

The psychosocial processes of aging affect interaction with friends, family, and occupational associates. The disengagement theory of aging states that desire and ability to maintain numerous complex relationships decrease with age, though this is disputed by some investigators.

While it is generally believed that old people fear death more than anything else, studies reveal that the majority of them consciously fear dependence more. Older people's increased isolation resulting from the death of their family and loved ones, from the fact that their children are grown, and from their retirement from jobs causes some of them to feel their dignity is diminished. Older people are more likely to look back than ahead. Their stories of the good old days may be a type of daydreaming back to the past. Further, their stories are sometimes part of an important life review, a process whereby they redefine existing attitudes and values in preparation for death.

The gravest problem for older people is society's tendency to stereotype them, thus overlooking what is really important to them. Discrimination against old people is called "agism." It is detrimental because, like other types of discrimination, it makes a given group of individuals (old people, in this case) feel less than human.

Part V Questions for Thought and Discussion

1. An alert 92-year-old patient who has been in your care for several days arrives late for treatment one morning. You begin to converse with her in your usual manner and very quickly realize that something is wrong; she does not answer your questions appropriately. Once or twice, she mentions her young son (who, you know, was killed in World War I), but her sentences are disconnected and incomplete.
   (a) What possible reasons may there be for her apparent confusion?
   (b) What will you do to try to help her?
2. You are hurrying down the hospital corridor when you notice an acquaintance of the family, a bricklayer in his middle forties. You express surprise at seeing him there, since he has always been the picture of good health. He tells you that he has had a heart attack. Suddenly be begins to pour out a blow-by-blow description of the incident. As he talks, he becomes increasingly agitated and finally bursts into tears, sobbing, "It's all over. I'll never be able to go back to my job or anything. What am I going to do?"
   (a) What can you say or do right then to calm this man's immediate anxious state?
   (b) Will you report this incident? To whom, and why?
   (c) How can health professionals work together to "treat" the middle-aged person's anxiety about the long-term effects of illness on family, job, and self-esteem?
3. Which stereotypes of elderly people do you think are most damaging to their self-esteem?
4. What do you dread most about growing old? What do you look forward to most? How do you think an older person's role will have changed by the time you grow old?

Part VI

EFFECTIVE INTERACTION: WORKING WITH PATIENTS IN LIFE-AND-DEATH SITUATIONS

Part VI

Part VI focuses on the life-and-death situations confronting every health professional at some time during his or her career, and considers the components of effective interaction in such situations.

Chapter 17 begins by drawing a fundamental distinction between "terminal illness" and the period during which the patient is "imminently dying"; it then describes the confusion surrounding the concepts of the *process of dying* and the *death event* in most discussions of the terminally ill patient. Specific fears that develop during the process of dying are considered by some psychiatrists only to reflect fear of the death event itself—a position that is examined in some detail. These fears and other responses to knowing that one has a terminal illness are described. There is emphasis on how health professionals can adequately meet the patient's treatment needs while attending to these specific fears.

Chapter 18 continues to focus on interactional components; specific suggestions for interacting with the terminally ill patient arise from the context developed in Chapter 17. A major section is devoted to "truth-telling" as an issue with which health professionals will have to deal. The other sections of Chapter 18 discuss the importance of including the family and involved health professionals in the support system surrounding the terminally ill patient.

Chapter 19 provides suggestions for the health professional at the time when a patient is about to die. The chapter then explores some broader ethical dilemmas created by present-day health-care practices. The distinction between life-prolongation and death-prolongation is offered as a first step toward being better able to assess the dilemmas, but the fact remains that in certain instances no clear resolutions exist at present. Some suggestions are offered for formulating a sound moral policy with regard to these issues. The chapter—and book—concludes with a brief discussion about the "quality of life."

Chapter 17

TERMINAL ILLNESS AND THE PROCESS OF DYING

Only in recent years has "terminally ill" come into use as a label for people having fatal diseases. Like all labels, "terminally ill" is a double-edged sword:

> Emphasis on the notion of radical differences [between the needs of patients having terminal illnesses and those of patients having non-terminal illnesses] and the social involvement accompanying this emphasis have played a prominent role in identifying some special needs of dying persons and raising the consciousness of our society regarding discriminatory treatment toward them. The invisible dying are suddenly visible and the importance of their newly won place among the living is not to be underestimated. As is often the case, however, the dove of human progress carries an albatross on its back. The stride toward increasing our insight into better care for terminally ill persons carries the possibility of further removing those persons from our caring by the fact that we have created a new category or label, "the terminally ill," and we have endowed the label with the possible shortcomings of all labels.[1]

The shortcomings of a label are those aspects of it that create stigma (as discussed in Chapter 4) and cause the labeled person to be treated as less than human. We have seen in previous chapters how the labels "physically disabled," "elderly," and even "sick" can threaten a person's well-being. "Terminally ill" has similar power.

One difficulty with the term is its generality. The person afflicted with a malignant lymphoma who may live for years and one who almost certainly will die within weeks or days are both labeled "terminally ill." Many health professionals, as well as others, immediately place both people on the "critical" list. A friend who has lived for more than ten years with a malignant lymphoma recently went into the hospital for his periodical blood test. A health professional who had come back to work after five years away greeted him cheerfully, "Are you still around?" She was apparently astonished that this "terminally ill" patient had not died long ago! He told me that although he knew her intentions were probably good, he has been fighting the most severe depression of the entire illness in the weeks since she said that.

There have been efforts to clarify terms important to the discussion of terminal illness. Consider the following distinctions:

Terminal illness

| X
Diagnosis
of fatal
disease | Imminently dying
(within weeks/days) | Brain dead |

The period of terminal illness, which can last for only a few days or many years, extends from the time of the diagnosis until the person dies. When it appears that the person is about to die (is imminently dying), then new considerations about what to do in the form of treatment may become appropriate. (Should most treatment be discontinued? Should the person go home?) The concept of a "brain dead" person enters into discussions of life-prolongation, transplantation, and other issues in which the moment of death—by no means a clearly defined event—is an important consideration. "Brain death" is the most recent way of thinking about the conditions necessary in order to declare that a person has died, because it is possible to continue the person's heartbeat and respirations almost indefinitely by artificial means. It is to be hoped that, as clarification of these terms increases, some of the stigmatization of the terminally ill resulting from the general use of the label will decrease.

The Process of Dying and the Death Event

There are two distinct aspects of terminal illness that must be understood. First, the person is going through *a process of dying*, which means that a known pathological condition is progressing and eventually will lead to almost certain death. In the minds of many, a known etiology and somewhat predictable range of symptoms distinguish terminal illness from the lifelong "natural" process of aging and eventually of dying. Terminal illness brings into focus a number of new fears, concerns, and hopes, and evokes some particular kinds of responses from persons.

Second, the person is going to *be dead*. The death event creates its own hopes, concerns, and fears, many of which are rooted in religious and philosophical understandings of life and death. All too often in discussions of "death and dying," the concept of dying and that of death are not separated, leading to confusion.

While much attention in recent years has been devoted to the subject of *dying*, for most people the concept of *death* remains a great mystery, and as such is still a taboo topic. Therefore, in spite of laudable progress in the care of dying people, the process of dying is still considered distasteful and socially unacceptable because of its Siamese twin connection with the death event itself.

Most childhood portrayals of the life-death continuum show no continuity between the two. A notable exception is the nursery rhyme "Solomon Grundy."

In contrast, the following excerpts recalled from childhood fairy tales are one source of clue as to why so many of us shrink from contact with people who are soon going to be dead.

> Down climbed Jack as fast as he could, and down climbed the giant after him, but he couldn't catch him. Jack reached the bottom first, and shouted out to his mother, who was at the cottage door, "Mother! Mother! Bring me an axe! Make haste, Mother!" For he knew there was not a moment to spare. However, he was just in time. Jack seized the hatchet and chopped through the beanstalk close to the root; the giant fell headlong into the garden, and was killed on the spot.
> So all ended well. . . .[2]

> Then Grethel gave her a push, so that she fell right in, and then shutting the iron door she bolted it. Oh how horribly she howled! But Grethel ran away, and left the ungodly witch to burn to ashes.
> Now she ran to Hansel, and opening his door, called out, "Hansel, we are saved; the old witch is dead!" . . .*[3]

Sleeping Beauty and Snow White were both put to death by wicked fairies (and later resurrected by good princes), and greedy King Midas turned his beautiful young daughter into a gold statue.

In many early fairly tales and nursery rhymes, death comes only to bad people and is inflicted upon them by someone else. Presumably, if they had been good, and escaped the evil forces or persons, they would have lived forever. Indeed, neither is death necessarily a permanent condition, particularly if the dead person is good or beautiful enough to attract the attention of a handsome prince!

Both the health professional and the patient share with past generations the superstitions and myths about the "unnaturalness" of death that are rooted in these childhood memories and are retained, in many cases, throughout life. One of the hardest misconceptions to correct is the subconscious belief that the patient's terminal illness is an enemy that must be overcome or the inevitable retribution for some wrong he or she committed. If it is impossible to stave off death, both health professional and patient may give up in despair, and the health professional may flee (at least emotionally) because he or she simply cannot face the fact of being unable to rescue the patient from death.

However, in some respects, the health professional and the patient in modern society also view death differently than did their predecessors. For instance, many peoples throughout history have had their apocalyptic visions of the destruction of the entire universe, but persons of today are the first to live with the belief that sudden annihilation of the earth, the power of total nuclear destruction, has been transferred from the hands of the gods to those of human beings. Ancient concern about appeasing the gods has become a modern-day concern about building a "fail-safe" defense system.

---

*From *The Arthur Rackham Fairy Book.* Copyright 1950 by Arthur Rackham. Reprinted by permission of J. B. Lippincott Company.

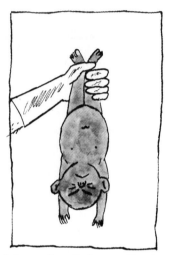

Solomon Grundy, Born on Monday,

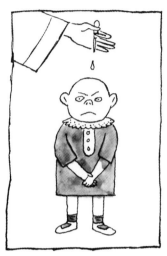

Christened on Tuesday,

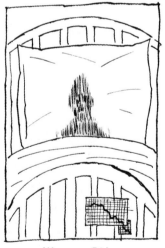

Worse on Friday,

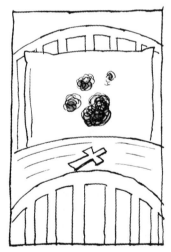

Died on Saturday,

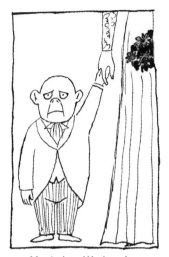

Married on Wednesday,

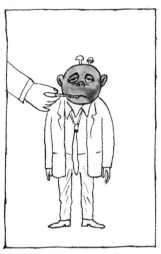

Took ill on Thursday,

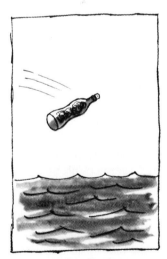

Buried on Sunday.

This is the end
of Solomon Grundy.

People who are currently 30 years of age and under in the Western world, as compared with young people in other historical periods and in other parts of the world, have had little experience in witnessing death at first hand. Young people do witness death in accidents, suicide, and war. But persons dying of disease are so successfully isolated from the living that, in the United States today, more than 60 per cent of them die in institutions, very often alone at the moment of death, in an environment that is technically sound but may lack means of moral support.[4] The bomb and the Intensive Care Unit of the hospital make strange bedfellows; together they suggest that death is simultaneously omnipresent and nowhere to be found, that it is in the hands both of human beings and of gods, and that in all cases it is inflicted.

Because there is so much that is not understood about death itself, ours is still primarily a death-denying society. A few years ago we were blatant about our denial. Geoffrey Gorer, in a book published in 1965, reflects on the state of affairs then:

> The natural processes of corruption and decay have become disgusting, as disgusting as the natural processes of birth and copulation were a century ago; preoccupation about such processes is (or was) morbid and unhealthy, to be discouraged in all and punished in the young. Our great-grandparents were told that babies were found under gooseberry bushes or cabbages; our children are likely to be told that those who have passed on (fie! on the gross Anglo-Saxon monosyllable) are changed into flowers, or lie at rest in lovely gardens. The ugly facts are relentlessly hidden; the art of the embalmers is an art of complete denial.[5]

Today, more than a decade later, some of the same outright denial still exists. Our treatment of the dead body is one expression of it. The dead body is painted, stuffed, and dressed to make it appear alive, while one live gesture such as a sigh or fluttering eyelash would cause most people to rush out of the room screaming; for those wealthy enough, the Life Extension Society offers the option of having one's body frozen until some later date, with the suggestion that it may be possible to reinstitute the life process in the individual as soon as modern science discerns how this can be done.

For the most part, however, denial has simply become more subtle. For example, a subtle denial of death is manifested in films and on television. A child sees the culprit killed but knows that the same culprit will be on next week's show, lurking in dangerous places. Death must seem a very exciting and not very permanent condition.

It should be emphasized here that denial as an important and useful coping mechanism is underestimated in much that is currently being written on the topic of "death and dying."[6] Rushing headlong into an apparent acceptance of death is encouraged today; some workshops are even set up with the explicit intent of helping people achieve this in a weekend, and the workshops are crowded with health professionals who

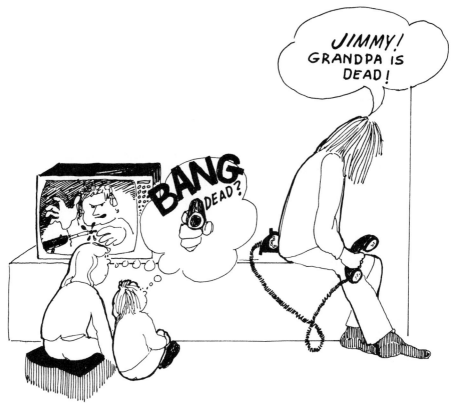

TV's influence on the child's perception of reality.
From: Swedish translation of *HPPI: Vård Vårdare Vårdad.* Page 242.

believe they can be of no help to a dying patient unless they have completely come to grips with the fact of their own death. Such efforts are to be applauded to the extent that self-reflection can enable them to sort out their own feelings about dying and thereby better prepare them for their reactions to certain aspects of the patient's process of dying. In some instances, this self-reflection will also lead to insights about the mystery of the death event itself. But to insist that denial must be entirely eradicated in order to help terminally ill patients at all is not reasonable.

This drive to eliminate all denial would be more appropriate if it instead primarily served to encourage persistent self-examination. Desire to move beyond denial toward a greater understanding seems to be the best way of actually gaining that understanding, especially of the death event itself. Jeremy Taylor suspected as much 300 years ago when he said, "In order to die well, look for death. Everyday knock at the gates of the grave, then the grave cannot do you a mystery."[7] To be sure, the health professions would be more effective in caring for terminally ill persons if the denial of death were less pervasive. The function of denial and its limitations are expressed well by a woman who is examining her own experience of having lung cancer:

Our fear of death makes it essential to maintain a distance between ourselves and anyone who is threatened by death. Denying our connection to the precariousness of others' lives is a way of pretending that we are immortal. We need this deception—it is one of the ways we stay sane—but we also need to be prepared for the times when it doesn't work. For doctors, who confront death when they go to work in the morning as routinely as other people deal with balance sheets and computer printouts, and for me, to whom a chest x-ray or a blood test will never again be a simple, routine procedure, it is particularly important to face the fact of death squarely, to talk about it with one another.

Cancer connects us to one another because having cancer is an embodiment of the existential paradox that we all experience: we feel that we are immortal, yet we know that we will die. To Tolstoy's Ivan Ilyich, the syllogism he had learned as a child, " 'Caius is a man, men are mortal, therefore Caius is mortal,' had always seemed ... correct as applied to Caius but certainly not as applied to himself." Like Ivan Ilyich, we all construct an elaborate set of defense mechanisms to separate ourselves from Caius. To anyone who has had cancer, these defense mechanisms become talismans that we invest with a kind of magic. These talismans are essential to our sanity, and yet they need to be examined.[8]*

Health professionals may unwittingly encourage a family's denial that a loved one is going to die. Consider the story of Beth Rice.

When Beth Rice, a woman with amyotrophic lateral sclerosis, began to experience discomfort from her symptoms, the health professional advised her husband, "Better bring her to the hospital, where she can get better care!" Beth was admitted to the hospital, but despite the best of care, the disease continued to run its debilitating course. The doctor then sent the patient to the Intensive Care Unit, where she could get constant attention.

At the Intensive Care Unit, many professional services were discontinued and adult visitors were allowed to be with her for only a few minutes at a time. The nurses were kind, but firm, in restricting the family's visits. Eventually the son and husband began to come less often, explaining to each other, "It's better for her, for there's really nothing more we can do for her and she needs her rest." In addition, her two grandchildren were kept from her, as is the case in most intensive care settings. The adults rationalized this too, saying, "It's better for them to be protected from this pathetic sight...." When finally Beth lapsed into unconsciousness, the family realized that for all practical purposes they had already disengaged from having her be a full part of their lives. All this was done by well-meaning or grieving people who simply could not cope with the reality of death and believed that they were doing what was most helpful for Beth.

What do you think could have been done differently?

---

*Excerpted by permission of The New England Journal of Medicine, 304:699, 1981.

Fears Associated with Dying and Death

Much research is being conducted to discover the fears faced by persons who learn that they have a terminal illness. Most people can vaguely imagine what they would dread most; once the diagnosis is made, however, harsh reality intrudes and forces them to become acutely aware of their fears. The patient's previous notions about the particular disease and the known experiences of others who have had the disease combine to create a vivid picture of what the patient believes to be ahead. Since nearly all of us dread the thought of gradual and certain loss, the news of a fatal diagnosis is almost always disquieting. Some people experience utter shock or panic. A number of specific fears associated with dying have been recognized, and a discussion of three of the most widespread follows.

FEARS OF DYING

Fear of Isolation. The fear of separation from loved ones is often realistic. This isolation, shown in the story of Beth Rice, who is first placed in a hospital, then in the Intensive Care Unit, is familiar to many health professionals. The theme is used in contemporary literature and developed to its macabre end, as in the excerpt from Albee's "The Sand Box" (Chapter 15), in which Mommy and Daddy take Grandma to an isolated beach, dump her into the sandbox, and sit out of earshot. At the end of the play, the Angel of Death comes and takes Grandma while Daddy and Mommy make small talk to the sound of the musician's violin.

A striking parallel between this scene and those at some hospitals becomes obvious in this excerpt from David Sudnow's definitive report on the care of the imminently dying in hospitals, *Passing On: The Social Organization of Dying*. Although the report was of a study conducted in 1967, unfortunately enough of it remains valid today to merit attention by the reader:

> During a "death watch," the phrase used by nursing personnel to refer to guarding a dying patient in anticipation of his death, the patient is treated as in a transitory state, the relevant facts about him being the gradual decline of clinical life signs. As death approaches, his status as a *body* becomes more evident in a manner in which he is discussed, treated, and moved about. Attention shifts more and more away from caring for his possible discomforts and instituting medically advised treatments, to the sheer activity of "timing" his biological events. . . .
>
> The technical feasibility of phasing out the treatment of dying patients is enhanced by the character of the ward's social structure. While "posted patients" theoretically have the right to round-the-clock visitors, in actuality nurses strive to separate relatives from those patients whose deaths are regarded as imminent. They urge family members to go home and await further news there or, at best,

insist that they wait outside in the corridors and not in the patient's room. At least part of their concern in doing so is to handle the forthcoming death within the context of other ward responsibilities. It is common for a patient to die unattended and be discovered as dead only considerably later, when a nurse, aide or doctor happens into his room. . . .[9]

In some instances, contact with most health professionals is discontinued long before the person is imminently dying. In most cases the person is aware of the practice of being placed in the hospital to die. (It is not unusual for patients who have had several admissions to the hospital during a lengthy terminal illness to announce during one of them that they will never leave the hospital again, and they are usually right.) This awareness alters their response to those around them long before the final separation from life is imminent. Chapter 18 lists some specific suggestions for working with patients who are in this situation. Suffice it to say here that the health professional will understand the patient better if he or she recognizes that the latter's anxiety about being abandoned may be shown in complaints like the following: "They are starting to ignore me"; "they skipped my medication this morning, so they probably are giving up on me"; "they spend more time with the woman in the next bed, but of course they know I'm dying." This extreme insecurity about being abandoned when facing the greatest, or at least the final, event of physical life should be the health professional's cue to spend as much time with, and lend as much support to, this patient as to one who will likely recover. This may mean fostering greater self-understanding and spiritual growth even though the person cannot repay the health professional with a long period of renewed functioning. If a terminally ill person's friends and relatives are withdrawing, the health professional can continue to treat him or her as a living, worthwhile human being.

Fear of Pain. Fear of pain is also common in patients with terminal illnesses. In one study, 96 per cent of the subjects said they wanted to die quickly without suffering, preferably in their sleep.[10] John Hinton observes: "The image of dying reflected in such a phrase as 'death agony' with its spectacular but distorted picture, is far too extreme, built up in part by the significance of the occasion rather than the reality of the situation and often deliberately embellished for the sake of drama. Nevertheless, many do suffer a lot in their mortal illness. It justifies some anxiety, and those who have known or witnessed a distressful end to life cannot be sure that their own dying will not be equally painful or worse.[11] Fortunately, modern medicine has the potential to nearly obliterate the physical pain in dying. The health professional should be mindful that even in those cases in which *pain* is persistent, the patient's *suffering* may be decreased by the health professional's compassion and caring. Also, it is well documented that the experience of physical pain is influenced negatively or positively by psychological states. For example, anxiety and depression have a heightened effect on suffering, whereas distraction and feelings of security tend to diminish suffering.[12]

Fear of Dependence. In previous chapters, the loss of independence during old age and in sickness or injury was examined. The attention already given to these issues should signify the importance of independence. With rare exceptions, terminally ill people face certain and increasing dependence. Proof that they have thought about this is shown in their expressions of astonishment at having reached the point they had previously felt would be totally unbearable. Indeed, everyone has ideas of what he or she believes to be the "outer limits": loss of bowel and bladder control; inability to feed oneself, to communicate verbally, or to think straight; unconsciousness; or something less obviously debilitating. The health professional who is aware of his or her own worries about dependence in some area of functioning will be better able to understand why certain patients with dreaded losses are repulsive or frightening. Very often the health professional will be horrified at what is happening (or has happened) to a patient and will wonder how one could possibly face such a loss. Consider the following story recently reported in a medical journal under the title "Coping with Sudden Blindness":

> Mr. W is a 20-year-old, white, college student, born to a close-knit middle-class family solidly anchored in religious beliefs and rural traditions. The family history is negative for mental illness. The father, a salesman, is described as gentle and cautious, the mother, a dietician, as realistic, courageous, the disciplinarian of the family, fair in her judgments and comfortable in her role as a mother. Her principle for child rearing is, "Give them enough rope, never let go 100 per cent." Mr. W has a brother 3 years younger than he for whom he has always had protective, almost paternal feelings.
>
> Mr. W's birth and early development were entirely normal. His scholastic record was good and his social adjustment very satisfactory. He was active in sports, always something of a leader. He entered college to study economics and planned to earn a master's degree in this field. He became active in his fraternity and recalled with pride introducing social events which included faculty and members of the community instead of the usual beer-drinking parties.
>
> Mr. W worked part-time since the age of 13. He hates to loaf. The summer before his accident, he worked as an assistant manager of a supermarket.
>
> He started dating at 15. He is a nonsmoker, but drinks occasionally in moderation.
>
> Before the accident, he was an active, outgoing person with good social skills and strong leadership ability. He was somewhat impatient with shirkers, a doer rather than a thinker, optimistic, and future oriented. He preferred problem solving to lengthy analysis and rumination.
>
> On May 6th, shortly before midnight, while the patient was resting in his lodgings, a bullet discharged from the gun of a drunken roisterer outside his house pierced the wall and entered his lateral canthal area, destroying both globes without disfiguring his face or damaging his brain. The bullet had traveled through the ethmoid

sinuses but there was no evidence of CSF leak. Except for total blindness, the only other effect was temporary impairment of the sense of smell which improved subsequently. He arrived at Johns Hopkins Hospital by helicopter at 2:00 A.M. At 8:00 A.M. he was told that bilateral enucleation would be necessary, and he signed consent. The operation was performed at 1:30 P.M. the same day.[13]*

In this case, Mr. W. suddenly, in a freak accident, lost both of his eyes. In the case of the terminally ill patient, increasing dependence in many areas often is the inevitable outcome, with death at the end of the losses. The health professional should realize that although the feelings of extreme pity or repulsion are common, the consequences of having them must be dealt with wisely. Some health professionals have to ask a colleague to assume responsibility for a patient because the health professional finds the patient's condition so horrible that his or her effectiveness is hindered. Usually such a radical measure is not necessary, but it may be the best alternative in this difficult situation.

Fear of isolation, pain, and dependence is basic, but there are other fears as well: for instance, the dread of suffocation and the fear that one's loved ones will not be adequately provided for. A person who dies suddenly in a car accident or plane crash, or from a myocardial infarction, may have long harbored these fears but did not have a period of terminal illness during which they intensified. The sudden deaths just mentioned, along with suicide, are more difficult to accept by those left behind, partly because the expression of fears during a period of terminal illness also often serves as an expression of caring. For example, the man who has had trouble openly expressing affection to his wife may be able to do so by sharing his fear that she will not be adequately provided for. An indirect means of communication, such as writing a letter or telling a friend how wonderful she is, can serve the same purpose. The health professional should not conclude from this that such fears will be overtly expressed only during terminal illness. Every illness is a reminder of one's vulnerability and impending death; the prospect of surgery, for example, almost always produces fears. In fact, fears may surface whenever dying is thought about. At any of these frightening times, but especially during terminal illness, people must rely on their own best inner resources and the support of family, friends, and health professionals to sustain them.

FEAR OF DEATH ITSELF

Some people suffer from a neurotic preoccupation with death (thanatophobia), and most at least agree with François de La Rochefoucauld's observation, "Neither the sun nor death can be looked at with a steady eye."[14]

---

*Reprinted by permission of Hoehn-Saric, R., Frank, E., Hirst, L., et al.: J. Nerv. Mental Dis. 169:662, 1981. ©1981, The Williams & Wilkins Co., Baltimore.

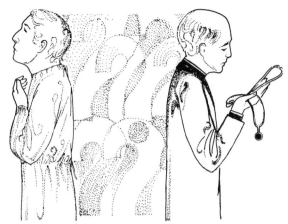

In dealing with the dying patient, the doctor begins to sound more and more like a chaplain while the chaplain sounds more and more like a doctor.

Why are we so afraid of the death event? There are many possible reasons why we dread being "dead and gone": the separation from loved ones, unfinished business, concern for the welfare of those left behind, the fear of being totally alone in some other world, and other uncertainties about life after death, to name a few.

Probably the greatest fear arises from the uncertainty of what death *is*. It's not only what we know but what we don't know that scares us! The author has observed that in discussions about death in the hospital, the chaplain sometimes tends to resort to medical and psychological terms while the health professional begins to sound very religious and philosophical. The mystery of death evades us all, and we are left groping for meaning beyond that provided by our own knowledge and experience. Herbert Marcuse warns that we should be careful not to oversimplify in seeking contemporary definitions of death: "In the history of Western thought the interpretation of death has run the whole gamut from the notion of a mere natural fact, pertaining to man as organic matter, to the idea of death as the *telos* of life, the distinguishing feature of human existence."[15]

Death and Immortality. The majority of people in the Western world are taught that after this life there is another, and that one's actions in this life will help to determine the type of existence one has in the next. One of the many variations of this concept—a personal, everlasting life after death—dominates Judaeo-Christian thought. It is sometimes believed that a person's attitude toward death is determined by his or her culture, age, and, especially, religious affiliation. However, most studies indicate little correlation between these factors and attitude. One study suggests that a person of firm Christian beliefs is more reconciled to dying and may even welcome death.[16] However, Feifel, long a research and clinical psychologist in the area of thanatology, disagrees, highlighting that at present one cannot count on strong religious belief to assure that one will not have last-minute worries:

> The religious person, when compared to the nonreligious individual, is personally more afraid of death. The nonreligious individual fears death because "my family may not be provided for," "I want to accomplish certain things yet," "I enjoy life and want to continue on." The emphasis is on fear of discontinuance of life on earth— what's being left behind—rather than on what will happen after death. The stress for the religious person is two-fold: concern with afterlife matters—"I may go to hell," "I have sins to expiate yet"—as well as with cessation of present earthly experiences. . . .[17]

Besides that of an individual eternal life, other concepts of immortality may affect one's attitude toward death. Historian Arnold Toynbee traces, from a historical perspective, the ways in which people have tried to circumvent the finality of death and achieve immortality.[18] In addition to an individual physical immortality, these ways include:

1. *Physical countermeasures.* Physical life is prolonged by providing the corpse with food, wives, drink, and so forth. This practice was common in ancient times and still exists in some parts of the world.

2. *Fame.* The dead person's image is preserved in poetry or inscription; war monuments, memorial rolls, and names inscribed in tree trunks are all examples. Plato encouraged his followers to achieve immortality through the fame of (1) heroic deeds or (2) scholarly pursuit, as well as through procreation.[19]

3. *Procreation.* Immortality is achieved through one's offspring. An example of this is found in James Agee's novel, *A Death in the Family.* When Jay Follet is killed, one sees him emerging again in the person of his son, Rufus; in a sense, Jay is reincarnated in his son. The possibility of procreation beyond one's own lifetime has recently been realized in the form of sperm banks. Cloning, though still in highly experimental stages, produces genetically identical offspring to succeed their parent.

4. *Passing down one's treasures.* Family heirlooms are constant reminders of their original owner, just as works of art such as paintings or books are reminders of their creator. Inanimate objects are the means of immortalizing a person.

5. *Submersion in ultimate reality.* Predominant in Indian philosophy and other forms of mysticism, in this process, births and rebirths are undergone until perfection (Nirvana) is attained.

6. *Resurrection of individual human bodies.* This is related to the concept of eternal life discussed earlier in this chapter. Some people believe in the resurrection of souls only, while others believe that the actual human body will be restored. Today one belief in the possibility of resurrecting the body is carried out in the practice of cryonic suspension. Here the corpse is frozen in liquid nitrogen—in a suspended, Rip Van Winkle–like state—and stored for later revival.

Any of these beliefs may influence the way in which an individual interprets his or her own death.

Death as the End. A significant number of people in today's society do not view death as a precursor of immortality in any form. Rather, in the language of existential theologian Paul Tillich, the courage to *be* (what one is) is the greatest in life, and death threatens *being* (in his words, "ontic self-affirmation"). The fear of death, then, is ultimately the fear of *non-being*.[20] This view is expressed in Stoppard's play *Rosencrantz and Guildenstern Are Dead*. The two attendants, who have believed through most of the play that they are accompanying King Hamlet to his death in Denmark, find out that instead *they* are going to be put to death. One of them reflects, "Death isn't romantic, death is not anything. . . . Death is . . . not. It's the absence of presence, nothing more . . . the endless time of never coming back . . . a gap you can't see."[21] From this standpoint, one may interpret a patient's fear of death as his or her dread of separation from family, bank account, or proposed cruise around the world, or regret over not knowing who will win the Super Bowl this year or whether there is life on Mars. To this person, death is viewed as an infringement on the right to continued life or "being."

These concepts of death are shared with the reader so that he or she can better understand the attitudes toward death in this society. Not all health professionals are psychotherapists or members of the clergy, but a patient nonetheless may choose one of them to share feelings with about his or her approaching death; this discussion will likely be in a philosophical or religious context. The health professional who can treat the terminally ill person with equanimity and express genuine interest in what the person wants or needs to say about death will significantly help the person. Some specific methods of helping will be presented in Chapter 18.

Having now discussed some basic sources of fear about dying and common interpretations of the death event, we will examine some other responses besides fear.

Patients' Responses to Knowing

What happens when a person learns that she or he has a terminal illness? As already noted, fears associated with dying and the death event may become more sharply focused and create new anxiety. But there are obviously other types of responses besides fear. For many, the first expressed reaction is acute shock or grief, followed very quickly by denial. It stands to reason that in a society that denies death to be a reality, the individuals in this society will not want to believe they are dying at that very moment.

Many people die with this attitude of denial, and others pretend to, because they are afraid those around them would be too upset if the truth were known. Unfortunately, loved ones (the husband or wife, in particular) too often play out a game of deception to the end because each is convinced that the other would not be able to stand the shock if he or she knew.

However, what happens to the person who finally cannot or does not want to deny it any longer? Such people may have some or all of the following other reactions; depression, anger and hostility, bargaining behavior, or acceptance. The reader probably recognizes these responses as Elisabeth Kübler-Ross' "stages of dying," introduced in the 1960's and now widely used in discussions concerning psychological aspects of terminal illness.[22] However, thinking of them as the *range* of responses a person will show rather than as stages he or she will pass through is more accurate. Patients who undergo a long process of dying are likely to feel *all* of these responses from time to time, and many times over: On one day a woman denies her impending death; on another she makes secret "bargains" with God about how long she should live; on the following day she feels the relief of acceptance, followed by a deep depression. Rainey and his colleagues have identified adaptive and "maladaptive" responses that can be expected of persons whose terminal illness is cancer. While the danger is that the health professional may tend to pigeonhole a patient according to the phase of treatment, expecting the patient to show only the behavior these authors have listed, the chart should be used as a helpful tool or referral for *likely* responses of a cancer patient during different phases of illness.

The patient's basic personality structure is an important factor in determining which of the responses will predominate. How did the person deal with stress before learning that he or she had a terminal illness? Similar coping responses will likely surface in both instances.[23]

Patients should be encouraged (but not harassed) to make their feelings known. Sometimes health professionals, in an attempt to reassure the patient that he or she is not alone in the process of dying, will continually compare that person with another "similar case." But ultimately patients *are* alone to the extent that it is their own death they must face, and no one else's. If such a person tries to express why the depression has settled in and the well-meaning health professional refers to "Mr. So-and-so, who had exactly the same feeling," the patient may feel robbed. That is, in order to know his own feelings and thoughts about an experience, the patient must be sure that this experience is wholly his own. Without this certainty, the struggle and suffering associated with it seem unreal. Charles Dahlberg, a physician who suffered a stroke and was temporarily aphasic, admits to the following reaction:

> People often tried to reassure me by partaking of my symptoms and in effect, sharing my burden. This was annoying. They said they also could not remember names or words, that they often forgot things, and so forth. Their intention was kind. I would reply, "Yes, but it happened to me suddenly." I soon got over this annoyance because what they were saying is partly true. . . . But their denial of my illness took away my uniqueness.[24]

ADAPTIVE AND MALADAPTIVE BEHAVIORAL RESPONSES
BY PHASE OF ILLNESS

Normal-Adaptive Behavior	Abnormal-Maladaptive Behavior
Prediagnostic Phase	
Constant or overconcern with the possibility of having cancer	Development of cancer's symptoms without having the disease
Denial of the disease's presence and delay in seeking treatment	
Diagnostic Phase	
Shock	Complete denial with refusal of treatment
Disbelief	Fatalistic refusal of treatment on the basis
Initial, partial denial	that death is inevitable
Anxiety	Search for other opinions or unproved
Anger, hostility, persecutory feelings	("quack") cures
Depression	
Initial Treatment Phase	
SURGERY	
Grief reaction to changes in body image	Postoperative reactive depression
Postponement of surgery	Severe, prolonged grief reaction to
Search for nonsurgical alternatives	changes in body image
RADIOTHERAPY	
Fear of x-ray machine and side effects	Psychotic-like delusions or hallucinations
Fear of being abandoned	
CHEMOTHERAPY	
Fear of side effects	Residual drug-induced psychoses
Changes in body image	Severe isolation-induced psychotic distur-
Anxiety, isolation	bances
Altruistic feelings and desire to donate body or organs to science	Severe paranoia
Follow-up Phase	
Return to normal coping patterns	Mild depression and anxiety
Fear of recurrence	
Recurrence and Retreatment Phase	
Shock	Reactive depression with insomnia, ano-
Disbelief	rexia, restlessness, anxiety, and irritability
Partial denial	
Anxiety	
Anger	
Depression	
At Point of Progressing Disease	
Frenzied search for new information, other consultants, and quack cures begins	Depression
Terminal-Palliation Phase	
Fear of abandonment at death by others, pain, shortness of breath, and facing the unknown	Depression
	Acute delirium
Personal mourning with anticipation of death and a degree of acceptance	

*From Rainey, L. C., Wellisch, D. K., Fawzy, I., et al.: Training health professionals in psychosocial aspects of cancer: a continuing education model. *J. Psychosoc. Oncol.* 1:41–60, 1983. Used with permission. Reprinted from the Journal of Psychosocial Oncology. © 1983, The Haworth Press, Inc. All rights reserved.

Terminally ill patients who are shortchanged in their attempts to claim the uniqueness of their dying experience a similar reaction. Those who are encouraged to view their own experience as unique are freer to search for some meaning and to maintain hope, which is vital to the well-being of such people. LeShan observes that "clinical experience seems to indicate rather strongly that in serious physical illness, the fear of death is not a very powerful tool. It does not appear to bind the resources of the individual together and to increase host resistance to pathological processes. The wish to live appears to be a much stronger weapon for this purpose and to bring more of the total organism of the patient to the side of the physician.[25] Thus, the knowledge that death is certain does not diminish the need for hope. More will be said of this in the next chapter.

In conclusion, death itself and the process of dying are two distinct phenomena. Although they cannot be entirely separated, they should not be considered identical either. Both evoke various fears and other responses. The health professional should remember that it is most important for the terminally ill person to maintain hope in spite of these fears and responses.

REFERENCES

1. Purtilo, R. B.: Similarities in patient response to chronic and terminal illness. *Phys. Ther.* 56:279–284, 1976.
2. Jack and the Beanstalk. In *The Arthur Rackham Fairy Book.* Philadelphia, J. B. Lippincott Company, 1950, p. 48.
3. Hansel and Grethel. *Op. cit.,* p. 276.
4. Cassell, E.: Dying in a technological society. In Steinfels, P. (ed.): *Death Inside Out.* New York, Harper & Row, 1976, pp. 43–49.
5. Gorer, G.: Appendix IV: The pornography of death. In *Death, Grief and Mourning.* New York, Doubleday & Company, 1965, p. 196.
6. Weisman, A. D.: Coping with illness. In Hackett, T., and Cassem, N. H. (eds.): *Massachusetts General Hospital Handbook of General Hospital Psychiatry.* St. Louis, C. V. Mosby Company, 1978, pp. 264–275.
7. Taylor, J.: *The Whole Works.* Rev. ed. 10 vols. Edited by R. Heber, 1847; rpt.: New York, Adler's Foreign Books, 1971.
8. Trillin, A. S.: Of dragons and garden peas: A cancer patient talks to doctors. *N. Engl. J. Med.* 304:699–701, 1981.
9. Sudnow, D.: *Passing On: The Social Organization of Dying.* Englewood Cliffs, N.J., Prentice-Hall, 1967, pp. 83–84.
10. Feifel, H.: Older persons look at death. *Geriatrics* 11:127, 1956.
11. Hinton, J.: *Dying.* London, Penguin Books, 1967, pp. 23–24.
12. Barker, J., and Adams, C. (eds.): *Psychological Approaches to the Management of Pain.* New York, Brunner/Mazel, 1982.
13. Hoehn-Saric, R., Frank, E., Hirst, L., et al.: Coping with sudden blindness. *J. Nerv. Mental Dis.* 169:662–665, 1981.
14. La Rochefoucauld, F. de: *Maxims of La Rochefoucauld.* Translated by L. W. Tancock. London, Penguin Books, 1959.
15. Marcuse, H.: The ideology of death. In Feifel, H. (ed.): *The Meaning of Death.* New York, McGraw-Hill Book Company, 1959, p. 64.
16. Swenson, W. M.: Attitudes toward death among the aged. In Fulton, R. (ed.): *Death and Identity.* New York, John Wiley & Sons, 1965, p. 110.

17. Feifel, H.: Attitudes toward death in some normal and mentally ill populations. In Feifel, H. (ed.): *The Meaning of Death*. New York, McGraw-Hill Book Company, 1959, p. 121.
18. Toynbee, A.: Changing attitudes toward death in the modern western world. In Toynbee, A. (ed.): *Man's Concern with Death*. New York, McGraw-Hill Book Company, 1968, pp. 74–89.
19. Plato: *The Dialogues of Plato*. Vol. 1. Translated by Benjamin Jowett. New York, Random House, 1900, pp. 332–334.
20. Tillich, P.: *The Courage to Be*. New Haven, Yale University Press, 1952, p. 41.
21. Stoppard, T.: *Rosencrantz and Guildenstern Are Dead*. New York, Grove Press, 1967, p. 126.
22. Kübler-Ross, E.: *On Death and Dying*. New York, The Macmillan Company, 1969, pp. 38–137.
23. Novack, D. H., Plumer, R., and Smith, R.: Changes in physicians' attitudes towards telling cancer patients. In Abrams, N., and Buckner, M. (eds.): *Medical Ethics: A Clinical Textbook and Reference for the Health Care Professions*. Cambridge, MIT Press, 1982, pp. 187–190.
24. Dahlberg, C. C., and Jaffee, J.: *Stroke: A Doctor's Personal Story of His Recovery*. New York, W. W. Norton & Company, 1977, p. 191.
25. LeShan, L.: Psychotherapy and the dying patient. In Pearson, L. (ed.): *Death and Dying: Current Issues in the Treatment of the Dying Person*. Cleveland, Case Western Reserve University Press, 1969, p. 32.

Chapter 18

WORKING WITH THE PATIENT WHO HAS A TERMINAL ILLNESS

Working with the patient who has a terminal illness involves basically the same considerations as working with any other patient. But the challenge of effectiveness may become greater in certain ways, some of which are discussed in this chapter.

Telling the Bad News

The issue of sharing information about diagnosis and prognosis has long haunted members of the health professions. Although "bad news" is not just limited to that concerning a fatal disease, much of the attention given to the topic of information-sharing has focused on whether or not the terminally ill person should be so informed.

INFORMATION-SHARING: DUTIES AND RIGHTS

Traditionally, the issue was kept alive by the conviction that the patient must not lose confidence in the health professional and, above all, must never give up *hope*. Therefore, one argument for withholding information from the patient is the possibility that in revealing certain information the health professional inadvertently takes away the patient's hope. Philosopher Nicoli Hartmann, writing in the 1930's, highlights that this position was being expounded outside the medical profession as well as within it. He proposed that sometimes it is necessary for a physician to lie to the patient "in order to ward off calamity," suggesting that in the context of the patient–health professional relationship there is such a thing as a "necessary lie"; the health professional must betray the truth and accept the guilt in order to protect the patient.[1]

The logic of such a proposal runs along the following lines: A primary dictum in the health professions is to *do no harm*; telling the whole truth to a patient may cause great suffering; therefore, it is incumbent on the health professional to withhold the truth or to lie outright in some situations. Truthfulness as a value may sometimes have to be sacrificed to the "higher duty" of preserving the patient from harm.

This position has been challenged on several grounds. First, the implicit assumption of a double moral standard is not justified to some, including many health professionals. They argue that the duty to be truthful applies as much to the health professional–patient relationship as to all others.

Closely related to that argument is one challenging the intent of such untruths. The belief here is that the health professional, rather than protecting the patient, is really shielding himself or herself from having to deal with the bad news. Maintaining the patient's confidence absolutely depends on being truthful, and any pretense to the contrary is not only paternalistic but also deceitful. Indeed, the position proposed by Hartmann regarding the necessity of the lie has by no means been accepted fully. Richard Cabot, a physician at the turn of the century, chided those of his colleagues who were defending the "necessary lie":

> We think we can isolate a lie as we do a case of smallpox and let its effect die with the occasion that brought it about. But is it not common experience that such customs are infectious, and spread far beyond our intention and beyond our control?[2]

The lie not only spreads beyond its intended use and boundaries but also may possibly produce the exact opposite of its intended effect. Few portrayals of the negative effects of the lie are more powerful than Tolstoy's glimpse at Ivan Ilyich's last days:

> Ivan Ilyich suffered most of all from the lie ... the lie adopted by everyone for some reason, which said that he was only ill and not dying, and that everything would be all right if he just kept quiet and did what the doctors told him to. He knew perfectly well that no matter what was done, nothing would change except that his sufferings would increase, and he would die. He was tortured by this lie, tortured by no one's wanting to acknowledge the lie, by his knowing the truth and everyone else's knowing the truth, and yet pressing this lie upon him because of the horror of his position, forcing him to become a party to the lie. This lie, the lie forced upon him on the eve of his death, the lie degrading the solemn, awesome act of his dying to the level of their social calls, porteries and oysters for supper, was an unspeakable torture to Ivan Ilyich. And, strangely enough, time and again when they went through the forms with him, he came a hair's breadth to shouting out, "Stop your lying! You know and I know that I am about to die. You might at least stop your lying!" But he never had the courage to do it.[3]

Ivan's response directly challenges the "necessary lie." Since Ivan's suffering seems to be related directly to the lie, the rule of preventing harm is violated. It appears that at least in this instance the truth would have been kinder to Ivan.

The debate over whether or not to tell the truth to patients continues today. It appears that the governing notion in most decisions today is a policy of disclosure based on the patient's right to information and a conviction that the duty not to harm is best realized by disclosure—the truth "sets free."

In recent years the health professional's duty to protect the patient has been challenged by the contention that the patient ought to assume more responsibility in the relationship and in order to do so must have all the necessary facts. The health professional no longer has unquestioned power to make decisions regarding the patient's welfare, especially in life-and-death situations. Federal law supports the patient's "right" to know with the Freedom to Information Act. In support of this Act, some states have passed laws that allow the patient to read the hospital chart, while several other states permit the patient's lawyer to do so. This trend toward immediate access to formerly confidential information will eventually eliminate the question of whether or not a patient ought to be "told."

Buttressing the argument that patients ought to be told the truth about their diagnosis is one maintaining that patients will find out anyway, and that of the two approaches the more direct information-sharing is less likely to cause more suffering on the part of the patient. Far worse for the patient and family is the uncertainty of not knowing. For example, in the early pages of *Endings and Beginnings*, a young woman's account of her husband's diagnosis of and eventual death from lymphosarcoma, the author recalls:

> The medical decision to do exploratory surgery after ten days of tests was a relief to us, as we were sure it would at last define the problem. We were still confident that once the doctors were able to identify the problem, a medical solution would follow. . . . It was, for reasons all too obvious later, a short operation. Within the hour I was startled to hear the surgeon speak my name. He had come directly to the waiting room, still in surgical dress. As I stood to meet him he said, "I'm afraid the news is not good." He explained that they had found a tumor in the abdominal cavity which could not be removed surgically. Then he went on to say that they needed to wait now for the biopsy reports . . .

The young woman does not translate "tumor" to "cancer." Instead her husband reassures her that since it was "lymphatic" it at least was not cancer.

> That evening, as I left the hospital elevator . . . I was startled to have the head resident under Dr. C (the surgeon) turn to me and say, "Try not to worry; we'll do everything we can." It was clear there was much more going on than any of us was admitting.[4]

Added to the suffering of uncertainty is the conclusion of the classic study by Glaser and Strauss. Their findings showed that eventually the actions of health professionals reveal to patients that their medical problem is life-threatening.

Despite the health professional's careful efforts at deception, the patient finds out about his or her condition within the *closed awareness* context. In this awareness context, several unusual events take place:

1. Most people who visit their physicians get a definite diagnosis and some idea of the duration of their illness; for the person with a terminal illness, this information will be vague or completely ignored, even if the physician has been with the family for years. Once the patient is hospitalized, stories sometimes vary from one person to the next.

2. The patient has a sense of being treated differently from other patients. In the hospital he or she has more tests, has several physicians, is given more medication, and is moved from room to room.

3. Medical personnel hastily give vague but reasonable-sounding explanations for all treatments. New symptoms are readily discounted; sometimes symptoms anticipated by medical personnel are explained away in advance!

4. Cheerful, noncommittal health professionals continually encourage the patient, directing conversation away from subjects related to the illness toward lighter topics.

5. The health professionals are careful to discuss the patient where he or she cannot hear them.

6. The time health professionals spend with the patient is gradually but markedly decreased.

7. Health professionals suddenly hesitate to talk about the future, whether the patient's or anyone else's. Instead, they tend to focus conversation on the immediate present.

Some people die in this context. Others pick up the clues and are thrust into the *suspicion awareness* context, in which they try to find out what they suspect. Still others progress to the *open awareness* context, in which the fact that they are dying is openly discussed by family, medical personnel, and themselves.[5]

Whatever combination of considerations go into the physician's decision, most physicians now are telling oncology patients their diagnosis, usually in direct terms.[6] Cassileth and co-workers suggest that this behavior is probably justifiable since patients they tested, using the Beck Hopelessness Scale, expressed a desire to be informed and actively involved in decisions about their cancer treatment.[7] Significant differences according to age were noted, the younger patients more strongly desiring involvement. This desire to know and participate in treatment decisions supports Waitzkin and Stoeckle's observation that withholding information creates a situation in which the patient feels (and is) powerless.[8]

THE WHAT AND HOW OF TELLING

Many discussions on truth-telling end with a decision about whether or not to tell. The reader knows well that the issue is complex; that the situation is not simply "give information—'yes' or 'no.'" When a patient *says* he wants that information, does he really mean it? Does he say he wants it because his wife is in the room and he wants to show that he can "take it"? Does he want the "truth"—provided it's the truth he wishes to hear? Is he depressed today and would he be better able to hear it tomorrow?[9]

Responsibility and Responsivity. The health professional may (1) withhold information until specifically asked, (2) withhold information even if specifically asked, and (3) offer information even if not asked. The first two practices are "responsive" in the sense that truth-telling becomes an issue only when the patient asks directly, "Am I dying?" or "Is it permanent?" or "What can I expect?" The health professional encounters a dilemma *only when he or she is asked* about the truth. The health professional does not further consider offering certain types of information freely.

The third practice, however, is more than simply "responsive," posing the question of whether or not some information ought to be voluntarily shared without waiting for the patient to ask about it. This practice is based on the conviction that withholding information is an unjustified way for one person to have power over another; sharing life-and-death information with the patient entails giving up some of this power. Some health professionals can actually *enable* patients to express their suspicions about the bad news, which the health professional can then confirm. Unfortunately, not many of us have this skill, either as a natural endowment or as a product of experience, and therefore must consider what type of information to offer the patient who does not ask for it. This point is something for the health professional to think about; there is no clear answer as yet.

Sharing Information: How Much and What Kind? The content of the information revealed is an important consideration that is often overlooked. Simply naming the diagnosis is one approach about which much is currently being written. To be sure, telling Mr. Olsen that he has a malignant myeloma does have a power of its own, and the truth has been told. In most cases, however, stopping there is rarely helpful to the person. In Chapter 14 we noted the woman who was told she had bone marrow disease and translated it as "bow and arrow" disease. She illustrates the point well. The significance of disclosing the diagnosis depends on the prognosis that is implied: In symbolic terms, this woman interpreted the disease as one that would shoot her down like an unsuspecting and helpless doe.

Of course, predicting a prognosis is tricky business. Except in the rarest circumstances, the prognosis is not definitely known; this has been one of the most persuasive arguments against giving a prognosis. Sounding the death knell for some given date in the future understandably would be disastrous to most patients. But the uncertainty attending statements about prognosis in the past has given way to confidently issued statements about probability: "You have a 50 per cent chance of a five-year survival." This approach allows certain information to be transmitted to the patient and therefore has salved the consciences of a great many health professionals. This statistical information does permit the patient to learn what usually happens to people in similar situations, but the information itself leaves a hollow feeling in the pit of the stomach.

The health professional must do more than simply reveal the diagnosis and prognosis; he or she must understand the *meaning* a diagnosis and prognosis holds for the individual patient. There are four major categories of meaning: For some it signifies a challenge, like any other vicissitude of life; some view it primarily in terms of the losses incurred; for a few it signals the relief or respite from unwelcome responsibilities; and for some it is viewed as punishment.[10] The patient who asks, "Am I going to die?" may be asking, "Do I have metastatic cancer of the breast?" (diagnosis) or "Where do I fall on the probability charts for a woman of my age?" (prognosis). But more likely the person is really asking, "Am I going to be dying in a slow, painful way for the next few months? Will I turn yellow and wrinkled like my Aunt Susan did?" "Will I be slowly abandoned by my family and friends?"

The last question is decidedly more challenging than the other two, and answering it requires more, and a different type of, information. It also calls for a response to this patient's request for conversation about her specific fears and suspicions; the pat answers provided in a diagnosis or a probability statement thus prove inadequate.

There are several suggestions health professionals might follow in such situations:

1. Disclosure of any information should come after careful consideration of the patient's need either to know or to not know at a given point in time. Someone must be attuned enough to the patient to perceive the person's mental and physical state at this given moment.

2. Different types of information are best provided by significant people in the patient's life. It takes a combination of insight into the patient's needs, a measure of courage, and ready sympathy for the person's situation in order to talk effectively about difficult aspects of what is ahead for the patient. Depending on the circumstances, the best person may, at any given time, be a member of the clergy, a family member, the physician, the health professional, or another person.

3. All communication should be expressed in a vocabulary that the patient can understand. Ways of expressing the same information will differ dramatically from person to person. Deciding what type of vocabulary is appropriate means getting to know the patient beforehand, at least to the extent of reading the hospital chart.[11]

All of these suggestions leave communication channels open. They also all focus on how knowledge can best be shared rather than on the question of whether it should be shared.

Any information must be incorporated into the entire context of the interaction with the patient in order for it to be effective. We will now consider some major components of that interaction.

CONFLICTS AMONG HEALTH PROFESSIONALS

If the diagnosis and prognosis are known, and the physician chooses to withhold them, another problem arises: Nurses, social workers, therapists, chaplains, and others who know the correct diagnosis get "caught in the middle" so that they must break faith with the physician in order to share such information with the inquiring patient.[12] House officers, too, sometimes are caught, in relation to attending physicians. This conflict of obligations—to one's colleagues versus to the patient—is present in the rare instance when the health professional believes the patient definitely is asking for the diagnosis (and not something else), has a right to know, and would be significantly harmed by not having the diagnosis in spite of the physician's continued refusal to disclose it. Jameton calls the psychological response on the caught health professional's part "moral distress": The distress arises when one knows precisely what ought to be done for the welfare of the patient but is unwilling or unable to act because of repercussions from doing so.[13]

Better procedures for fending off moral distress are needed: "Careful definition of roles, clear delineation of authority and responsibility, and forthright explanation to patients of the function of each team member" are suggestions for a reasonable starting point. Mechanisms for constructive solutions to conflicts that still arise are needed.[14]

The Family During Terminal Illness

At no time is effective interaction between health professional and patient more dependent on the patient's family than during terminal illness. The best and worst aspects of all family relationships are exposed at times of crisis, including terminal illness. During this period, the health professional is often the unwilling witness to both the lifelong destructive patterns and the most intimate, loving characteristics of family relationships. When family troubles have been extreme and deepseated, there is little the health professional can accomplish in terms of constructive intervention except to remember the commitment to provide care for the patient. The hostility that sometimes erupts can be extremely destructive. If the people involved seek the assistance of a chaplain or psychiatrist, the health professional can sometimes help them to find a suitable person. But to take sides in a power struggle that has latently or blatantly existed for years is an exercise in folly, more akin to meddling than to helping.

The great majority of families are brought closer together by the experience, and their mutual support during this time is touching to observe. Despite this, for some health professionals, the members of the terminally ill patient's family are viewed as intruders to be tolerated rather than as important people to be included. The experienced health professional definitely knows that the family's presence complicates the picture. At all hours of the day and night, they ask questions, peek in on the patient, disrupt schedules, and offer suggestions. If the patient has not been told of the terminal illness, they whisper to you in doorways, trying to involve you in elaborate schemes to ensure continued deception. At the busiest time of day, they stop you to tell you something, only to burst into tears.

Why is it important to allow them to be there, despite their omnipresence and their often erratic behavior? First, it is an important means of coping with their own grief. Toynbee, at the age of 79, could reflect on the sadness he experienced when his wife died, and he gave this insight: "That is, as I see it, the capital fact about the relationship between living and dying. There are two parties to the suffering that death inflicts; and in the apportionment of that suffering, the survivor takes the brunt."[15] Regardless of whether Toynbee overstates the point, being able to be in the presence of the loved one is comforting to the family. The astute health professional recognizes the agony the family experiences in anticipation of the loss of their loved one. The family sometimes goes through a series of reactions called "anticipatory grief" that parallel the symptoms usually seen in the acute grief that follows a death. The symptoms of acute grief include (1) a tendency to sigh, (2) complaints of chronic weakness or exhaustion, and (3) digestive distress. In addition, a family member may show (1) preoccupation with the person's image, (2) guilt, (3) hostility, and (4) loss of usual patterns of conduct.[16] As a result, the family's behavior in the presence of their loved one may appear (indeed, may be) altogether inappropriate for the welfare of the patient.

Some people with terminal illnesses, acutely sensitive to the needs of their grieving loved ones, try to make it easier for them by cheering them up! Some say they want to die at night because it would be easier on their loved ones.

Despite the difficulty that arises when such a person and his or her family have conflicting needs, it is of utmost importance that the health professional make every effort to comfort both. The great fear of isolation and the family's dread of the approaching separation make them unable to act more rationally, even though they sometimes acknowledge that their behavior is bizarre or annoying. The health professional's kindness and understanding are greatly appreciated by them at this time.

Second, the presence of the family is often a vital component of the care and treatment offered to the patient. The family members not only need comfort but also provide it; they need to receive communications about the patient's status but often are also the best source for providing information; and they need to do their own grieving but can assist both the health professional and the patient in theirs as well. Sharing decision-making power with the patient and the family is one way of helping them to maintain their dignity. They may respond to a health professional's suggestion by saying, "That's something you can judge better than we can," but having been given the option of deciding will help prevent them from feeling completely disregarded when important decisions are made. Those family members who recognize themselves as part of a supportive context that also involves the patient and the health professionals are likely to offer more, receive more, and continue to keep a better perspective on what is happening.

Interaction with Patients and Their Families

The idea of a supportive context is a useful starting point for considering some specific elements of interaction not yet elaborated.

The first task in this section is to define what is meant by "treatment" when a patient is terminally ill. The previous chapter suggested that different patterns of interaction may be appropriate when a person is terminally ill and when he or she finally is "imminently dying."

A terminal illness can go on for weeks, months, or years, so that hovering around the person as if the angel of death were just down the corridor can make the person's life unbearable! No one who is dying from a terminal illness can or wants to think about it all the time, and to force the person to do so is inhumane. However, this process of dying does bring to a conscious level certain fears, concerns, and hopes, some of which were discussed in Chapter 17. The health professional's ways of interacting during this period must indicate that these factors are being considered.

Then, when the person is apparently at the point of death, further alterations in treatment are necessary. All aggressive treatment is sometimes stopped, and the person is made as comfortable as possible. The types of interaction that involve what we typically regard as "treatment" are supplanted by a more general type of human caring. Of course, caring should have been expressed all along, but now it is the primary mode of interaction.

The following sections of this chapter focus on the elements of caring, especially as they are already present within the interaction that takes place during the process of dying. Chapter 19 will look more closely at some changes in care that may be appropriate as the moment of death approaches.

TREATING THE LOSSES AND FEARS

Previous sections of this book have emphasized the importance of recognizing and understanding the patient's losses. Those experienced by terminally ill people can span the whole range discussed in Chapter 4. However, the terminally ill patient is facing the prospect of losing everything associated with life, including physical identity. In *A Very Easy Death*, Simone de Beauvoir poignantly describes the effects of such losses on her mother, who has been dying from cancer over a period of several months. She reflects:

> I looked at her. She was there, present, conscious and completely
> unaware of what she was living through. Not to know what is
> happening underneath one's skin is normal enough. But for her the
> outside of her body was unknown—her wounded abdomen, her
> fistula, the filth that issued from it, the blueness of her skin, the
> liquid that oozed out of her pores. She had not asked for a mirror
> again; her dying face did not exist for her . . .[17]*

Most terminal illnesss are accompanied by gradual diminution of
strength, endurance, control of movement, and sensory acuity. Helping
the person, and the family, adjust to each of the "little deaths" as they
are experienced is a continuing challenge; the health professional must
be attuned to what at the time is being suffered as a loss.

The fears outlined in the previous chapter also call for attention.
The professional skills of health workers may well include techniques
that relieve pain, maintain bodily functions, and provide an ongoing
source of information about the course of the pathological process. The
application of these techniques can be said to "treat" (allay) the patient's
fears that dying will be painful, that loss of function will be profound,
and that an isolation from people and a curtailment of relevant information will occur. Moreover, the presence of the health professional
during the performance of a technique is proof that abandonment has
not occurred, at least not yet. The responsiveness of the health professional to the patient is a key factor in the patient's assessment of this
situation; if the health professional maintains only the barest amount of
contact required, the patient may fear abandonment more than ever. The
reader has to be reminded that all the fears, especially the fear of
abandonment, are potentially realized during the process of dying.

> . . . the first weeks following a person's [hospitalization] are attended
> by flowers, cards, numerous visitors, and constant encouragement.
> But the able-bodied grow weary. Their responsibilities are many and
> varied. They are disillusioned by the afflicted person's inability to
> return to the real world of involvement, independence, and respon-
> sibility. Sometimes they are even angry that the afflicted person
> "refuses" to come back home where she or he "belongs," or return to
> the job in order to lighten the work load. Then, just about the time
> the [terminally ill] person comes to full grips with the stunning reality
> . . . the room is bare, the phone silent, and the flowers have long
> since wilted.[18]

This tapering-off of supportive relationships is often the most trying
aspect of the entire dying process. Relationships are bound to be altered
during this time; some friends and relatives disappear because of neglect,
despair, or exhaustion, and those who don't become more cherished.
Health professionals often are eventually able to ascertain who, among
the many at the start of the long haul, will endure.

---

*From *A Very Easy Death* by Simone de Beauvoir. Copyright 1973. Reprinted by
permission of G. P. Putnam's Sons.

In addition to the interaction directly associated with the performance of technical skills, many health professionals choose to stop in and see a patient briefly or to talk with the patient's family from time to time after treatment has been discontinued. Sometimes a telephone call to the patient's home following discharge is a great source of comfort and encouragement to all there.

Of course, these means of maintaining human contact can present some difficulties. First, tension arises over the establishment of priorities. Spending extra time with a terminally ill person subtracts from the time left for all other patients. Furthermore, spending extra time with the terminally ill person outside the treatment or testing situation may encourage detrimental dependence (see Chapter 7). Judgment must be exercised in deciding how to proceed so that other patients receive their fair share of time and attention. Detrimental dependence *may* develop, but given that the patients (and their families) are in a time of great turmoil and need, the payoffs most often far outweigh the risks.

Another way to consider the treatment issue is to propose that in this situation, more than in any other, the differences between effects of competently applying a technical procedure and those of expressing human caring are less distinct. Treatment takes curious forms when a person is dying. I've thought many times of the following story, told to me by a physician friend.

When she was an intern, part of her day consisted of making rounds with the attending medical staff and residents. Each day for several weeks one of the patients they saw was a withered wisp of an old woman who was now semi-comatose in this stage of a long bout with cancer. The old woman had no known relatives and was never visited by anyone, but she lived on and on past the time the medical staff believed she would die. The group of physicians stood at the foot of the bed each day, glanced at her in bewilderment, read her chart, said a few words to each other, and left. The intern believed that the old woman would become tense during these discussions, and finally one day she mentioned it to her colleagues. They scoffed at the idea, saying she was too weak and too far gone to know what they were saying or that they were even there. The intern became increasingly troubled by the presence of this tiny lady, who was lying in what seemed to be a gigantic hospital bed. Finally, one time while on call, the intern was walking down the patient's corridor at 3 o'clock in the morning. For some inexplicable reason she was drawn into the patient's room. The woman looked no different than ever—very small, very alone, and very still. The intern shut the door, gathered the woman into her arms, and wept. Later that morning when the intern went to the front desk, she was told that the woman had died at about 5 o'clock. It seems to me that the intern "treated" the woman with the human contact that she somehow needed in order to be released from her suffering. We know very little about the process of dying, but such acts of basic human caring may be the key to helping the patient in these situations.

MAINTAINING HOPE

The previous chapter briefly mentioned the importance of allowing the patient to claim fully the uniqueness of his or her dying in order to begin the search for meaning in the experience. "Meaning" is related to maintaining hope, if hope is defined as belief in the desirability of continued survival.[19] Hope usually changes, at least in part, from a hope for cure to a hope for meaningful activities in the remaining period of life. The terminally ill person's hope is therefore often directed toward events such as seeing a loved one another time, visiting a favorite place, hearing a piece of music played. One patient told me that his only hope was never to use the bedpan, and his heroic attempts to avoid doing so proved that he meant it! Hopes are sometimes less tangible: that one will be able to keep a positive spirit or sense of irony to the end; that one will be remembered and missed; that a particular tradition will be carried on in one's absence. The previously sought long-term goals are put into perspective, and the patient focuses his or her hopes on the most important ones, knowing that they no longer will all be attainable.

The health professional can best help some important goals be realized by listening carefully to the patient express hopes and by taking them seriously. Hope itself depends significantly on the attitudes of health professionals as well as on those of family and friends when the patient dares to disclose a hope. The health professional can help to maintain the person's feeling of worth and thereby provide a human context in which hopes may be expressed. Of course, the health professional can also often play a significant role in actually helping the patient realize some specific hopes by making a few important telephone calls to the right people, by making the patient's wishes known to the family and others, or by other similar means. Too often, imagination fails at this crucial time when the health professional can use it to make a valuable contribution to the person's life.

All terminally ill patients implicitly hope that they will be treated kindly, that everything medically possible will be done for them, and that meaningful human exchange will not disappear. The health professional can assure the patient and family of these things by personally helping to effect them.

In recent years the *hospice* movement in England, Canada, and the United States has been one commendable attempt to provide treatment and care expressly designed to meet the needs of terminally ill patients and their families.

Hospice is a comprehensive program of management which eliminates or deemphasizes the institutional and technologic aspects of traditional care of the dying. It is interdisciplinary and palliative; focused on symptom relief and psychosocial support for the patient and family when cure or remission is no longer possible. Embodying a commitment to provide all necessary elements of care, hospice management includes pain and other symptom control, emotional and spiritual support, home care, and bereavement counseling. The family, not the patient alone, is the unit of care, and the primary caregivers are not physicians but family members, volunteers, nurses, social workers, and counselors.

Hospice is not for everyone. However, intrinsic weaknesses in the acute-care hospital's ability to tend the dying make it a viable option for many. When disease is beyond hope of remission, and palliation becomes the treatment goal, hospice broadens the opportunity to obtain appropriate and needed care.[20]*

Cancer patients constitute the vast majority of hospice patients; it is estimated that hospice programs now serve 25 per cent to 40 per cent of dying cancer patients in their service areas.[21] As hospices become better established and more widely recognized, greater numbers of terminally ill people will be able to benefit from their services, and health professionals will learn better methods of treatment in this difficult area. All readers of this book should acquaint themselves with the functions and structure of the hospice and with the hospice(s) in the communities where they work.

Supportive Interaction Among Health Professionals

A discussion centering on the health professional's role in treating the terminally ill person would not be complete without some mention of the need for health professionals to support each other in the working situation. All too often, emphasis is placed solely on helping the patient and the family cope with the patient's dying. Health professionals involved with the patient also need help; the health professional is going to "lose" the patient, too, and must mourn the anticipated loss. Furthermore, in the course of his or her work, the health professional experiences many such losses. These losses are cumulative; each one brings to mind losses of previous patients and loved ones.

Because it is difficult to grieve alone, I encourage new graduates, in applying for positions at various places, to consider whether there is anyone there who seems capable of sharing sad or angry feelings with them. Can they imagine any of the people they see there as someone whose shoulder they could cry on, either literally or figuratively?

All too often the physical setting works against the health professional's expression of feelings. There is seldom a room where health professionals can close the door to talk with each other privately, or to cry or even scream. One nurse told me that on the cancer ward where she works, the only place where she can have a good cry is the bathroom—a sorry comment on the priority given to satisfying the needs of health professionals in that setting.

Eaton maintains that the reasons we are not emotionally drawn to

---

one another more in such situations are many and complex: First, health professionals have learned to hide strong feelings and to value detachment; second, there is a deep-seated fear that inordinate anxiety about death will surface if any emotion is released; third, such a release of feeling is believed to be a sign of defeat in our struggle to preserve life; and finally, health professionals sometimes project feelings of self-blame about the situation onto colleagues, so that anger toward the colleagues precludes looking to them for support. Nonetheless, Eaton concludes that health professionals eventually may be able to progress beyond their divisiveness and create a support system.[22] This is already happening in some select settings.

The dividends for providing interprofessional support are great. Some of them are mentioned in the following excerpt:

> . . . the supportive context of shared-care diminishes some of the feeling of impotence we all have because of the time pressures under which we work. Sometimes we are afraid to get close to the person because we know that we are only with them for, at most, a few hours a day and feel there is nothing really significant we can do. Other times we find it hard to justify the time it takes to simply "be with" a person when there is no technical procedure to be accomplished. By sharing the care we can plan together so that the person is not alone except as he or she wishes to be, and the burden of maintaining human presence falls on the group as a whole.[23]

Health professionals can help each other learn to cope with patients who are dying. They must first agree that they all harbor anxieties about death and the process of dying. Until they learn to accept each other's fears or misconceptions, however, they cannot build healthier attitudes and provide mutual support. Sometimes seminars, workshops, or other structured activities provide adequate opportunity for sharing these anxieties with others. Some people may prefer to discuss them with a friend, or, if the fears are deep-seated and overwhelming, to work with a counselor, a psychiatrist, or a chaplain first.

The number of high-quality publications on the subject is increasing in university and hospital libraries. Reading followed by talking about the subject is one important way of understanding the basic, shared problems. Only when each person in a work setting feels free to reach out to his or her colleagues for support will it be possible to provide the patient with the best care possible during this difficult period.

REFERENCES

1. Hartmann, N.: Truthfulness and uprightness. Ethics 2:281–285, 1932.
2. Cabot, R. C.: The use of truth and falsehood in medicine: an experimental study. Am. Med. 5:344–349, 1903.
3. Tolstoy, L.: The Death of Ivan Ilyich. In Six Short Stories by Tolstoy. Translated by Margaret Wettlin. New York, Am-Rus Literary Agency, 1963, p. 264.
4. Albertson, S. H.: Endings and Beginnings. New York, Random House, 1980, pp. 19–22.

5. Glaser, B. G., and Strauss, A.: *Awareness of Dying.* Chicago, Aldine Publishing Company, 1965, pp. 29–46.
6. Novack, D. H., Plumer, R., Smith, R. C., et al.: Changes in physicians' attitudes toward telling cancer patients. In Abrams, N., and Buckner, M. (eds.): *Medical Ethics: A Clinical Textbook and Reference for the Health Professions.* Cambridge, MIT Press, 1982.
7. Cassileth, B. R., Zupkis, R. V., Sutton-Smith, K., et al.: Information and participation preferences among cancer patients. *Ann. Intern. Med.* 92:832–836, 1980.
8. Waitzkin, H., and Stoeckle, J.: The communication of information about illness. *Adv. Psychosom. Med.* 8:185–189, 1972.
9. Purtilo, R. B.: Ethical issues in cancer. *J. Psychosoc. Oncol.* 1:3–16, 1983.
10. Lipowski, Z. J.: Psychosocial reactions to physical illness. *Can. Med. Assoc. J.* 128:1069–1072, 1983.
11. Purtilo, R. B.: *Essays for Professional Helpers: Some Psychosocial and Ethical Considerations.* Thorofare, N.J., Charles B. Slack, 1975, p. 149.
12. Purtilo, R. B.: Ethical issues in cancer. *Op. cit.,* p. 6.
13. Jameton, A.: Nurses and moral distress in the hospital. In Gruzalski, B., and Nelson, C. (eds.): *Value Conflicts in Health Care Delivery.* Cambridge, Ballinger, 1982, pp. 131–147.
14. Subcommittee on Hospital Practice, New York Academy of Medicine: A cure for conflicts between physicians and residents? *American College of Physicians Observer,* May 1981.
15. Toynbee, A.: *Man's Concern with Death.* New York, McGraw-Hill Book Company, 1968, p. 271.
16. Siegel, K., and Weinstein, L.: Anticipatory grief reconsidered. *J. Psychosoc. Oncol.* 1:61–73, 1983.
17. de Beauvoir, S.: *A Very Easy Death.* Translated by Patrick O'Brien. New York, Warner Books, 1973, p. 89.
18. Purtilo, R. B.: Similarities in patient response to chronic and terminal illness. *Phys. Ther.* 56:282, 1976.
19. Weisman, A. D.: *On Death and Denying.* New York, Behavioral Publications, 1972.
20. Cassileth, B. R., and Donovan, J.: Hospice: history and implications of the new legislation. *J. Psychosoc. Oncol.* 1:59–69, 1983.
21. Gaetz, D.: The case for hospice from a hospital perspective. *Bull. Am. Prot. Hosp. Assoc.* 45:33–40, 1981.
22. Eaton, J. S., Jr.: Coping with staff grief. In Earle, A. M., et al. (eds.): *The Nurse as Caregiver for the Terminal Patient and his Family.* New York, Columbia University Press, 1976, pp. 140–146.
23. Purtilo, R. B.: *Essays for Professional Helpers. Op. cit.,* pp. 150–151.

Chapter 19

LIFE-AND-DEATH DECISIONS IN THE HEALTH PROFESSIONS

Thus far, Part VI has focused on life-and-death situations involving terminal illnesses. However, not all life-and-death situations are limited to interaction with patients who have terminal illnesses. For example, accidents, suicide attempts, and medical problems of premature infants who must be placed in a newborn intensive care unit cannot be regarded as "terminal illnesses" in the sense in which this term has been used so far. Therefore, this final chapter of the book includes further considerations about terminal illness as well as some that also encompass other life-and-death situations.

When Death Is Imminent

Throughout Part VI a distinction has been made between (1) the period of terminal illness and (2) the time when death is imminent. The fears, responses, and hopes associated with both the process of dying and death itself have been shown to occur primarily during the extended period of terminal illness. But at some point in the course of the fatal disease it becomes apparent that the person is "imminently dying," that is, will die soon. This point of imminent death is equivalent to that experienced by the moribund premature newborn, accident victim, or attempted suicide victim, though such deaths are not preceded by a terminal illness.

In some world religions, certain rituals designed to assist the person's passage into the other world are performed when death is imminent. Many people today do not have any customary rituals associated with the time of death, although it is obvious that new factors come into play at this point for the patient and his or her loved ones. These factors make it necessary for health professionals to alter their treatment procedures and attend to certain aspects of interaction previously not as important. One useful way of conceptualizing the change is to regard it as a move from providing *caring treatment* to providing *only care*.

Ramsey describes "care" as a duty simply to comfort and to be present with the person and the family. He contends that health professionals have lost—and must recover—the meaning of *only* caring for those who are imminently dying and that there is a moral obligation to protest some of the medical practices done today.[1] While Ramsey's

269

suggestions are excellent, they are not without complications of a legal, emotional, and practical nature. On the one hand, the patient who is in the hospital or health facility remains in an environment in which the health professional is legally bound, as well as emotionally committed, to take life-preserving measures that would perhaps not be required outside that setting. That is, the patient is there expressly for the purpose of receiving what we think of as "treatment." It would thus be awkward for the health professional to suspend treatment and associate with the patient as with a friend in more casual surroundings. On the other hand, the patient who leaves the environment and goes home is not readily accessible to the health professional, should the health professional wish to have friendly visits with him or her! Although these difficulties cannot be dismissed lightly, they are usually not insurmountable. Three of the many ways that caring can be expressed are explained in the following discussion, and the reader will surely think of others.

MAXIMIZING COMFORT

The patient who is imminently dying should not be barraged with routine requests and procedures that no longer matter. As one woman asked a group of health professionals, "Does it *matter* if your bowels haven't moved on the last day you are alive?"

Attempts to relieve pain by medication, massage, and other therapeutic means may have been started long before, and these should be continued unless the patient asks that they be withdrawn. Some people, if they know that they are experiencing the final days of their lives, find the torpor induced by heavy medication more troublesome than intense, unrelieved pain.

But maximizing comfort goes well beyond alleviating pain. It involves the relief of real or potential suffering. Suffering is a far more inclusive, personalized concept than pain, though pain may be one important ingredient. A friend relates that on the last day before her 29-year-old husband died of cancer, she read to him, bathed him, nursed their 2-month-old daughter (who had to be sneaked up to the hospital room under a friend's poncho), sang songs he loved, and filled the room with apple blossoms. Friends came in to have "communion," which consisted of brownies and ginger ale, and her husband shared in it, although he had been nourished only intravenously for days.[2] The specific activities would vary from person to person, but it seems to me that she had the right *idea* of how to care for her husband in significant ways during the last day they would be together. In addition, the health professionals who were involved helped the situation by allowing the family and friends their final day together. The woman says that one of the greatest gifts she received was being able to share this intimate time with her husband while still having the assurance that the health professionals were "on standby" if needed.

From this woman I learned that probably the most meaningful act of caring the health professional can do is to enable such loved ones to be with the patient and each other. This may mean breaking hospital rules and readjusting one's schedule. It also means knowing who should be called if the patient worsens and appears near death. Unfortunately, many patients die alone because the health professionals, in spite of good intentions, did not take the necessary steps to ensure that the family would be contacted at the appropriate time.

Another aspect of caring is to know whether certain rituals should be performed at the time of death, and whom to contact for that. Every health professional who deals with the patient for any length of time beyond the briefest encounter ought to have this information. On two occasions, patients have died during the time I was treating them in physical therapy, and to have called the rabbi immediately would have been a great source of comfort to the family of one of them.

SAYING GOOD-BYE

Many people find it hard to say good-bye to a friend or other loved one who is going away. It is harder still when the person is dying—so much so that good-byes are seldom said, especially by the health professional to the patient and the patient's family. But this is something meaningful the health professional can do when many other forms of interaction have been suspended. One psychiatrist offers this suggestion:

> What should be said is, I want you to know the relationship was meaningful, I'll miss this about you, or . . . it won't be the same, I'll miss the bluntness that you had in helping me sort out some things, or I'll just miss the old bull sessions, or something like that. Because those are things you value. Now what does that do for the other person? The other person learns that although it's painful to separate it's far more meaningful to have known the person and to have separated than never to have known him at all. He also learns what it is in himself that is valued and treasured by [you]. And some of those underlying, corrosive feelings of low self-esteem that plague people are shored up . . .[3]

This encounter also allows the patient and his or her family to express similar feelings. There is often a real sense of closeness and gratitude felt toward the health professional, and to be able to show it is a great relief.

In addition to what the exchange does for the patient and family, it is important to realize how much it can help in the health professional's own grieving. The previous chapter mentioned that the health professional's own resources become depleted because he or she does not look to colleagues for support. Expressing gratitude is one way in which the patient and the family themselves can be supportive. When they observe that the health professional receives their thanks humbly, they will appreciate this show of human caring. A young mother recently told my husband that one of the things that most sustained her was to notice one night, when it was apparent that her young son was going to die in spite of the efforts of my husband and other physicians, that my husband had tears in his eyes. Telling him that was a way of saying "thank you," and if he had not been able to receive it, she would have felt embarrassed or rejected.

ACCEPTING REJECTION

Having outlined some ways in which good-byes and thank-yous can be exchanged gracefully and meaningfully, we should now examine those instances in which the patient and family reject the health professional's attempts to interact. Obviously, the good-bye scene just described is rare in comparison with the chaos that attends many patients' last days in the hospital.

Even when there is no apparent chaos, the patient may not want to have anything more to do with the health professional. There are many reasons for this. First, there is great difficulty in saying good-bye or in showing affection under such trying circumstances. Second, there is the possibility that the person has accepted his death and no longer needs any of the people around him. That such acceptance does occur has been well documented by those who have worked with a large number of terminally ill people. Though not impossible, it seems unlikely to occur when the approaching death has not been preceded by a long illness. Third, the health professional simply is not as important as other loved ones, and the little energy the patient has is reserved for them. Fourth, the patient and his or her family may actually project any anger they feel about the death onto the health professional. The health professional who is the object of such anger may not even be the one who spent the lengthiest, or the most significant, time with the person, but rather one who happened in at some crucial moment. Such projections are complex subconscious phenomena that cannot be easily analyzed. Nonetheless, the possibility that rejection is based on projected anger must at least be kept in mind. Finally, the health professional is inextricably linked to the whole setting in which suffering and dying have taken place. So much anguish is associated with the health professional's role and environment that it is painful for the patient to be in the presence of the person. The patient handles this difficulty by rejecting the health professional along with other distressing aspects of the experience.

In short, the health professional's good intentions and willingness to be helpful are not the only factors to be considered. On some occasions the health professional will be hurt by these rebuffs and can do little more than forgive the person responsible for them. At times when hurt is present, interprofessional support becomes vital. Sharing feelings of failure, rejection, or bewilderment with an understanding colleague can be a balm for injured feelings and can give one the courage to try again in another such situation.

When Imminent Death Is Not Inevitable

From the beginning of time, human beings have interfered with their physiological and psychological functioning by using herbs and other medicines, spas, massages, and surgical techniques. These earlier kinds of interference, however, were aimed at relieving pain (psychological or physical), at spiritual transcendence, and at increasing physical, spiritual, or sexual power; they all aimed at improving the *quality of existing life.* For the first time in history, modern modes of interference are aimed at *prolonging life,* with the quality of that life being sometimes a secondary or neglected consideration.

Earlier means of interference were: (1) removal of part of the body (e.g., amputation and excoriation); (2) biochemical changes due to medicines; and (3) external application of physical agents to affect internal functioning (e.g., mud or mustard packs and hot springs).[4] Besides these three, modern means of interference include: (1) *replacement* of defective parts of the body (e.g., an organ transplantation and synthetic tubing for arteries) or (2) *artificial substitution* for defective body functions (e.g., a renal dialysis unit, respirator, or cardiac pacemaker).

The renal dialysis unit, positive intermittent pressure respirator, and cardiac pacemaker will be shown in future Smithsonian Institutions as curious artifacts or relics of the twentieth century. Today these kinds of equipment are used to prolong or alter life, so that normal physiological and psychological processes no longer completely determine the length of life. In some cases, then, the time when death occurs is no longer beyond control. That is, when respiration or heartbeats stop, death is not necessarily the only alternative. Accepting the "inevitable" is too simple. Rather than receiving the Last Rites, today's patient may instead receive a new heart.

Technology: Blessing or Behemoth?

Many questions have arisen in regard to how health professionals can act wisely in the face of such awesome possibilities. To show the complexity of such situations, the case of a patient with chronic renal failure will be examined. In chronic renal failure, death will inevitably result unless the person periodically undergoes renal dialysis, a process that removes excretory wastes from the blood stream in much the same way that the kidney ordinarily would. If the patient withdraws from the course of treatment, death will follow. The patient may eventually receive a kidney transplant, but the chance that the body will reject the kidney is high; if rejection occurs, the choices are to return to dialysis indefinitely, to submit to another transplant attempt should a kidney become available, or to die.

A 54-year-old man, Mr. Crawford, has been kept alive with a renal dialysis unit for 1½ years.* One day while Mr. Crawford is receiving treatment, he tells the nurse, Anna Young, that he has made an important decision: He no longer wants to use the dialysis unit. He knows this means certain death. The nurse, who has known Mr. Crawford during the entire treatment, is surprised. She has heard other patients make similar statements, but Mr. Crawford seemed to be entirely adjusted to the process. Anna asks Mr. Crawford why he has arrived at this decision, and Mr. Crawford, with a deep intake of breath, replies: "Well, I know now that I made the wrong decision when I gave my consent to begin dialysis. Believe me, I've thought about this plenty. . . . You know there's not much else to do during those long hours on the machine but think!

"I consented originally because, well, for one thing, I'm as scared of dying as anyone else. But the wife begged me to do it, and my son. And Dr. Cassel too. I mean I felt like it wasn't fair to refuse her after all she's done for me. . . .

"But now I know I am being kept alive at a cost that is too great. My wife has had to go to work because I can't work anymore, and now her health is failing. I am killing her, you might say, with my nonfunctioning kidney. My children are grown and don't need me. I am sick and tired of being imprisoned—I cannot go more than a hundred miles from home because of my life-long appointment with the dialysis unit. I am not what you would call 'healthy' anyway. There are constant aches in my joints and I am tired, tired, tired all the time.† Even on the nights I am home instead of on the machine I have to go to bed immediately after supper. In short, I have lost my will to go on."

As Anna listens to Mr. Crawford tell his story, she recalls Mr. Crawford's decision to begin dialysis treatment. She also recalls Mrs. Crawford's joy at the news and wonders now if she has any idea that her husband has decided to end his life.

She knows that it has cost at least $12,000 a year to keep Mr. Crawford alive (primarily because of the high cost of laboratory testing necessary to ensure continuing metabolic balance after dialysis) and that most of this money has come from federal and local funds. She also remembers the number of patients who have made similar announcements during especially low periods and wonders whether Mr. Crawford will go home and sleep off his depression or, like others before him, will die in the dreamy delirium caused by uremic poisoning.

The nurse senses that it has taken tremendous courage for Mr. Crawford to come to his present decision. He has finally succumbed to the extreme frustration, experienced by most patients, caused by his dependence on the dialysis machine, the necessity to adhere to a strict diet, and his continuous discomfort.

---

*Patients have to spend about 30 hours a week on the dialysis unit at the renal center from the time they begin treatment until they die or have a kidney transplant. Today, some are treated at home.

†George Schreiner and John Maher cite the following as central nervous system manifestations of uremia: fatigue, apathy, drowsiness, inability to concentrate for a long time, depression, and instability. From *Uremia: Biochemistry, Pathogenesis and Treatment.* Springfield, Ill., Charles C Thomas, 1961, pp. 237–239.

Mr. Crawford could have been spared the agony of making the original decision. Dr. Cassel could have ordered Mr. Crawford to accept dialysis, a police guard could have enforced the order, and Anna Young and other health professionals in the dialysis unit could have administered treatment. But health professionals and a concerned society have made sure that such events cannot happen and that patients like Mr. Crawford will make, or at least participate in, their own life-and-death decisions.

Assurance that Mr. Crawford will be included in the deliberation about life-and-death decisions affecting him is given in the sound, humane principles of the Declaration of Geneva (1948), the Nuremberg Code (1949), and the Declaration of Helsinki (1964). These international codes of ethics state that a patient must always (1) be informed of the procedures to be performed, (2) be told of the known consequences, and (3) be allowed to accept or reject the procedure.

Of course, the physician or other health professional who wishes to perform a procedure can greatly influence the patient's decision by wording the explanation in a certain way. Friends and relatives sometimes place pressure on the patient, and religious convictions concerning acceptable treatments further limit what finally appear to be the real alternatives.

Sorting out the appropriate role of the family in the final decision may be very difficult for the health professional to do. For example, if the wife wishes her husband to continue, she may not dare to say so because she is so sympathetic to his suffering. However, she knows that his decision to stop dialysis will not relieve her present distress: She will have lost his companionship and may be left with the feeling that he betrayed her by discontinuing treatment after she had invested so much in his continued survival.

As highlighted in the recent report of the President's Commission for the Study of Ethical Problems in Medicine, nearly every decision about life-sustaining treatment involves persons other than the patient, and those who act as agents for patients' decisions will have their own decisions to make. Therefore, the health professional must first try to assure that communication channels are kept open, with the patient being the focus of concern and decision-making.[5]

Mr. Crawford has something else to consider. He must decide whether or not he has a moral obligation to continue dialysis; after all, the original decision to go on dialysis has cost society thousands of dollars.

The health professional most immediately involved in the situation is Anna Young, the nurse. She will probably first try to make contact with Dr. Cassel, the physician who has been following Mr. Crawford's progress. Together they can discuss the situation and then check closely with the many other health professionals who have been interacting with Mr. Crawford. The questions they will ask include: What has Mr.

Crawford's attitude been? Have they noticed profound changes in his mood that might suggest a decrease in his will to continue? Do they know of traumatic incidents in his home or on his job? Is there reason to believe that Mr. Crawford is primarily testing the nurse, as patients are wont to do? Answers to such questions will help them further understand Mr. Crawford. These answers will not, however, solve the difficult ethical quandaries implicit in the situation:

1. Does Mr. Crawford have the right to suspend treatment after so much has been invested in him—his wife's health, thousands of dollars of society's money?

2. Is it possible that the doctor has no right to comply with his wishes but should try to encourage him to continue treatment?

3. Is it reasonable to honor Mr. Crawford's will not to live, no matter what the circumstances under which he made his decision?

These questions cannot be easily answered, although there is a compelling argument in favor of urging Mr. Crawford to continue treatment because the decision affects not only him but also his wife and son. Moreover, he should take into account that he, like all of us, is an inseparable part of society, linked especially to certain people whose lives have been and will be influenced by his. Therefore, the moral significance of his decision encompasses much more than his "right" to do what he will with his own life.

However, urging him to continue puts a great burden of responsibility on all involved as well. Mr. Crawford is, at the very least, calling for help in a situation that has become unbearable.

Everyone, including family and friends, will have to figure into his final assessment. But the nurse and the allied health professionals can play a critical role at this point. They are more likely to have been involved with Mr. and Mrs. Crawford over a long period of time, and their continued willingness to support them now may make the situation easier. The Crawfords are faced with a life-and-death situation, and their present anxiety will undoubtedly be followed by other periods of anxiety, no matter what Mr. Crawford ultimately decides to do. If he chooses to stop dialysis, death will ensue; and the previously offered suggestions for treating the imminently dying patient apply. If he decides to continue, both he and his wife will be shaken by his temporary loss of confidence in his original decision to accept dialysis, and they may worry that it will happen again. The ongoing support of all those concerned, even if their involvement is for only a few moments of each treatment period (such as when the medical technologist is performing some laboratory work), is crucial.

Life—or Death—Prolongation

Mr. Crawford and other patients on dialysis must face the life-or-death question in a manner not experienced by most people. Their anxieties are revealed in the comments of a male patient undergoing renal dialysis: "We're sort of zombies . . . sort of close to death . . . I guess we're like the living dead . . . somebody who should be dead but who isn't. . . . We're just marking time. In essence, we're dead anyway. I'll never have the feeling of being a whole human being. Even if I have a [kidney] transplant one of these days, I'll never get over the feeling I'm already dead."[6]

Health professionals would quickly affirm that the man undergoing dialysis is indeed alive. However, it is sometimes difficult for the health professional to decide whether a person is dead or alive. Commonly used terms such as "artificially maintained vital signs," "life sustainers," and "spontaneous functioning" warn people seeking an uncomplicated definition of where life ends and death begins that old, oversimplified ideas about it are no longer useful.

When patients are in a comatose state, the agonizing question arises of when to "pull the plug," as it is often phrased in lay terms. The consent of the family is almost always sought, and, in the absence of such persons, others who can show themselves to have the best interest of the patient in mind will be sought for their counsel. That there is much confusion about the matter is verified by almost weekly newspaper reports of court rulings made on individual cases. Some years ago, Karen Quinlan became a "case" when her parents requested that artificial maintenance of her life functions be stopped. When it finally was, she continued to breathe on her own, thus illustrating with awesome clarity the complexity of such situations and the dilemmas we have created for ourselves by introducing extensive technological measures. Several other similar perplexing situations have reached the courts in ensuing years.

One difference between Karen Quinlan and Mr. Crawford is that the latter was still able to participate in the decision, at least to the extent of expressing his wishes. During the hearing about Karen Quinlan, there was much effort to assess what Karen would have wanted were she able to express her wishes. "Did she keep a journal?" the judge asked. Had she ever discussed her wishes with friends? Did anyone have an old letter that might provide insight?

The "Living Will" movement, as I will call it, is one of several attempts to deal with this problem. Basically, the Living Will document, as well as certain legislation passed or pending in several states, is designed to allow people to make their wishes known at a time when they are still able to do so. The voluntary document begins with the following statement:

> If the time comes when I, _____, can no longer take part in decisions for my own future, let this statement stand as an expression of my wishes, while I am still of sound mind.[7]

This voluntary document requests the withholding of treatment in certain conditions. It is not a legally binding document, so the physician may choose not to honor the request. The document does not ask for euthanasia: No permission is given to inject a fatal dose or actively bring about death in any other way. It is a source of communication between physician and patient, and does allow the patient to exercise some control over the situation, at least to the extent of making his or her wishes known.

The recent Living Will type of legislation being passed in several states does much more than the voluntary document, whose role is strictly advisory. The first, California's Natural Death Act (The Keene Bill, California Assembly Bill No. 3060), binds the physician and others to comply with the wishes of the patient as stated in the form that is provided in the bill. Today, 11 states have passed similar "Natural Death" Acts.[8]

Certain aspects of the Living Will movement are to be commended. First, if more can be done to understand a person's wishes, it is less likely that decisions will be made haphazardly and in violation of the patient's desires. Second, the Living Will documents and legislation remind some physicians and other health professionals that technological competence is not automatically compatible or synonymous with compassionate treatment. Thus the Living Will documents are one effective means of protecting vulnerable members of society who have lost their decision-making power through illness or accident.

To be sure, there are some troublesome aspects to the legislation that is being passed. One major problem is the tendency of some such laws to minimize or confuse the distinction between withholding extraordinary life-prolonging measures (which thereby allows the person to die naturally) and taking more active steps to end the person's life. Health professionals from all disciplines are being asked to help clarify the issues concerning life-prolongation and euthanasia, particularly in regard to the direction that public policy should take. Only when all relevant terms and concepts are rigorously distinguished and completely understood will society be certain about what it is condoning.

The Living Will movement is widespread. Underlying it is an assumption that there may be a difference between *life*-prolongation and *death*-prolongation. In signing a Living Will, one is saying, "I want you to stop trying to save me when I have, for all practical purposes, 'died,' that is, stopped living what I consider *life*. Anything you do beyond that point will be simply prolonging my death event."

Ernlé Young maintains that there *is* a distinction between extending life and prolonging death, in spite of the difficulty in locating the precise moment when one becomes the other. On the continuum between birth (X) and death (Y), a point (Z) is located.

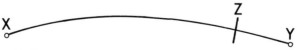

From Young, Ernlé W. D.: Reflections on life and death. *Stanford M.D.* 15:20, 1976. Used with permission.

Where is point (Z)? Young suggests that from a medical viewpoint, it may be said to have arrived "when irreversible damage is observed in any one of the life support systems." From some theological viewpoints, it might be said to have occurred when the capacity for responsiveness to others in faith, hope, and love is irrevocably lost.[9] The important point is to acknowledge the possibility that a distinction exists, thereby enabling the health professional and loved ones to choose a humane course of action when faced with the problem of whether to sustain a patient indefinitely by technological means. The Living Will is the patient's attempt also to participate in the decision of how to proceed during the period from (Z) to (Y).

The Quality of Life

The fact that life and death can be prolonged, sometimes indefinitely, produces an awareness that *life* may not necessarily be synonymous with *significant life*. Indeed, we are all aware that the quality of life is important, and we work to maintain meaning in our relationships, commitments, and lifestyle.

In part, the prolongation of life has brought us closer to the possibility of immortality. We are captivated by the idea of living longer, maybe forever, but do not fancy the notion of immortality for everyone; besides the probability of the earth becoming more quickly overcrowded than it now is, the idea of all relationships lasting forever produces ambivalent feelings in us!

We should, perhaps, also heed the warnings that have come down to us through mythology, literature, and folklore. The immortal Prometheus was doomed to eternal physical suffering for stealing some of the sun's fire and giving it to the human race. The fate of Merlin was made more tragic because he was immortal. He pleaded with the beautiful Niniane to imprison him in her hair, and she complied with his request. But even when she grew tired of him, he was still forever imprisoned because of his immortality. The myth of the overcrowded earth is found in the lore of many ancient and tribal peoples. It expresses the necessity for replacement of the old generation by the new.[10] In short, it would seem that the quality of a good life has to include a great deal more than the possibility of living forever. Jonathan Swift, too, portrays the dilemmas of immortality in the splendid section in *Gulliver's Travels* in which Gulliver meets the Struldbruggs. They have been marked with a sign on their foreheads that means they are immortal. Gulliver is ecstatic about meeting them, believing they will embody the knowledge of all ages. Instead, he finds a society of babbling old people whose immortality is a curse. Advances in the health sciences have opened up so many new possible modes of existence that the health professional, theologian, jurist, social scientist, and others are compelled to consider not only what makes an individual's life worthwhile but also, in a broader sense, what makes life worthwhile to all humans.

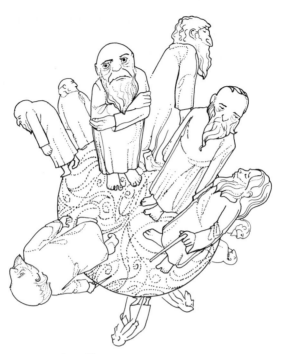

A problem caused by immortality.

The extent to which this question is being explored is illustrated by theologian Herbert Richardson, who asks: "What is the value of life? Reverse the question: When is life utterly without value? When is it worthless? A man lies in a hospital bed. His heartbeat is maintained by artificial stimulation and his brain has by now lost all reactive power. His illness is irreversible. He will never again regain consciousness. Why do we hesitate to pull the switch?"

The author goes on to suggest several life values that must be considered when there is the possibility of "pulling the switch." Briefly, these are: (1) the value of life's happiness; (2) the value of freedom, including the intellectual understanding that makes choice possible; (3) the value of reverence for life, including the care that expresses it; (4) the value of justice, which aims at a simultaneous realization of values in such a way that none must be sacrificed; and (5) the value of peace, in which both justice and caring are maximally operant.[11] Note that Richardson's discussion of life qualities has little to do with the extent to which the patient's physiological function is maintained!

Sometimes a patient concludes that his or her life is no longer rich enough to merit continued and considerable effort to stay physically alive. Mr. Crawford came to this decision. But even after this decision is made, a person such as Mr. Crawford still has the hardest decisions ahead of him. These must be made independent of the many influences around him, including: (1) technology, beckoning him to prolong his life; (2) society, demanding he take advantage of his rights; (3) duty, reminding him of obligations; and (4) emotion, expressing relief, fear, love, pain, or self-pity. The health professional who wishes to understand the problems such patients face must be aware of these influences. Furthermore, he or she must know that technology will likely have a part in determining the quality of the patient's remaining life.

The responsibility for maintaining a reasonably high quality of life for a patient falls not on one person but on all those involved in his or her care, including the patient. One possible result is that, like water that flows into a river and is forever lost, the responsibility will be dispersed into oblivion. However, responsibility can, and should, remain intact. In this way, the burden is made lighter for each individual because it is shared by a cohesive group of human beings bound by a common concern.

Most patients, whether or not they need sophisticated technical measures, are aware that they have placed their health in the hands of the health professional. They expect to be helped with the problems that arise from their illness. However, they are often surprised and delighted that an effort is being made to understand some of their personal problems—their search for the will to live, their evaluation of life values, the difficulty of making decisions, the pressures of society, and the weight of obligation. Once the patient is convinced that the health professional understands some of these problems, the quality of the patient's remaining life improves immeasurably just because of that assurance.

REFERENCES

1. Ramsey, P.: The Patient as Person. New Haven, Yale University Press, 1970, p. 120.
2. Albertson, S. H.: Endings and Beginnings. New York, Random House, 1980, pp. 19–22.
3. Cassem, N. H.: The caretakers. In Langone, J. (ed.): Vital Signs: The Way We Die in America. Boston, Little, Brown & Company, 1974, p. 255.
4. Majno, G.: The Healing Hand. Cambridge, Harvard University Press, 1976.
5. President's Commission for the Study of Ethical Problems in Medicine: Deciding to Forgo Life-Sustaining Treatment: Ethical, Medical, and Legal Issues in Treatment Decisions. Washington, D.C., U.S. Government Printing Office, 1983, pp. 91–92.
6. Abrams, H. S.: The psychiatrist: the treatment of chronic renal failure and the prolongation of life. Am. J. Psychiatr. 126:157–166, 1969.
7. Questions and Answers About the Living Wills. Pamphlet. New York, Concern for Dying, undated.
8. President's Commission for the Study of Ethical Problems in Medicine. Op. cit., p. 138.
9. Young, E.: Reflections of life and death. Stanford M.D. 15(1):20–24, 1976.
10. Schwartzenbaum, J.: The overcrowded earth. Numen 4:59–71, 1957.
11. Richardson, H. W.: What is the value of life? In Cutler, D. R. (ed.): Updating Life and Death: Essays in Ethics and Medicine. Boston, Beacon Press, 1969, pp. 168–177.

Part VI Summary

In today's technological society, the health professional must invest his or her own life with meaning and should try to understand the meanings patients assign to their lives. This is not a simple task in a society in which advances in health care have complicated traditional definitions of life and death. More is being done today than ever before to keep more people alive longer. What, one may ask, is the quality of each of these lives? In what ways, if any, does the quality of each life affect the quality of society as a whole?

Some changes that have taken place in recent years include: (1) the means whereby physiological functioning can be sustained for weeks or months after the end of normal mechanisms; (2) the increasing interest in the *quality* of life; (3) the sharing and possible diffusion of responsibility for difficult decisions; (4) the astounding increase in the number and difficulty of decisions to be made; and (5) the realization that one advantage to recognizing the patient's will to live is that it gives the health professional a positive attitude toward the individual patient; it creates an atmosphere conducive to effective interaction in the health care environment.

Age or physical condition has very little to do with a person's readiness to die. Rather, there are people of all ages in all conditions who have a tremendous will to live, while others are aware they will soon die and are terrified of the knowledge; still others know and accept it.

The initial reaction of most people on realizing or being told they have a terminal illness is that of profound denial. The overt reactions vary from denial to anger, bargaining, and depression. The health professional's approach to the terminally ill patient should be life-affirming, not death-denying, and should emphasize ways in which hope can be maintained.

Fear can be associated with either the process of dying or the death event itself. Components of the fear of the dying process usually include: (1) fear or isolation, (2) fear of pain, and (3) fear of increasing dependence. None of these is entirely unrealistic. Fear of the death event is related to fear of the unknown.

What information to supply, as well as how to share it, is an important issue in life-and-death situations. Refusal to tell the patient of his or her condition (working within the *closed awareness* context) usually interferes with effective interaction. The emphasis of health care should be on (1) decreasing the patient's suffering and maximizing comfort, (2) maintaining physical function, (3) providing reassurance that everything possible is being done, and (4) *supporting him emotionally rather than abandoning him.*

The Western person's attitudes toward death itself, learned very early, usually persist into adult life. It is impossible to understand the person's experience without at least superficially exploring the religious and philosophical interpretations given to the death experience. In Judaeo-Christian thought, immortality is achieved through the resurrection of individual souls or bodies. In Far Eastern thought, the individual soul is eventually submerged into the Ultimate Reality. Others feel that immortality is achieved through one's offspring, creative works, and material goods. A secular point of view is that death is the final and irreversible end of existence.

Part VI—Questions for Thought and Discussion

1. You are in a patient's room performing a procedure. The patient, who has a type of cancer that is always terminal, has been told of his condition. While you are there, a man visiting a patient in the next bed begins to describe the horror of his wife's last days before she died of cancer. Your patient becomes increasingly tense and finally begins to sob.

   (a) What can you do to console or reassure this patient?

   (b) How could you have helped prevent this situation?

   (c) Should you report this incident? To whom, and why?

2. A patient with a terminal illness is being treated in your department. During her treatment, she begins talking with the other patients, and when one of them asks why she is there, she replies, "The doctor is trying to devise a new method of torture. I have a fatal disease and he won't let me die like a common ordinary human being. . . . He wants to try all these new things on me that he knows won't help me. I would be lucky if I lived 500 years ago—they used to throw people like me to the lions."

   How will you respond when one of the people to whom the patient addressed these comments draws you aside and asks, "Is it really right to force a person like that, who is suffering and wants to die, to be experimented on by the doctor?"

3. Under what conditions would your life seem no longer worth living? What course would you take if you must treat a patient whose life is very much similar to these conditions?

INDEX

Note: Page numbers followed by *t* indicate tables.